ADVANCES IN
MEDICAL ONCOLOGY, RESEARCH
AND EDUCATION

Volume VII

LEUKEMIA AND
NON-HODGKIN LYMPHOMA

ADVANCES IN MEDICAL ONCOLOGY, RESEARCH AND EDUCATION

Proceedings of the 12th International Cancer Congress,
Buenos Aires, 1978

General Editors: A. CANONICO, O. ESTEVEZ, R. CHACON and S. BARG, Buenos Aires

Volumes and Editors:

I - CARCINOGENESIS. *Editor:* G. P. Margison

II - CANCER CONTROL. *Editors:* A. Smith and C. Alvarez

III - EPIDEMIOLOGY. *Editor:* Jillian M. Birch

IV - BIOLOGICAL BASIS FOR CANCER DIAGNOSIS. *Editor:* Margaret Fox

V - BASIS FOR CANCER THERAPY 1. *Editor:* B. W. Fox

VI - BASIS FOR CANCER THERAPY 2. *Editor:* M. Moore

VII - LEUKEMIA AND NON-HODGKIN LYMPHOMA. *Editor:* D. G. Crowther

VIII - GYNECOLOGICAL CANCER. *Editor:* N. Thatcher

IX - DIGESTIVE CANCER. *Editor:* N. Thatcher

X - CLINICAL CANCER - PRINCIPAL SITES 1. *Editor:* S. Kumar

XI - CLINICAL CANCER - PRINCIPAL SITES 2. *Editor:* P. M. Wilkinson

XII - ABSTRACTS

(Each volume is available separately.)

Pergamon Journals of Related Interest

ADVANCES IN ENZYME REGULATION
COMPUTERIZED TOMOGRAPHY
EUROPEAN JOURNAL OF CANCER
INTERNATIONAL JOURNAL OF RADIATION ONCOLOGY, BIOLOGY, PHYSICS
LEUKEMIA RESEARCH

ADVANCES IN MEDICAL ONCOLOGY, RESEARCH AND EDUCATION

Proceedings of the 12th International Cancer Congress, Buenos Aires, 1978

Volume VII
LEUKEMIA AND NON-HODGKIN LYMPHOMA

Editor:

D. G. CROWTHER

Cancer Research Campaign Department of Medical Oncology
Christie Hospital and Holt Radium Institute
Manchester

PERGAMON PRESS

OXFORD · NEW YORK · TORONTO · SYDNEY · PARIS · FRANKFURT

LMLOM JCM)

U.K.	Pergamon Press Ltd., Headington Hill Hall, Oxford OX3 0BW, England
U.S.A.	Pergamon Press Inc., Maxwell House, Fairview Park, Elmsford, New York 10523, U.S.A.
CANADA	Pergamon of Canada, Suite 104, 150 Consumers Road, Willowdale, Ontario M2J 1P9, Canada
AUSTRALIA	Pergamon Press (Aust.) Pty. Ltd., P.O. Box 544, Potts Point, N.S.W. 2011, Australia
FRANCE	Pergamon Press SARL, 24 rue des Ecoles, 75240 Paris, Cedex 05, France
FEDERAL REPUBLIC OF GERMANY	Pergamon Press GmbH, 6242 Kronberg-Taunus, Pferdstrasse 1, Federal Republic of Germany

First edition 1979

British Library Cataloguing in Publication Data

International Cancer Congress, 12th,
Buenos Aires, 1978
Advances in medical oncology, research
and education.
Vol.7: Leukemia and non-Hodgkin lymphoma
1. Cancer - Congresses
I. Title II. Canonico, A III. Crowther, Derek
616.9'94   RC261.A1   79-40547
ISBN 0 08 024390 8
ISBN 0-08-023777-0 Set of 12 vols.

In order to make this volume available as economically and as rapidly as possible the authors' typescripts have been reproduced in their original forms. This method unfortunately has its typographical limitations but it is hoped that they in no way distract the reader.

*Printed and bound at William Clowes & Sons Limited
Beccles and London*

Contents

Non-Hodgkin's Lymphomas

Foreword

This book contains papers from the main meetings of the Scientific Programme presented during the 12th International Cancer Congress, which took place in Buenos Aires, Argentina, from 5 to 11 October 1978, and was sponsored by the International Union against Cancer (UICC).

This organisation, with headquarters in Geneva, gathers together from more than a hundred countries 250 medical associations which fight against Cancer and organizes every four years an International Congress which gives maximum coverage to oncological activity throughout the world.

The 11th Congress was held in Florence in 1974, where the General Assembly unanimously decided that Argentina would be the site of the 12th Congress. Argentina was chosen not only because of the beauty of its landscapes and the cordiality of its inhabitants, but also because of the high scientific level of its researchers and practitioners in the field of oncology.

From this Assembly a distinguished International Committee was appointed which undertook the preparation and execution of the Scientific Programme of the Congress.

The Programme was designed to be profitable for those professionals who wished to have a general view of the problem of Cancer, as well as those who were specifically orientated to an oncological subspeciality. It was also conceived as trying to cover the different subjects related to this discipline, emphasizing those with an actual and future gravitation on cancerology.

The scientific activity began every morning with a Special Lecture (5 in all), summarizing some of the subjects of prevailing interest in Oncology, such as Environmental Cancer, Immunology, Sub-clinical Cancer, Modern Cancer Therapy Concepts and Viral Oncogenesis. Within the 26 Symposia, new acquisitions in the technological area were incorporated; such acquisitions had not been exposed in previous Congresses.

15 Multidisciplinary Panels were held studying the more frequent sites in Cancer, with an approach to the problem that included biological and clinical aspects, and concentrating on the following areas: aetiology, epidemiology, pathology, prevention, early detection, education, treatment and results. Proferred Papers were presented as Workshops instead of the classical reading, as in this way they could be discussed fully by the participants. 66 Workshops were held, this being the first time that free communications were presented in this way in a UICC Congress.

The Programme also included 22 "Meet the Experts", 7 Informal Meetings and more than a hundred films.

METHODOLOGY

The methodology used for the development of the Meeting and to make the scientific works profitable, had some original features that we would like to mention.

The methodology used in Lectures, Panels and Symposia was the usual one utilized in previous Congresses and functions satisfactorily. Lectures lasted one hour each. Panels were seven hours long divided into two sessions, one in the morning and one in the afternoon. They had a Chairman and two Vice-chairmen (one for each session). Symposia were three hours long. They had a Chairman, a Vice-chairman and a Secretary.

Of the 8164 registered members, many sent proferred papers of which over 2000 were presented. They were grouped in numbers of 20 or 25, according to the subject, and discussed in Workshops. The International Scientific Committee studied the abstracts of all the papers, and those which were finally approved were sent to the Chairman of the corresponding Workshop who, during the Workshop gave an introduction and commented on the more outstanding works. This was the first time such a method had been used in an UICC Cancer Congress.

"Meet the Experts" were two hours long, and facilitated the approach of young professionals to the most outstanding specialists. The congress was also the ideal place for an exchange of information between the specialists of different countries during the Informal Meetings. Also more than a hundred scientific films were shown.

The size of the task carried out in organising this Congress is reflected in some statistical data: More than 18,000 letters were sent to participants throughout the world; more than 2000 abstracts were published in the Proceedings of the Congress; more than 800 scientists were active participants of the various meetings.

There were 2246 papers presented at the Congress by 4620 authors from 80 countries.

The Programme lasted a total of 450 hours, and was divided into 170 scientific meetings where nearly all the subjects related to Oncology were discussed.

All the material gathered for the publication of these Proceedings has been taken from the original papers submitted by each author. The material has been arranged in 12 volumes, in various homogenous sections, which facilitates the reading of the most interesting individual chapters. Volume XII deals only with the abstracts of proffered papers submitted for Workshops and Special Meetings. The titles of each volume offer a clear view of the extended and multidisciplinary contents of this collection which we are sure will be frequently consulted in the scientific libraries.

We are grateful to the individual authors for their valuable collaboration as they have enabled the publication of these Proceedings, and we are sure Pergamon Press was a perfect choice as the Publisher due to its responsibility and efficiency.

Argentina   Dr Abel Canónico
March 1979   Dr Roberto Estevez
                                   Dr Reinaldo Chacon
                                   Dr Solomon Barg

                                   General Editors

Introduction

This volume is devoted to papers on acute leukaemia and non-Hodgkin's lymphoma presented at the XIIth International Cancer Congress in Buenos Aires (1978).

The first section of the volume is devoted to papers on acute leukaemia. J. Clemmerson reviews the evidence for an increase in leukaemia incidence using international data. The next two papers deal with the relationship between prognosis, cell surface markers and genetic markers in acute lymphoblastic leukaemia. The Houston group present their data on agar culture in acute myeloblastic leukaemia. This is followed by several papers on the treatment of acute leukaemia.

The second section is devoted to the non-Hodgkin's lymphomas with the first paper on the aetiology and epidemiology and the next series on factors important in the classification and prognosis. The Toronto group present their experience in determining prognostic factors and there are several papers on the role of different histopathological classifications. The Kiel classification is dealt with by several German groups.

The final section is concerned with the treatment of the non-Hodgkin's lymphomas. A group from the NCI present a summary of current clinical trials and the remaining papers are devoted to the role of chemotherapy and radiotherapy.

D. CROWTHER
March 1979

Acute Leukemia

Leukemia — Change of Pattern

Johannes Clemmesen

The Danish Cancer Registry, Strandboulevard 49, Copenhagen 2100, Denmark

ABSTRACT
An analysis of Leukemia incidence in various countries shows that an increase limited to groups aged over 60, which groups also account for international differences. Results from Denmark and other countries suggest that the increase is due mainly to more efficient diagnosis among the old.

KEYWORDS
Leukemia incidence. Age Groups. Geographical distribution. Leukemia Increase with time.

Since the first experimental approach by Ellermann & Bang, 1908 leukemia has taken a special position different from other neoplastic diseases. In fact it took several decades before it was recognized as such. Characteristic it was that the virus etiology has always been more under consideration for leukemia, and for **related** diseases, such as the juvenile African lymphoma, called Burkitt's tumor, and also the socalled lymphoepithelioma, whatever its true nature.
In animals confirmation of a viral etiology has been collected gradually for a number of species, beginning with chicken in 1908, and continued with mice in 1951 (Gross), with Cats 1964 (Jarrett et al.) and with cattle in 1972 (Olson et al.)

On epidemiological evidence the viral etiology of e.g. cattle leukemia had been suspected for long, and Bendixen had in Denmark taken the consequences, gradually eradicating the cattle leukemia, and so producing the final evidence of its contagiousity.

The old argument, why virus should play a different part in the etiology of malignant neoplasms in Man, from what is the case in animals may be answered by the one word Hygiene. It seems too modest to assume that the difference between our and other species is negligible, and nobody would ask a corresponding question in relation to chemical carcinogenesis. It may still be questioned to which extent racial factors may play a part. For instance, it seems significant that pharyngeal lymphoepithelioma is frequent in South East Asia as well as among the inhabitants of Greenland, which have racial features in common with the Chinese.

Registration and viruses
It may be argued that cancer registration has failed to reveal clusters or similar features supporting an infectious pathogenesis for leukemia. Usually cancer registries are established in regions with highly developed medical facilities, where

Johannes Clemmesen

a virus may be supposed to have relatively less facilities for spreading. One exception may have been the Cancer Registry of Kampala, Uganda, established by J.N.P. Davies, which provided the basis for the clarification of the Burkitt' tumour and contributed to the discovery of the Epstein-Barr virus, related to this tumour as well as to the nasopharyngeal socalled lympho-epithelioma.

Clusters
During later years the studies of clusters reported from various places have never provided very striking evidence of a viral spread, but it may be wise no to engage statisticians too ddeply in such studies, because they may be inclined to regard statistical significance as identical with medical significance.

An example is a cluster in New Zealand which statisticians explained away by epidemiological assumption of biological factors like many children or migration of unpredictable influence on analysis data.

All these data on clusters, which seem to have no parallel in other neoplastic diseases present clinical evidence - but during recent years we have come no further to any clue.

Chemical Leukemogenesis
Since no decisive changes seem to have been observed on the virus front, it should not be overlooked that there has been a number of statements on chemical leukemogenesis from various sides, but they do not seem to have made any overall change in the picture.

Radiation
At the time after World War II, there was general concern in some circles about a possible leukemogenic effect from nuclear radiation on the overall level of leukemia incidence but in the Danish Cancer Registry, which was established in 1942 we found no evidence of a general rise in incidence.

It applies, of course, both to chemical leukemogenesis and to radiation leukemia that we may expect some cases, secondary to antineoplastic treatment, and such cases have in fact been reported, although with the reveration that they may be due to a late leukemogenic effect from the carcinogen resulting in the neoplasm under therapy. It will be the task of workers in the near future to clarify this issue as far as possible.

Countries
In a previous study we compared the age distribution of leukemia mortality rates for a number of countries based on WHO data for the year 1953. It appeared that international differences in rates are limited to the age groups beyond 60 years. We were under the impression that the effort dedicated to the diagnosis of causes of death among the aged might influence these rates differently in the various countries.

On the basis of registry data for various countries published by the U.I.C.C. in its volumes on Cancer Incidence in Five Continents we have worked out corresponding age curves for incidence. It should be kept in mind that since the larger countries are represented only by regional registries their curves will tend to be more irregular than for mortality data. Nevertheless the curves leave an impression of similarity, except for the age groups beyond 60.

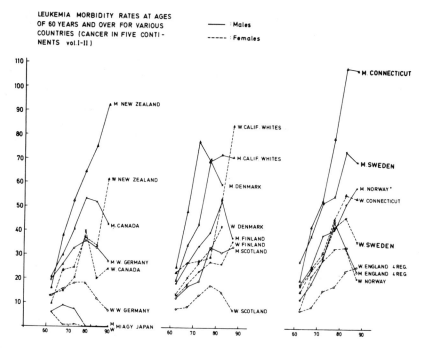

Fig.1.

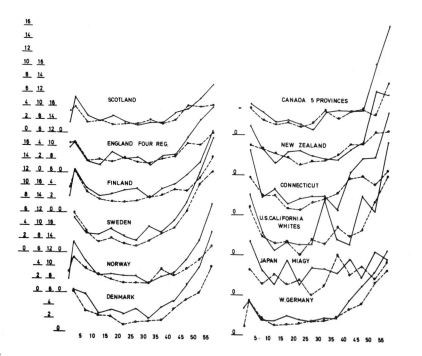

Fig.2.

Johannes Clemmesen

A study of Danish rates based on registration since 1942 shows an increase in overall rates, but when we study to which age groups we should ascribe this increase, we find it limited to the older age groups. For lymphatic leukemia it seems that the increase is limited to persons aged beyond 70 while for myeloid leukemia it starts no later than 60 years. Table I.

Since the age curve for lymphatic leukemia in general has its decisive rise later in life than the myeloid type has, this finding suggests that there may be no increase in the causative factors rather than just improved diagnosis among the aged.

Table I.

CANCERREGISTERET DENMARK

MEN PR.100,000	LYMPHATIC LEUKEMIA		MYELOID LEUKEMIA	
	1943-47	1968-72	1943-47	1968-72
00 - 04	3.8	4.0	2.1	1.1
05 - 09	1.1	2.2	0.9	0.5
10 - 14	1.3	1.2	1.3	0.5
15 - 19	1.2	1.6	0.9	1.6
20 - 24	1.0	0.4	1.5	1.2
25 - 29	1.3	1.2	1.6	1.5
30 - 34	0.7	0.3	1.7	1.7
35 - 39	0.9	1.7	2.2	2.4
40 - 44	1.0	1.0	1.2	2.4
45 - 49	2.7	2.3	2.4	3.3
50 - 54	5.8	3.8	2.6	4.8
55 - 59	9.8	8.1	4.5	5.7
60 - 64	12.2	12.4	4.5	7.9
65 - 69	19.4	18.0	6.7	11.0
70 - 74	21.7	34.7	6.1	16.1
75 - 79	15.0	45.4	5.0	22.9
80 - --	11.2	56.4	0.0	21.2
ALL AGES EUR.STAN.	4.6	6.3	2.4	4.0

A Biological Approach to the Diagnosis of Leukemias

L. Borella, J. T. Casper, A. E. Hodach and S. J. Lauer

The Midwest Children's Cancer Center, Department of Pediatrics,
The Medical College of Wisconsin, Milwaukee Children's Hospital,
Milwaukee, Wisconsin, U.S.A.

ABSTRACT

The approaches to the diagnosis of leukemia can be divided into 3 groups. The first group consists of procedures, such as cytomorphology and cytochemistry, which are required to reach an immediate therapeutic decision and are accessible to the hematologist. The second group involves more specialized methology that helps in the immediate diagnosis, but in addition may provide new concepts and experimental data. Examples are electron microscopy and the identification of cell membrane phenotypes. The third group is concerned with the biological diagnosis, which is available only in specialized centers integrated with multidisciplinary teams and enhances our knowledge regarding the pathogenesis of the disease. The biological diagnosis does not stop after therapy is initiated. It includes a longitudinal and multifactorial analysis of changes in leukemia and normal cells under the selective pressures of therapy. This knowledge is essential for the development of more specific and effective anti-leukemia treatments. To develop this concept of biological diagnosis we will include a short outline of leukemia cell differentiation and genetic markers and discuss data from our laboratory on prospective analysis of cell characteristics at various stages of the disease.

KEYWORDS: Diagnosis, leukemia, genetic markers, differentiation, phenotypes.

INTRODUCTION

"Diagnosis" implies a certain urgency to classify a patient within a disease category and to initiate a specific therapy. In this sense, establishing the diagnosis does not necessarily require a basic understanding of the disease's etiology and pathogenesis. Although this approach is valid for practical reasons, it may obscure the thinking needed to develop different and more effective therapeutic strategies.

The 50% cure rate of childhood ALL achieved almost a decade ago has not changed during recent years (Pinkel, 1977). Basic understanding of the leukemic process is a pre-requisite for improving these therapeutic results. We doubt that the challenge to cure the other one-half of ALL and to find effective treatments for other forms of leukemia will be met unless we define biological differences between individual patients. This can be accomplished if we think in terms of a biological diagnosis rather than on a limited pre-therapy decision.

APPROACHES TO THE DIAGNOSIS OF LEUKEMIA

Based on this reasoning we have divided the approach to the diagnosis of leukemias
into 3 groups (Table 1).

TABLE 1 Diagnosis of Leukemias

Group I	Procedures For An Immediate Therapeutic Decision	Clinical Features Cytomorphology Cytochemistry
Group II	Specialized Methodology	TEM and SEM Cell Membrane Phenotypes
Group III	Biological Diagnosis	Cell Differentiation and Virus Associated Antigens Genetic Markers Cytokinetics Functional and Pharmacological Characteristics Host Response

The first group consists of diagnostic procedures that are accessible to the hematologist and serve to classify the leukemia as acute or chronic, lymphoid or non-
lymphoid. These procedures are required to reach a therapeutic decision and include the differential clinical diagnosis, complemented by cytomorphology and cytochemistry. Although these tools would likely provide the diagnosis to the experienced hematologist, their limitations were emphasized in a recent comment by Profes-
sor Galton (1978). He stated that in the first leukemia trials of the Medical Research Council (MRC) only 18 of 100 slides reviewed by the MRC typing party received
the same diagnosis from all 8 observers. Hopefully, the development of new cytochemical techniques coupled with immunologic assays should provide more consistent
results.

In the second group we have included methods that although still in the experimental
phase, have already provided important information to establish or confirm a diagnosis before starting treatment. They are in the interphase or transitional phase,
i.e., are used as routine diagnostic procedures only in certain specialized centers
and the data obtained has both therapeutic and biological relevance. Within this
category is the study of cell ultrastructure using transmission and scanning electronmicroscopy, and the identification of cell membrane phenotypes with immunological
techniques. Electronmicroscopy has been useful in distinguishing leukemia or lymphoma cells from other tumor cells and identifying leukemic cell types, e.g., hairy
cell leukemia. The diagnostic and therapeutic implications of membrane phenotypes
are discussed in another section of this volume.

The rest of this discussion will be centered on the third type of diagnosis, the biological approach. The biological diagnosis of leukemias is based on methodology
which is only available at specialized centers possessing multidisciplinary teams.
The questions being asked relate to the origin and genetic make-up, proliferative,
functional and pharmacological characteristics of the tumor cells and their inter-
relationship with host responses, (Table 1). More importantly, this diagnosis does
not stop after initiation of treatment. It involves a multifactorial and prospective
analysis of the selective effects of therapy upon tumor and host cells. Our premise
is that the biological diagnosis of leukemia should provide the basis for the de-

velopment of more specific and effective leukemia therapy.

To emphasize this point we will briefly discuss the biological significance of cell
differentiation and genetic markers in relation to human leukemia, and present data
from our laboratory illustrating the importance of a prospective, longitudinal analysis of cell characteristics at various stages of the disease.

GENETIC AND CELL DIFFERENTIATION MARKERS

Newer concepts and methodology are being applied to the biologic diagnosis of leukemia. Areas which have greatly expanded in the 4 years since the last International Cancer Congress are genetic and differentiation markers of leukemic cells.
Table 2 summarizes some recent genetic developments.

TABLE 2   Genetic Markers

	Enzymes	Chromosomes	Hybridization
Example	G-6-PD in Females	1. Philadelphia 2. 14 q$^+$	1. DNA-RNA 2. Somatic Cell Hybrids
Significance	Clonal Origin	1. Pathogenesis 2. Pre-leukemia 3. Relapse	Membrane Structure and Gene Loci
Limitation	Patient Selection	Few Mitosis	Technical

The work of Fialkow et al. (1978) demonstrates an original approach in the study
of the biology of leukemias and lymphomas. It is based on the genetic fact that
women who are heterozygous for gene A and B of the enzyme glucose-6-phosphate
dehydrogenase (G-6-PD) have two cell types, one that synthesizes (A)G-6-PD, the
other (B)G-6-PD. These investigators have successfully applied this genetic information to establish if tumor cells originate from one or more cell types i.e.,
the presence of only one type of G-6-PD within the neoplastic cell population
suggests the monoclonal origin of this tumor. The main limitation of this method
is that it can be used only in a selected group of patients, heterozygous females.

Advanced cytogenetic techniques, such as chromosome banding employing Giemsa and
fluorescent dyes have provided a fresh impetus to chromosome analysis in hematopoietic neoplasias. The recent discovery of a chromosome 14 translocation not only
in Burkitt's lymphoma (Kaiser-McCaw, 1977) but also in the few B-cell leukemias
that have been studied (Cimino, 1978) suggest a genetic linkage between these types
of B-cell diseases. In addition, chromosome markers are useful tools in identifying neoplastic cells in the pre-leukemic phase and establishing the relationship
between initial and recurrent tumors. Unfortunately, many leukemias have few
mitotic figures, limiting this technique to neoplasias with high mitotic indices.
To partially overcome this problem the tumor cells can be fused with other cells
capable of active proliferation. This hybridization results in cells carrying
genotypes and phenotypes from both parental cell lines (Jones, 1977). Fusion of
mitotic cells with interphase cells has also allowed the visualization of premature chromosome condensations in the interphase cells (Sperling, 1974).

For simplification we have included under "Hybridization" (Table 2) two methods
which are conceptually and technically different. One method searches for gene
homologies using DNA and RNA as molecular probes; the degree of hybridization

L. Borella *et al.*

between genetic material from two sources, e.g. virus and cell, establishes the
degree of homology. Although this approach has been applied successfully to the
study of experimental leukemias, the results in human leukemias have been generally
disappointing. The reason for this failure is that human experimentation still
lacks specific probes, similar to those expressed in virus-induced leukemias. The
other form of hybridization involves fusion of two cells of different origin, e.g.,
human-hamster somatic cell hybrids (Jones, 1977). Using this approach, specific
cell surface components can be identified and their corresponding genetic elements
can be established. Somatic cell hybrids should play an important role in future
research related to the pathogenesis of leukemia.

TABLE 3   Cell Differentiation Markers

	Marker	Normal Expression	Leukemic Expression
A. Intracellular			
	Terminal-D Transferase	Thymocytes, Stem Cells?	ALL, CML in blast crisis
	Acid Phosphatase	T-Cell Subpopulation?	T-Leukemias
	Hexosaminidase Isoenzymes	?	Different Distribution in ALL
	Cytoplasmic Ig	Pre-B-Cells	Some ALL
B. Cytoplasmic Membrane			
	E-Receptors Thy Antigens μ and Fc Receptors	T-Cells	T-Leukemias
	mIg	B-Cells	B-Leukemias
	cALL Ag	Stem Cells?	"Common" ALL
	Ia-Like Ag	B-Cells, Monocytes, Myeloid Progenitors	Non-T-Leukemias
	C' Receptors	Lymphocytes, Monocytes Granulocytes	?
	Monocyte Ags	Monocytes	Mono-leukemias

An important step towards a better understanding of human leukemia biology has been
the recognition that leukemic cells possess differentiation markers which are also
expressed by their normal counterparts. Furthermore, the clinical features and
response to therapy of certain types of leukemia correlates with these normal cell
phenotypes (Borella, 1977; Brouet, 1976; Janossy, 1977; Sen, 1975). These differentiation markers are summarized in Table 3. Some are detected intracellularly
while others are expressed on the outer cell surface. Among the intracellular
markers are 3 enzymes: terminal-D-transferase, acid phosphatase and hexosaminidase
isoenzymes. Although the functional role of these enzymes are still unclear, they
are useful markers in identifying leukemic cells and in distinguishing leukemic
subtypes (Catovaky, 1978; Ellis, 1978). An additional intracellular characteristic
of leukemic cells recently described is the presence of cytoplasmic Ig (cIg). The
distribution of cIg in blasts from children with ALL is similar to that described

for normal pre-B-cells, suggesting a common origin (Vogler, 1978). Although this finding needs to be confirmed and extended, it provides additional evidence supporting the biological heterogenity of childhood ALL.

The majority of cell membrane markers are differentiation antigens. Some, such as T-cells (Thy) antigens, are restricted to a normal cell subpopulation, thus providing reliable information on the origin of leukemic cells. Based on the presence of Thy antigens on neoplastic cells a new clinical and biological entity: T-like leukemia/lymphoma has been established (Borella, 1977: Brouet, 1976; Janossy, 1978). Similarly, monoclonal membrane Ig synthesized by the tumor cell identifies B-like leukemia/lymphoma (Brouet, 1976). Obviously this is a simplified picture because leukemic cells also reflect other antigenic shifts that occur during normal T and B cell differentiation. Human T-cell leukemia may possess one or more different T-antigens normally expressed at various stages of maturation, similar to the murine system. Membrane receptors for sheep erythrocytes (E), the Fc portion of Ig and complement components are expressed on normal cells and leukemic cells. However, with the exception of E-receptors, a T-cell marker, they are not specific for a single cell population. It has recently been recognized that not only B, but also T-lymphocytes possess Fc receptors. The differential binding of μ Fc and γ Fc to functionally different human T-cell subpopulations provide an additional marker in the study of leukemias (Webb, 1977).

DIAGNOSIS AFTER INITIATION OF TREATMENT

Leukemias that appear similar before treatment may differ when subjected to the selective pressures of therapy. For this reason the biological diagnosis continues throughout the whole course of the disease. When the patient relapses, the leukemic cells may be phenotypically different from those present at initial diagnosis. This information is important not only to understand the pathogenesis of leukemia relapse, but for therapeutic reasons.

During the last 2 1/2 years we have conducted a prospective study of membrane phenotypes on neoplastic lymphoid cells at the time of diagnosis and relapse. Of 52 children with lymphoid malignancies who were initially studied, 19 have had tumor recurrence. The initial immunological diagnosis of these 19 children is shown in Table 4.

TABLE 4   Membrane Phenotypes at Diagnosis and Relapse in
Childhood Lymphoid Malignancies

Phenotype at Diagnosis		Phenotype at Relapse	
		No Change	Shift
Common Ag	11	11	0
T-Like	4	3	1
B-Like	3	2	1
"Null" Cell	1	0	1
Total	19	16	3

The objective of this study was to establish if leukemic cells that had been exposed to multiple antileukemia agents, expressed the same membrane differentiation markers that were present at diagnosis. Sixteen of these 19 patients have the same pheno-types at diagnosis and first relapse. The same results were obtained in 4 patients who were studied again in their second and third relapses. We conclude that in most children with lymphoid malignancies, chemotherapy does not affect the expression of membrane markers on recurrent tumor cells. There were, however, 3 exceptions (Table 5).

L. Borella *et al.*

TABLE 5   Membrane Phenotype Shifts in Childhood
Lymphoid Malignancies

Patient	1	2	3
Diagnosis	E^+ Thy^+	mIg $\mu\partial/\lambda$	Thy^- mIg^- $^cAg^-$
1st Relapse	E^- Thy^+	mIg μ/λ	Thy^- mIg^- $^cAg^-$
2nd Relapse	E^- Thy^+		Thy^+ mIg^- $^cAg^-$

At diagnosis the bone marrow blasts from the first patient formed E-rosettes and
expressed thymic (Thy) antigens. At relapse, the leukemic cells did not form
E-rosettes although they still possessed Thy antigens. The second patient had a
B-cell lymphoma. Most of the cells from the initial specimen expressed both IgM
and IgD, but when the tumor recurred only IgM bearing cells were detected. The
third patient was tentatively classified as "Null" cell ALL because her lymphoblasts did not possess any of the lymphoid markers (E^-, Thy^-, mIg^-, and $^cAg^-$). In
her first bone marrow relapse the leukemic cells were still "Null", but the phenotype shifted to Thy^+ with the second relapse. At this time 90% of bone marrow
blasts expressed Thy antigens. An attractive hypothesis to explain these findings
is that chemotherapy has selected a subpopulation of cells which may have been
present, though in small numbers, within the initial leukemic cell population or
that the drugs had altered an existing population.

Electronmicroscopy has added another dimension to the cytomorphological diagnosis
of leukemias. At the Midwest Children's Cancer Center we have initiated a prospective comparison of ultrastructural features of neoplastic cells at diagnosis
and relapse.   Fig. 1 illustrates the striking changes observed in the tumor cells
obtained from the same patient at time of diagnosis and at subsequent relapse.

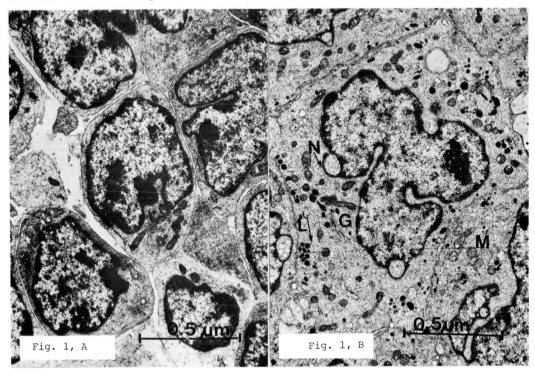

Fig. 1, A

Fig. 1, B

This child presented with a retroperitoneal tumor which invaded the kidney. By light microscopy and transmission electronmicroscopy the cells resembled lymphoblasts (Fig. 1A), though they did not possess any of the lymphoid differentiation markers (E^-, Thy^-, $^CAg^-$ and mIg^-). This patient was treated with anti-leukemic combination therapy, but multiple lymph node recurrence was observed 9 months after initial diagnosis. Again, no lymphoid markers were detected, but at relapse the ultrastructural features of the tumor cells were compatible with the diagnosis of histiocytic lymphoma (Fig. 1B). These cells were 2 to 3 times larger than the original tumor cells, with a high cytoplasm-to-nucleus ratio, the cytoplasm contained aggregates of lysosomes (L), numerous mitochondria (M) and prominent Golgi (G). Of interest was the peculiar infolding of the nuclear membrane and the appearance of nuclear blebs (N) in all cells examined. It is likely that this patient represents another example of a neoplasm containing cells at various stages of differentiation and with different sensitivity to chemotherapy. Following the selective destruction of lymphoblasts by the drugs, the tumor recurred but it was composed mainly of drug-resistent malignant histiocytes. This is not a unique finding as other cases of malignant histiocytosis occurring in patients with ALL have been described previously((Karcher, 1978).

Prospective analyses of changes in cell properties should not be limited to leukemic cells. To establish whether a neoplastic cell shares characteristics with normal cells, this cell should be compared with control populations undergoing the suppressive and regenerative changes induced by chemotherapy. An abnormal proliferation, differentiation and migration of normal cells may lead to the appearance of a neo-population or an expression of unexpected phenotypes. This has been demonstrated in a recent study comparing the presence of cells bearing DRw alloantigens in the blood of non-leukemic controls and children with leukemia in remission during and after cessation of therapy.

DRw alloantigens are expressed on non-T acute leukemia blasts and on normal B-cells, monocytes and myeloid progenitors. They are HLA antigens which are distinct from HLA-A, B and C and have physicochemical and amino acid sequence homologies with murine B-cell antigens (Ia) (Janossy, 1977); Schlossman, 1976). The cytotoxic assay using specific alloantisera to detect DRw antigens gives negative results against normal blood cells, unless the samples are selectively enriched for B-cells.

The results of 62 cytotoxic assays using blood mononuclear cells from controls and leukemic patients are shown in Table 6. These cells were separated from granulocytes and red cells using Ficoll-Hypaque.

TABLE 6   DRw Alloantigens on Blood Cells from Children with
Leukemia in Remission After Stopping Therapy

	Non-Leukemics	On Therapy	Leukemics in Remission Off Therapy (Months)		
			0·4	5-8	⩾9
Total	7*	13	11	18	13
DRw Positive	0	0	1	9	1

*
 Number of observations

All samples obtained from normal controls and patients with leukemia in remission
undergoing therapy were negative with the specific DRw alloantisera. In contrast,
9 of 18 cytotoxic assays using peripheral blood cells obtained 5 to 8 months after
cessation of therapy from leukemic children in remission were positive for specific
DRw antigens. DRw positive samples were also detected in 2 other children off
therapy for 2 and 9 months. Additional studies indicated that the high proportion
of DRw positive cells in these samples was not due to the presence of leukemic
cells or an increased number of B-cells or monocytes. Thus, a population of cells
bearing DRw antigens increased in the circulating pool during the regenerative
phase that followed cessation of therapy. We postulate that these cells are either
pluripotent stem cells or committed myeloid and lymphoid progenitors (Richman, 1976).
Although it is not clear whether these DRw-bearing cells may express other leukemia-
associated antigens, this possibility should be considered when phenotype markers
are used to identify early leukemic relapses.

ACKNOWLEDGEMENT

This work was supported by Research Grant CA 18602 and Cancer Center Grant CA 17700,
from the National Cancer Institute, by American Cancer Society Research Grant
IM-100C and by the Faye McBeath Foundation. J.T.C. and S.J.L. are recipients of a
Junior Faculty Award from the American Cancer Society. The authors gratefully
acknowledges the technical assistance of Ms. Jeanne Finlan, and Ms. Vicki Burke and
the secretarial assistance of Betty Carabello Cronan.

REFERENCES

Borella, L. , Sen, L., Dow, L. W., and Casper, J. T. (1977). Cell differentiation
    "versus" tumor related antigens in childhood acute lymphoblastic leukemia
    (ALL). Clinical significance of leukemia markers. In S. Thierfelder, H.
    Rodt, and E. Thiel (Ed.), Immunological Diagnosis of Leukemias and Lymphomas.
    Springer-Verlag, Heidelberg. pp. 77-84.
Brouet, J. C., Valensi, F., Daniel, M. T., Flandrin, G., Preud'homme, J. L., and
    Seligmann, M. (1976). Immunological classifications of acute lymphoblastic
    leukemias. Evaluation of its clinical significance in a hundred patients.
    Br. J. Haematol., 33, 319-326.
Catovsky, D., Greaves, M. F., Pain, C., Cherchi, M., Janossy, G., and Kay, H. E.
    (1978). Acid-phosphatase reaction in acute lymphoblastic leukaemia. Lancet,
    1, 749-751.
Cimino, M. C., Roth, D. G., Golomb, H. M., and Rowley, J. D. (1978). A chromosome
    marker for B-cell cancers. N. Engl. J. Med., 298, 1422.
Ellis, R. B., Rapson, N. T., Patrick, A. D., and Greaves, M. F. (1978). Expression
    of hexosaminidase isoenzymes in childhood leukemia. N. Engl. J. Med., 298,
    476-480.
Fialkow, P. J. Denman, A. M., Singer, J. Jacobson, R. J., and Lowenthal, M. N.
    (1978). Human myeloproliferative disorders: clonal origin in pluripotent
    stem cells. In Fifth Cold Spring Harbor Conference on Cell Proliferation
    (in press).
Galton, D. A. G., and Kay, H. E. M. (1978). Leukaemia clinical trials for
    children and adults. In Leukemia Research Fund 13th Annual Lecture.
Janossy, G., Goldstone, A. H., Capellaro, D., Greaves, M. J. Kulenkampff, J.,
    Pippard, M., and Welsh, K. (1977). Differentiation linked expression of p 28,
    33 (Ia-like) structures on human leukaemic cells. Br. J. Haematol. 37,
    391-402.
Jones, C., and Puck, T. T. (1977). Further studies of hybrid cell-surface antigens
    associated with human chromosome 11. Somatic Cell Genetics 3, 407-420.
Kaiser-McCaw, B., Epstein, A. L., Kaplan, H. S., and Hech, F. (1977) Chromosome
    14 translocation in african and north america Burkitt's lymphoma. Int. J.
    Cancer 19, 482-486.

Karcher, D. S., Head, D. R., and Mullins, J. D. (1978). Malignant histiocyto-
    sis occurring in patients with acute lymphocytic leukemia. Cancer 41, 1967-
    1973.
Pinkel, D., Simone, J., Aur, R. J., Borella, L., and Hustu, O. H. (1977). Per-
    spectives in diagnosis, prognosis and therapy of childhood acute lymphocytic
    leukemia. In Bentvelzen (Ed.), Advances in Comparative Leukemia Research.
    Elsevier/North Holland Biomedical Press. pp. 375-382.
Richman, C. M., Weiner, R. S., and Yankee, R. A. (1976). Increase in circulating
    stem cells following chemotherapy in man. Blood, 47, 1031-1039.
Schlossman, S. F., Chess, L., Humphreys, R. E., and Strominger, J. L. (1976).
    Distribution of Ia-like molecules on the surface of normal and leukemic cells.
    Proc. Natl. Acad. Sci. U. S. A., 73, 1288-1294.
Sen, L., and Borella, L. (1975). Clinical importance of lymphoblasts with T-mark-
    ers in childhood acute leukemia. N. Engl. J. Med., 292, 828-823.
Sperling, K., and Rao, P. N. (1974). The phenomenon of premature chromosome con-
    densation: its relevance to basic and applied research. Humangenetik. 23,
    235-258.
Vogler, L. B., Crist, W. M., Bockmam, D. E., Pearl, E. R., Lawton, A. R., and
    Cooper, M. D. (1978). Pre-B leukemia, a new phenotype of childhood lympho-
    blastic leukemia. N. Engl. J. Med., 298, 872-878.
Webb, S. R., Lydyard, P. M. Moretta, L. Ferrarini, M., Mingari, M. C., Moretta, A.,
    and Cooper, M. D. (1977). Proliferative responsiveness of two distinct human
    T-cell subpopulations to ConA, PHA and alloantigens. In D. O. Lucas (Ed.),
    Regulatory Mechanisms in Lymphocyte Activation. Academic Press, Inc., New
    York. pp. 512-514.

Cell Surface Markers in Acute Lymphoblastic Leukemia

Stephen Davis

*Oncology Section, Veterans Administration Medical Center, East Orange,
New Jersey, and the CMDNJ-New Jersey Medical School, Newark,
New Jersey, U.S.A.*

ABSTRACT

Membrane receptor analysis have been used to separate human lymphocytes into distinct populations. Thymus-derived (T-cell) lymphocytes can be identified by their
ability to form rosettes with sheep erythrocytes; bone marrow-derived (B cell)
lymphocytes bear characteristic surface markers of immunoglobulin, complement, and
the Fc portion of Ig. Recently, populations of lymphocytes having multiple markers (D cell) or no markers (null cell) have been observed. In addition to providing insights into cellular development, classifying the membrane characteristics
of the immature cells of acute leukemia seems to be important diagnostically and
prognostically. Present data suggest that T-cell markers on the lymphoblasts of
childhood acute lymphoblastic leukemia (ALL) is associated with a poor prognosis.
Aggressive induction therapy appears justified in this sub-group of ALL patients.
KEY WORDS: lymphoblastic leukemia, membrane markers, T cells, B cells, null cells,
             leukemic Ia antigens

PRESENTATION

Techniques for analyzing specific membrane receptors on human lymphocytes has added
valuable information to our understanding of the structure-function relationship of
these cells. The presence of surface immunoglobulin (Ig) determinants and the
ability to secrete Ig are characteristic of the B-cell. In addition, the human B-
cell has receptors for complement as well as the capacity to bind aggregated Ig and
antigen-antibody complexes, by means of surface receptors for the Fc portion of the
Ig molecule; however, these are not specific for lymphocytes and are detectable on
myeloid and monocytoid tissue. Human T cells are identified by their ability to
form rosettes with sheep erythrocytes. More recent studies have identified populations of lymphocytes having multiple markers (D cell) or no detectable markers
(null cell) by these techniques. These later cells cannot be precisely classified
as T or B, suggesting transitional forms (Davis, 1975).

The scheme shown in Fig. 1 depicts the hypothetical differentiation of the lymphocyte from a bone marrow stem cell based on the above cell surface markers (Davis,
1975). The scheme utilizes the concept of progressive and regressive change in
surface alloantigens, a phenomenon well described in mice (Raff, 1971). In man,
both T and B cells appear to arise from a common precursor which bear no detectable
surface markers. The first step in the maturation of this stem cell is the production of a null cell. The transition of stem cells to null cells has not been

17

documented experimentally; however, the finding that null cells form colonies of mature T- and B-cells in vitro suggests that they represent a lymphocyte precursor cell (Geha, 1973). The proposed model assumes that the null cell represents a single population of uncommitted cells; however, the null cell could conceivably be comprised of two cell populations, phenotypically similar, which are destined to reveal a distinct population of small lymphocytes (2%-13%) bearing no detectable markers.

Continued differentiation of the null cell results in a cell capable of expressing both T- and B-cell markers (D cell). The most consistently detectable B-cell marker is the complement receptor. Maturing lymphocytes subsequently fall under the influence of the central lymphoid organs. Cells destined for the T cell compartment migrate to the thymus and undergo alterations both in functional capacity and in cell surface markers. B cells mature in a fashion similar to T-cells by developing from a multiple marker cells into cells endowed with Fc and complement markers. Because these cells do not secrete Ig they cannot be definitively classified as B-lymphocytes. Recent investigations (Gathings, 1977; Owen, 1977) have characterized a B-cell precursor containing no surface Ig and small amounts of cytoplasmic IgM. Occasionally, complement receptors have been detected on these cells. It appears reasonable to consider these "pre-B" cells as intermediary forms between D cells and cells expressing Fc and complement receptors. These "pre-B" cells precede the appearance of B cells bearing Ig markers, i.e., IgD, IgM, IgG, IgA (Fig. 1).

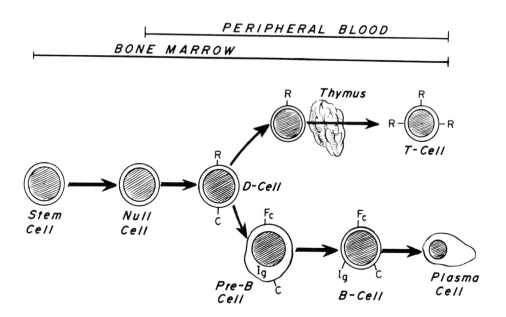

Fig. 1. Hypothetical differentiation of the lymphocyte from a bone marrow stem cell. R, receptor for sheep erythrocytes; Fc, receptor for Fc portion of immunoglobulin; C, complement receptor; Ig, immunoglobulins

Recognizing the hazards of extrapolating data obtained from normal lymphocytes we may speculate about the origin of childhood ALL blasts in the context of the differentiation scheme described above. ALL has long been appreciated to be a heterogeneous disease based upon clinical presentation, response to chemotherapy, and prognosis. Many investigators (Hardisty, 1968; Lampkin, 1972) have reported a poor prognosis in patients who have the following findings at the time of diagnosis: age less than a year or greater then ten years; white cell count greater than 50,000; hepatosplenomegaly; mediastinal mass; central nervous system involvement. Tsukimoto and his associates (1976), Sen and Borella (1975), and Glick and co-workers (1978) have studied surface markers in cases of childhood ALL. In the majority of cases (75%) lymphoblasts had no detectable markers (null cells), the remaining cases form rosettes with sheep erythrocytes (T-cell). Greaves and associates (1975) have confirmed these data using an antiserum rendered specific for null-ALL blasts. The membrane antigens that this antiserum recognizes are not present on normal lymphocytes nor T- or B-cell leukemias. In the studies of Tsukimoto,and Sen and Borella patients with T-cell receptors on the blasts, in general, were characterized by a mediastinal mass and massive leukemic infiltra-- tion of body tissues. Tsukimoto and associates (1976) observed 36 patients for periods greater than six months; 60% of patients with T-cell ALL had relapsed; compared with 14% for null cell ALL. Belpomme and co-workers (1978) have confirmed these findings. Glick and his co-workers (1978) found that all patients went into remission with vincristine and prednisone and that mean survival in the null- and T-cell groups was identical (15.6 months). However, mean remission duration was significantly decreased in the T-cell subgroup. Thus, the ability of ALL blasts to form rosettes with sheep erythrocytes seems to connote a poor prognosis. Our own experience is in agreement with these investigators. Because of the poor prognosis of T-cell ALL we are presently using four-drug multimodal therapy for remission induction. Survival data is preliminary but suggest increased survival over standard vincristine and prednisone therapy. In my opinion, this subgroup of ALL patients should, for therapeutic considerations, be considered as having poorly differentiated lymphocytic lymphoma. Further studies, however, are obviously needed.

Conceptually, failure of lymphocytes in the bone marrow to mature properly might result in null cell ALL, a disseminated disease. Similarly, maturation arrest in the thymus results in T-cell ALL, a disease localized to the mediastinum initially but whose clinical course in its late stages may be indistinguishable from null cell ALL (Fig. 1). The clinical similarities between what is called T-cell ALL and mediastinal lymphoma of childhood are striking. At the present time, it is perhaps wiser to consider them a spectrum of the same disease process. Such an analogy has been drawn for Sezary syndrome and mycosis fungoides, two T-cell lymphoproliferative diseases (Davis, 1975).

The presence of B-cell markers on ALL blasts is reported to be a rare event (Seligmann, 1973) using routine immunofluorescent methodology. Many investigators believe that B--cell ALL actually represents the leukemic phase of poorly differentiated lymphoma (Flandrin, 1975). Catovsky and associates (1978) recognized two morphologic types of B-cell leukemia: the Burkitt's type and the lymphosarcoma type. In my opinion and that of other investigators (Tsukimoto, 1975), there is no morphologic, histochemical or immunologic evidence to support the fact that B-cell ALL represents lymphoma variants. Furthermore, using technics designed to characterize cytoplasmic Ig, recent studies in mice and man have characterized a B-cell precursor containing minute amounts of cytoplasmic IgM and no surface Ig, Vogler and his associates (1978) found 4 of 22 consecutive patients with childhood ALL had the appearance of these "pre-B" cells. If these findings are confirmed, it would appear that a sizeable proportion of previously catogorized null cell ALL blasts are actually of B-cell lineage. Preliminary data suggest that remission induction in this subset of patients is easily achievable with vincristine and

prednisone not unlike what has been observed in null cell cases; however, more
data is needed to see if this ALL subset is different in response to therapy and
prognosis (Fig. 2).

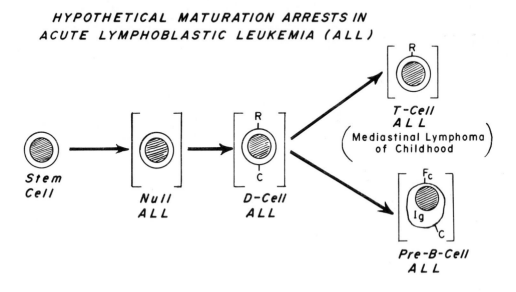

Fig. 2. Lymphoblastic leukemia vaiants based on cell surface
markers.

Recently, an antiserum was prepared from a glycoprotein complex of 23,000 to 30,000
daltons (p23,30) obtained from a human lymphoblastoid B cell line (Schossman, 1976).
This antiserum reacts specifically with B cells but fails to recognize HLA antigens,
Fc and complement receptors, or surface Ig. Schlossman and his associates (1976)
found that p23,30 antibody reacted with ALL blasts in 90% of their patients and
100% of blasts from patients with AML. The remaining 10% of their ALL cases were
p23,30-negative; however, these cases clearly reacted with an anti-T cell serum.
Thus, all their ALL cases could be shown to possess either B- or T-cell markers.
Fu, Winchester, and Kunkel (1975) obtained similar results using anti-sera against
HL-B alloantigens. In the six ALL cases they studied, four were null cell by
classic cell marker criteria; however, all four reacted with anti HL-B serum. Both
p23,30 and HL-B alloantigens are thought to be related to the human counterpart of
murine Ia antigens which are preferentially expressed on normal B cells. According
to these findings all cases of childhood ALL are of B cell origin. The significance of p23,30 and HL-B antigens is unknown at the present time; however, one can
hypothetically view them as early differentiation antigens in a fashion similar to

that described in Fig. 1. Lymphoid cells destined to be T cells lose detectable p23,30 and HL-B antigens whereas B cells retain these characteristics. Alternatively, p23,30 and HL-B antigens are recognizing different antigens on myeloid and lymphoid cells. One must interpret these data with caution. Because these Ia-like antigens are found in so many different cell types, they actually may represent differentiation antigen of all hemopoietic cells (myeloid, erythroid, and lymphoid) and not necessarily represent evidence for a B-cell lineage. No data is available using p23,30 or HL-B antigen markers as to prognostic significance.

Experience with ALL of adulthood suggests this to be a disease distinct from the childhood variety. Not only is there marked heterogenecity in the morphology of the blast population but the remission rate is lower (70-80%) than in children (Scavino, 1976) using vincristine and prednisone therapy and early relapse and shorter median survival duration (about 15 months) is seen. Reasons for this difference might involve the inherent cell biology of the blast or that adult ALL blasts represent an undifferentiated blast not characterizeable by current methodology. Using classic cell markers 60-70% of adult ALL cases are null cell. However, when tested with the anti-null cell sera of Greaves (1975) only 75% of the later cases are positive. The remaining adult ALL cases are classified as T-cell (Catovsky, 1978). Chromosome analysis of adult ALL blasts has demonstrated a significant number of cases to be Ph^1-positive. If one realizes that the cells in chronic myelogenous leukemia (CML) in blast conversion also have Ph^1-positivity acute ALL and CML might actually represent stem cell leukemias (Tsukimoto, 1975; Catovsky, 1978). I believe it is safe to say that adult ALL is a heterogenous disease distinct clinically and immunologically from childhood ALL; more patients must be analyzed with current techniques to further subdivide the disease in order to formulate definitive conclusions. Future studies on adult ALL should be performed and analyzed independent of the childhood variety.

In summary, it is clear that the heterogeneity of ALL is now being redefined by the use of cellular probes. As our knowledge advances further substets of ALL will emerge leading to a better prognosis and a greater appreciation of normal and neoplastic cell biology.

REFERENCES

Belpomme, D., and colleagues (1978). Cytological and immunological types: Two factors of prognosis of acute lymphoid leukemia. In J.V. Gutterman and colleagues, Rationale and Application of Immunotherapy for Human Cancer; Current Problems in Cancer, Vol. 2, No. 11, Year Book Medical Publishers, Chicago. pp. 50-52.

Catovsky, D. (1978). Immunologic markers in acute leukemia. In H.R. Gralnick (moderator). Classification of acute leukemia. Ann. Intern. Med., 87, 743-746.

Davis, S. (1975). Hypothesis: Differentiation of the human lymphoid system based on cell surface markers. Blood, 45, 871-880.

Flandrin, G., and colleagues (1975). Acute leukemia with Burkitt's tumor cells: a study of six cases with special reference to lymphocyte surface markers. Blood, 45, 183-188.

Fu, S.M., R.J. Winchester, H.G. Kunkal (1976). The occurrence of the HL-B alloantigens on the cells of unclassified acute lymphoblastic leukemia. J. Exp. Med., 142, 1334-1337.

Gathings, W.E., A.R. Lawton, M.D. Cooper (1977). Immunofluorescent studies of the development of pre B cells, B lymphocytes and immunoglobulin isotype diversity in humans. Eur. J. Immun., 7, 804-810.

Geha, R.S., F.S. Rosen, E. Merler (1973). Identification and characterization of subpopulations of lymphocytes in human peripheral blood after fractionation on discontinuous gradients of albumin. The cellular defect in X-linked

agammaglobulinemia. J. Clin. Invest., 52, 1726-37.
Glick, A.D., and colleagues (1978). Ultrastructural study of acute lymphocyte
    leukemia: Comparison with immunologic studies. Blood, 52, 311-322.
Greaves, M.F., and colleagues (1975). Antisera to acute lymphoblastic leukemia
    cells. Clin. Immunol. Immunopathol., 40, 67-84
Hardisty, R.M., M.M. Till (1968). Acute leukemia 1959-64: factors affecting
    prognosis. Arch. Dis. Child, 43, 107-115.
Lampkin, B.C., N.B. McWilliams (1972). Treatment of acute leukemia. Pediatr.
    Clin. North Am., 19, 1123-1140.
Owen, J.J.T., and colleagues (1977). Studies on the gonoration of B lymphocytes
    in fetal lives and bone marrow. J. Immunol., 118, 2067-2072.
Ruff, M.C. (1971). Surface antigenic markers for distinguishing T and B lympho-
    cytes in mice. Transplant Reo., 6, 52-64.
Scavino, H.F., J.N. George, D.A. Sears (1976). Remission induction in adult acute
    lymphocytic leukemia. Use of vincristine and prednisone alone. Cancer, 38,
    672-677.
Schlossman and colleagues (1976). Distribution of Ia-like molecules on the sur-
    face of normal and leukemic human cells. Proc. Nat. Acad. Sci. (USA), 73,
    1288-1292.
Seligman, M., J. L. Preud'homme, J. C. Bronet (1973). B and T cell markers in huma
    proliferative blood diseases and primary immunodeficiencies with special
    reference to membrane bound immunoglobulin. Transplant. Rev., 16, 83-113.
Sen, L., L. Berella (1976). Clinical importance of lymphoblasts with T markers in
    childhood acute leukemia. New Eng. J. Med., 292, 828-832.
Tsukimoto, I., K.Y. Wong, B.C. Lampkin (1975). Surface markers and prognostic
    factors in acute lymphoblastic leukemia. New Eng. J. Med., 294, 243-248.
Vogler, L.B., and colleagues (1978). Pre-B-cell leukemia. A now phenotype of
    childhood lymphoblastic leukemia. New Eng. J. Med., 298, 872-878.

The Heterogeneity and Clonal Evolution in Preleukemic States and Oligoleukemia: Results with in vitro Agar Culture

G. Spitzer, D. S. Verma, K. A. Dicke, A. Zander and K. B. McCredie

Department of Development Therapy,
University of Texas System Cancer Center,
M.D. Anderson Hospital and Tumor Institute, Houston, Texas

ABSTRACT

Nineteen patients with a diagnosis of preleukemia and 65 patients with a diagnosis of oligoleukemia, were studied by in vitro agar culture. Five in vitro growth patterns were recognized (1) Category (Cat) I-A with low colony and cluster incidence, normal cluster/colony ratio and normal cellular differentiation in colonies, (2) Cat I-B with normal to high number of colonies and clusters, normal cluster/ colony ratio and normal cellular differentiation in colonies, (3) Cat II with low colony and high cluster incidence and normal granulocytic colonies, (4) Cat III-A with growth of excessive clusters (3-20 cell size) and (5) Cat III-B with excessive numbers of clusters of >20 cells size with or without colonies consisting predominately of blast cells. Growth patterns II, III-A and III-B are characteristic of acute myeloid leukemia, and are therefore celled leukemic growth patterns. In preleukemia, progression to leukemia was uncommon in patients with Category I-A patterns, but common in patients with other categories. As in preleukemia, patients with oligoleukemia Cat I-A appeared to have a benign course and seldom developed progressive leukemia. Sequential cultures detected changing in vitro culture patterns frequently in advance of changing clinical status. Preliminary experiments also suggest that these methods can be used to study cell regulation of both normal and leukemic growth in these conditions.

Key words: Preleukemia, oligoleukemia, agar culture, in vitro subdivision, clinical prediction, and cellular regulation.

INTRODUCTION

Prelekemic states are manifested by cytopenia of the peripheral blood elements and dyshematopoiesis in the marrow without evidence of increased marrow blast cells. This diagnosis has been increasingly recognized. Approximately 30% of these patients will develop overt leukemia within 6 months, 71% by the end of 2 years, and some may never. A complete morphological and clinical description of these states, has been described by Linman and Saarni, 1974. Possibly these conditions consist of patients who (a) truely do have leukemic clones of cells, and may develop leukemia within a relatively short period of time, (b) have a marrow dysplasia with an increased tendency to clonal evolution to a degree clinically recongniz-

able as leukemia, or (c) have bone marrow dysplasia without the differentiation
block classical of leukemia and who do not show progressive clonal evolution
during clinical observation. A number of publications (Dreyfus, 1976; Geary,
1975; Jacquillat, 1975; Rheingold, 1963) emphasize the variable clinical behavior
of leukemic states with a low percentage of myeloblasts in the bone marrow. We
have termed this condition oligoleukemia, but this term embrases such entities
as chronic myelomonocytic leukemia, refractory anemia with excess myeloblast and
smoldering leukemia. Some patients have an indolent history, others display
aggressive leukemic growth and still others die early due to hematological compromise. There is no available methodology to determine patients with aggressive
disease, who should be treated immediately from those destined to have relatively
benign clinical course who maybe harmed by aggressive therapy.

It is well recognized that the vitro growth pattern of leukemic myeloid progenitor cells is different and distinctive from that of normal myeloid progenitor
cells (CFU-c). Instead of colonies (40 cells or greater), with clusters (3-39
cell aggregates) in a frequency of approximately 5 times greater, bone marrow
from leukemic patients usually grows in vitro as only clusters frequently with
an increased incidence (Moore, Williams, Metcalf, 1973; Moore and others, 1974;
Spitzer and others, 1976a; Spitzer and others, 1976b). Since we have shown previously (Spitzer and others, 1976a; Spitzer and others, 1976b) that these assays
appear to measure cells biologically relevant to leukemia behavior, it appeared
logical to examine the different in vitro growth patterns in both preleukemia and
oligoleukemia. The initial primary question in the preleukemic state was whether
these methods are sensitive enough to detect leukemic clones in patients with an
immediate risk of leukemic transformation. Our second question was in oligoleukemia, could we identify patients with differing clinical behavior. Lastly we wished to examine it these methods could be used to examine such important biological
questions as, (1) possible cell mediated control of leukemic growth and (2) leukemia inhibition of normal myelopoiesis so we may modify this inhibition of normal
growth preventing death in patients with indolent disease.

MATERIALS AND METHODS

Extensive definitions of preleukemic states and oligoleukemia are given in other
publications (Spitzer and others, 1978; Verma and others, 1978). For the diagnosis of a preleukemic state, we required involvement of all cell lines (cytopeni-
as, plus morphological abnormalities), a normal to hypercellular bone marrow with
less than 5% blast and the elimination of secondary causes of such a hematological picture. Oligoleukemia was defined as a leukemic condition with less than
50% leukemic cell infiltrate.

The absolute marrow blast cell infiltrate is calculated as follows:

$$\frac{\% \text{ Blast + Promyelocytes} \times \% \text{ Clot Section Cellularity}}{100}$$

The methods of culture, culture scoring, colony and cluster morphological analysis, statistical methods, follow-up and criteria for chemotherapy intervention,
are given in other publications (Spitzer and others, 1978; Verma and others,1978).

RESULTS

Some of these results are a summary of those that are to appear more extensively

in other publications (Spitzer and others, 1978, Verma and others, 1978). In all
19 patients with a diagnosis of preleukemia and 65 with a diagnosis of oligoleukemia were studied. Examination of the culture dishes under the dissecting micro-
scope revealed three types of growth patterns. (a) a lower than normal incidence
of colony and clusters, with normal cluster/colony ratio, (b) a growth of excessive clusters with or without colonies in low numbers, and finally, (c) the growth
of colonies and clusters in normal to high numbers with normal cluster to colony
ratio and normal colony morphology. The first growth pattern was termed Category
(Cat) I-A. Colonies were of normal granulocytic differentiation. The second
type of growth pattern was further subdivided into Cat III-A, consisting of only
clusters of 20 cells or less, Cat III-B consisting of variable number of clusters
of greater than 20 cells and sometimes colonies of blast cell morphology and Cat
II which in addition to the excessive number of clusters, also had normal granulocytic colonies. The group with the high number of granulocytic colonies was
termed Cat I-B. These subdivisions are diagramatically represented in Fig. 1.
Table 1 gives a distribution of these categories in preleukemia and oligoleukemia.
The most common growth pattern in oligoleukemia was Cat III, a pattern classical
of acute leukemia. In preleukemia the most common growth pattern was Cat I-A
(non-leukemic).

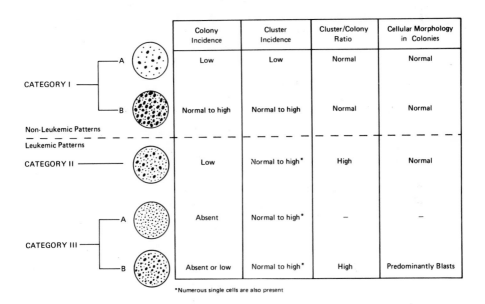

Fig. 1. In vitro culture patterns in preleukemia and
oligoleukemia. Reproduced with kind permission from:
Verma, D.S. and others. In vitro agar culture patterns
in preleukemia and their clinical significance. Leuk.
Res. - (In Press).

TABLE 1 Distribution of Patients According to In Vitro
Culture Pattern.

	Category	Numbers of Patients	
		Preleukemia	Oligoleukemia
Non-Leukemic Growth Patterns	I-A	12 (63)*	12 (18)
	I-B	2 (11)	5 (8)
Leukemia Growth Patterns	II	2	5
	III-A	2 (26)	28 (74)
	III-B	1	15
TOTAL		19	65

*Percent

The follow-up date of patients with preleukemia is given in Table 2. As can be
seen from this Table, progression to acute leukemia is more common and survival
is shorter in patients with preleukemic states and Cat I-B, II, III-A and III-B
compared to Cat I-A. Only 1 patient with Cat I-A progressed to leukemia and this
clinical change was preceded by change in culture pattern to III-A, a leukemic
culture pattern.

TABLE 2 Preleukemia: incidence of Progression to Oligo or
Acute Leukemia.

Reporduced with kind permission from Verma and others, In
vitro agar culture patterns in preleukemia and their clinical significance. Leuk. Res. - (In Press).

Category	Total Patients	Progressed to Leukemia	Period of ‡ Follow-up (weeks)	Time to Change (weeks)
I-A	12	1	38*(4-104)+	40
I-B	2	2	32, 32	16,32
II	2	1	14,18	8
III-A	2	2	34, 2	
III-B	1	1	36	28

*Median + Range   ‡ values in all categories except
I-A, represent individual pat-
ents.

In oligoleukemia, survival was significantly longer in Cat I-A (P value = <0.04), progression to acute leukemia slower (P = <0.02), and rate of increase in leukemic cell infiltrate lesser (P = <0.02) (Fig. 2) than in patients with a Cat III pattern.   Of particular interest was that the large majority of those with the leukemia culture pattern of Cat III showed progression to acute leukemia compared to those with a Cat I-A pattern (approximately 50% vs. 17%). The number of patients with Cat I-B and II, were too small to make any meaningful comparisons.

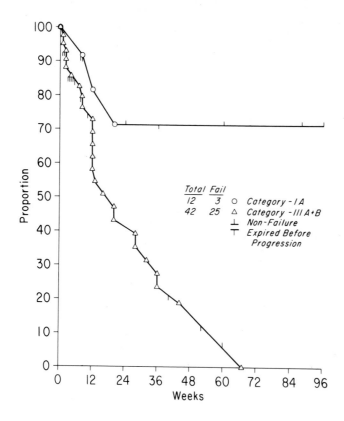

Fig. 2.   Progression by 15% increase in leukemic inflit-rate (Oligoblastic Leukemia)
Reproduced with kind permission from Spitzer, G., and others, Subgroups of oligoleukemia as indentified by in vitro agar culture. Leuk. Res. - (In Press).

Sequential cultures in preleukemia and oligoleukemia of patients with Cat I-A, I-B and II culture patterns, showed changes such as loss of diffentiated colonies (Cat II ⟶ Cat III), or loss of coloneis and the appearances of excessive clusters (Cat I-A and I-B ⟶Cat III).   These changes occurred frequently in advance of the appearance of excessive myeloblast (Preleukemia) or sudden change in leukemic cell infiltrate or worsening hematopoietic status (Oligoleukemia). A worsening hematopoietic status may represent increasing leukemic clonal expansion or development of a new leukemic clone not morphologically recognizable, but with secondary effects on normal hematopoiesis.

G. Spitzer *et al.*

It is possible that the majority of Cat I-A and I-B patients with preleukemic
states may not, in fact, be at immediate risk of leukemic transformation. Methods
to increase the sensitivity of leukemic clone detection, might identify these
patients more accurately. The discontinuous albumin density gradient was pre-
formed on an oligoleukemia patient with a I-B growth pattern (Table 3). Culture
features of acute leukemia (excessive cluster formation) was detected in fraction
3 and 4. These and other separation methods may be applicable to more accurately
detect leukemic transformation in Cat I-A and I-B patients. Further investigations to understand why a leukemic clone may be suppressed or relatively inhibit-
ed in growth potential was performed by examining leukemic cluster growth before
and after E-rosette positive cell removal from the peripheral blood of a case of
oligoleukemia. Both placental conditioned media stimulated and spontaneous cluster growth was enhanced by removal of T-cells (Table 4). Further experiments are
needed to examine more closely the possible presence of regulatory cells modify-
ing leukemic growth in these conditions. To examine the possible leukemic inhibition of normal hematopoiesis, cell incubation experiments were performed using
cells from oligoleukemia and normal bone marrow. Figure 3 gives an illustration
of the experimental design and Fig. 4, the data from such experiments. The range
of suppression or stimulation with mixes of normal bone marrow was within a narrow
range of that expected ($\pm$ 20). However, variable effects were seen in mixes of
leukemic and normal bone marrow. It will be interesting to correlate these in
vitro inhibitory and stimulatory effects with the degree of hematopoietic compromise observed clinically.

TABLE 3 Discontinuous Gradient Separation of Cat I-B oligoleukemia (Blasts = 9%)

Fraction	Colonies	Cluster	Ratio
1 + 2	430	1960	3.8
3	29	690	23.7*
4	1	123	123*
5	0	2	2

* Abnormal: Upper limit of normal = 17.

TABLE 4 Enhancement of In Vitro Leukemia Cluster Growth by
E-Rosette Cell Removal

	+ PCM	- PCM
Without E-Rosette Cell Removal	280 $\pm$ 9.6*	0
With E-Rosette Cell Removal	1350 $\pm$ 21.2	93 $\pm$ 5.5

PCM = Placental conditioned media
     * Standard error

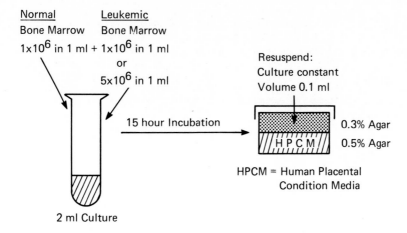

Fig. 3. Schema of experiment for suppression of normal hematopoiesis.

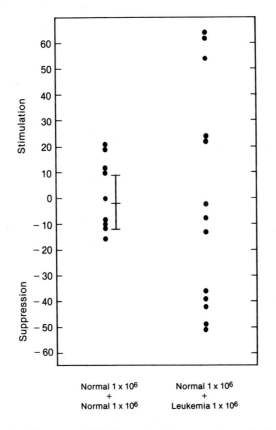

Fig. 4. Change of CFU-C compared to expected after mixing combinations of normal or normal and leukemic bone marrow for 15 hours in liquid culture.

CONCLUSIONS

In vitro agar culture identifies subgroups of preleukemic states and oligoleukemia consistant with the heterogeneity of these diseases. Patients with preleukemia and Cat I-A growth pattern show a generally benign course and seldom transform to acute leukemia. Patients with other growth patterns and preleukemia show a high tendency to leukemia transformation. It also appears from this data, that patients with oligoleukemia and a Cat I-A in vitro growth pattern, irrespective of any morphological description have a relatively benign course and a long survival and seldom have progression to leukemia. Patients with Cat III, the majority of patients, are associated with more progressive disease and shorter survival. The behavior of Cat I-B and II are still uncertain, but these patients as mentioned previously, frequently change their growth pattern to that of Cat III, with time. Why a leukemic growth pattern is not initially expressed in culture in oligoleukemia with Cat I-A pattern, is uncertain, but the possibility of a suppressor cell is under investigation. In the attempt to synthesize the culture findings in preleukemia and oligoleukemia, we have come up with a tentitive scheme of clonal evolution as detected by culture patterns. In preleukemia, Cat I-A because of the rarity of leukemic transformation in this group, represent an early stage of preleukemic states. Cat I-B, despite no obvious leukemia growth pattern, behaves similarly to patients with leukemic growth patterns (II, III-A and III-B), and may therefore, represent a transitory or intermediate state between I-A and II and III. In fact, of recent, we have seen two patients change from Cat I-A and I-B and subsequently to III. Finally, in preleukemia, Cat II and III, represent more aggressive disease with relatively rapid transformation to leukemia. Similarly, in oligoleukemia, there may be 3 such groups of patients, (1) those with an initial indolent course and a Cat I-A culture pattern, which may later change to a more aggressive leukemic disorder and then reveal a Cat III culture pattern. (2) those beginning with a moderately slow clinical course occasionally with monocytosis in the peripheral blood and a Cat I-B culture pattern who may progress to a more aggressive leukemic disorder and similarly change their culture pattern to that of II or III and (3) those who from the very beginning present with a rather aggressive disease and a leukemic culture pattern (II, III-A or III-B). These possibilities are depicted in Fig. 5.

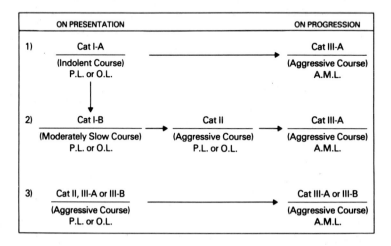

Fig. 5. Changing in vitro agar culture patterns as observed during the clinical course of oligoleukemia and preleukemia.

P.L.:   Preleukemia
O.L.:   Oligoleukemia
A.M.L.: Acute Myeloid or myelomonocytic leukemia

It is possible by the use of these techniques that we may be better able to understand the biology of (a) leukemic growth control in these conditions and (b) suppression of normal hematopoiesis by leukemic cells. Such understanding may help
us better manage other preleukemic conditions such as actue myeloid leukemia in
remission and CML benign phase.

REFERENCES

Dreyfus, G. (1967). Preleukemic states. I. Definition and classification. II,
    Refractory anemia with an excess of myeloblasts in the bone marrow (smolder-
    ing leukemia). Blood Cells, 2, 33-55.
Geary, C.G., D. Catovsky, E. Wiltshaw, G.R. Milner, M.C. Scholes, S. van Noorden,
    L.D. Wadsworth, A. Muldal, J.E. MacIver and D.A.G. Galton (1975). Chronic
    myelomonocytic leukemia. Br. J. Haematol., 30, 289-302.
Jacquillat, C.I., V. Izrael, M. Weil., C.I. Chastang, M. Boison, and J. Bernard
    (1975). A study of 120 patients with oligoblastic leukemia (OBL). Am. Assoc.
    Cancer Res., # 413, 103.
Linman, J.W., and M.I. Saarni (1974). The preleukemia syndrome. Semin. Hematol.
    11, 93 -
Moore, M.A.S., N. Williams, and D. Metcalf (1973). In vitro colony formation by
    normal and leukemic human hematopoietic cells: characterization of the colony
    forming cells. J. Natl. Cancer Inst., 50, 603-623.
Moore, M.A.S., G. Spitzer, N. Williams, D. Metcalf and J. Buckley (1974). Agar
    culture studies in 127 cases of untreated acute leukemia: The prognostic
    value of reclassification of leukemia according to in vitro growth character-
    istics. Blood, 44, 1-18.
Rheingold, J.J., R. Kaufman, E. Adelson and A. Lear (1963). Defective in vitro
    colony formation by human bone marrow preceeding overt leukemia. N. Eng. J.
    Med. 268, 812-815.
Spitzer, G., K. Dicke, E.A. Gehan, T. Smith, K.B. McCredie, B. Barlogie, and E.J.
    Freireich (1967a). A simplified in vitro classification for prognosis in
    adult acute leukemia; the application of in vitro results in remission - pre-
    dictive models. Blood, 48, 795-807.
Spitzer, G., K.A. Dicke, E.A. Gehan, T. Smith and K.B. McCredie (1976b). The use
    of the Robinson in vitro agar culture assay in adult acute leukemia. Blood
    Cells, 2, 139-148.
Spitzer, G., D.S. Verma, T. Smith, K.A. Dicke and K.B. McCredie (1978). Subgroups
    of oligoleukemia as indentified by in vitro agar culture. Leuk. Res. (In
    Press).
Verma, D.S., G. Spitzer, K.A. Dicke, and K.B. McCredie (1978). In vitro agar
    culture patterns in preleukemia and their clinical significance. Leuk. Res.
    (In Press).

Acute Lymphoblastic Leukemia Treatment

Federico Sackmann-Muriel

Hospital de Niños de Buenos Aires, Gallo 1330, Buenos Aires, Argentina

INTRODUCTION

Acute lymphoblastic leukemia (ALL) is the most common type of cancer in children. Within a single generation, the prognosis for children with ALL has changed tremendously. Really, there are very few malignant childhood diseases which have shown such a gratifying response to improved therapy in such short period of time, as has the ALL. A steady progress in outlook rather than a breakthrough characte—rizes this improvement. This reality has also changed the therapeutic approach from one of palliation of almost universally fatal disease to approaches aiming at long-term disease-free survival and cure.

The first specific chemotherapy was introduced by Farber in 1948. Subsequently other effective agents appeared but the disease remained fatal. The introduction of multiple-drug chemotherapy, preventive measures against leukemic infiltration of CNS and vigorous supportive care have added impetus in recent years. In some selected studies 50% of children with ALL have remained disease-free for at least 5 years (Simone and colleagues, 1975). There are good reasons to hope that most of the children who remain in continuous complete remission (CCR) for 4 to 5 years will prove to be cured of their disease. However, many problems have emerged like the avoidance and control of opportunistic infections, the toxic side-effects of aggresive therapy (such as, undernutrition, visceral fibrosis, neurological com-plications, hematopoietic and immunological suppression, skeletal, oncogenic and genetic late side-effects) and more accurate identification of those children who are unlikely to have such favourable prognosis and for whom a different approach of therapy may be needed.

In this review we shall discuss some relevant facts in the prognosis and treatment of ALL occurred in the last years and we will emphazise some experiences gathered by the Grupo Argentino de Tratamiento de la Leucemia Aguda (GATLA).

PROGNOSTIC FACTORS

Nowadays, it is becoming increasingly clear that ALL is an heterogeneous group of diseases. The criteria for the classification of acute leukemias in the basis of Romanowsky and cytochemical staining methods are well established (Hayhoe, Quagli

no, Doll, 1964). However, at present there is no general agreement in classification or even on the methods for distinguishing myeloblastic from lymphoblastic
leukemias. A very recent effort has been made by the French-American-British-
Cooperative Group to define more accurately this problem (Bennett and colleagues,
1976). Two groups of acute leukemia were established (lymphoblastic and myeloblastic) and further subdivided into 3 (L1, L2,L3) and 6 (M1, M2, M3, M4, M5, M6)
groups, respectively. What has to be observed is whether this classification is
useful as regards prognosis and if it has any correlation with other well known
prognostic factors. A very preliminar and unpublished observation shows that L2
has a worse prognosis though it is not related with the initial WBC count.

Several cytological characteristics have been claimed to be of prognostic significance. Laurie (1968) has suggested that PAS positivity of high proportion of
lymphoblasts was a good prognostic feature (Laurie, 1968). However, this opinion
was disputed by Bennett and Henderson (Bennett, Henderson, 1969) and supported by
Feldes and colleagues (1974). In our experience, the PAS positivity is not a
useful indicator of prognosis (Campuzano Maya and colleagues, 1976). Mathé and
colleagues (1971) subdivided cases of ALL into four types in the grounds of blast-
cell morphology and claimed prognostic value for their classification, but other
workers have found it less useful in this respect (Bernard, Weil, Jacquillat,1975).
Pantazopoulos and Sinks (1974), using a simpler but more objective classification
according to the size of blasts, found that patients with not more than 10% of
blasts greater than 12μ in diameter had a better prognosis than those with a
higher proportion of larger cells. Other investigators (Murphy and colleagues,1975;
Oster and colleagues, 1976; Wagner and Baehner, 1977) and ourselves (Campuzano
Maya and colleagues, 1976), however, found no correlation between blast-cell size
and prognosis in larger series of children.

Nevertheless, if there is a poor general agreement on various cytological characteristics, there is more agreement in the presenting features of most value to
assess prognosis as accurately as possible in individual cases. In this respect,
age, initial WBC count, the presence of mediastinal mass, initial CNS leukemia
infiltration, the degree of clinical organomegaly and race are useful prognostic
indicators (George and colleagues, 1973; Hardisty and Till, 1968; Sackmann and
colleagues, 1978; Simone and colleagues, 1975c).

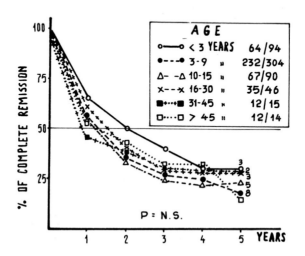

Fig. 1   Duration of complete remission in acute
lymphoblastic leukemia according to age (GATLA)

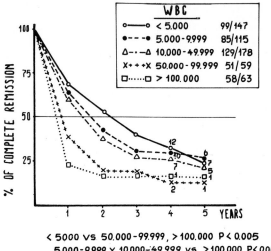

Fig. 2   Duration of complete remission in acute lymphoblastic
         leukemia according to WBC count (GATLA)

Curiously, a recent study has shown that age and WBC count - the most important
prognostic indicators - lose their significance at 24 months of CCR but possibly
reappear to predict worse prognosis after that time. This analysis suggests that
children remaining in CCR for 18-24 months after diagnosis have the same possibility of subsequent relapse regardless those prognostic indicators (Sather and
colleagues, 1978).

Most recent advances in this field have come from the application of immunological
techniques (Brouet and colleagues, 1976; Catovsky, 1977; Sen and Borella, 1975)
and have resulted in a major advance in the study and classification of ALL.
Lymphoid cells can be divided into two major subpopulations based upon their
differentiation pathway, function and cell surface characteristics. Human thymus-
independent (B) lymphocytes are usually distinguished by the presence of surface
immunoglobulins, B-lymphocyte antigens, and surface receptors for Fc, C3 and
Epstein-Barr virus, while human thymus-dependent (T) lymphocytes spontaneously
form rosettes with sheep erythrocytes at 4° and possess thymus-associated antigens.

In the majority of patients with ALL (about 70-80%), neither B nor T cell markers
can be detected on the leukemic cells; these are commonly called as "null"-cell
ALL. In the minority of cases (about 20-30%), lymphoblasts have characteristics
of T-lymphocytes. Only occasional cases (not more than 1-2%) are due to proliferation of a B-cell alone, and these have peculiar cytology and sometimes, clinical
features closely resembling those of Burkitt's lymphoma. Obviously, this immunological classification has no distinguishing feature on Romanowsky staining but
T-lymphoblasts can be identified by the positive staining reaction for acid
phosphatase (Catovsky, 1977). A recent paper (Dow and colleagues, 1977) has shown
that children with ALL whose lymphoblasts have formed rosettes (called E +) are
significantly associated with mediastinal enlargement, WBC count over 100.000/ml,
large lymph nodes, age over 5 years, hemoglobin level over 8 g%, hepatomegaly,
male sex and lymph node enlargement outside of the cervical area. They suggested
that E + ALL may result from a leukemic transformation of a non-Hodgkin lymphoma.

This subdivision of ALL into T-, B- and "null"-cell varieties is of practical as

well as academic importance, since the first two carry a poorer prognosis than
the third and largest group.

TREATMENT

Remission induction. Currently the strategy for remission induction is designed
to take advantage of drug combinations which are most quickly effective in killing
leukemic cells and have the least degree of suppressive effect on normal bone
marrow cell proliferation. There is a widespread agreement that vincristine and
prednisone are the principal drugs of choice for the initial treatment. Remission
rates of 80-95% have been achieved in several large series. Although, it is
difficult to improve this rate, the addition of L-asparaginase and/or daunorubicin
have sometimes produced still better results. In this respect, it is worth mentioning that in earlier controlled studies the combination of daunorubicin-vincristine
prednisone had no advantage over vincristine-prednisone alone (Holland, 1971;
Verzosa and Fite, 1971). However, in our experience, it is noteworthy that the
combination of daunorubicin-vincristine-prednisone from the onset of therapy
achieved better results than vincristine-prednisone for four weeks plus daunorubicin added on day 28 (if the patient is not yet in CR) in any of the three categories, standard and high risk children and adults (Pavlovsky and colleagues, 1975;
Sackmann and colleagues, in press).

TABLE 1 Results of Induction Treatment According to Initial Chemotherapeutic
Regimen Employed (Number of Patients)

		CHILDREN		ADULTS
		"Standard Risk"	"High Risk"	
(A)	VCR-PRED	244	50	27
	# C.R. (%)	170 (69)	27 (53)	9 (33)
	After day 29: VCR-PRED-DNR	61	17	10
	# C.R. (%)	40 (66)	9 (53)	5 (50)
	TOTAL C.R. (%)	210 (86)	36 (72)	14 (52)
(B)	From onset: VCR-PRED-DNR	36	59	48
	# C.R. (%)	34 (94)	47 (80)	32 (67)

(A) = VCR-PRED for 4 weeks followed by VCR-PRED-DNR if day 29 a M1 bone marrow
      was not achieved.
(B) = VCR-PRED-DNR from the onset.

VCR: vincristine; PRED: prednisone; DNR: daunorubicin; C.R.: complete remission.

Bernard and colleagues (1975) have published the results obtained at St. Louis
Hospital between 1964 and 1968. A total of 205 patients were induced with the
combination of vincristine-prednisone and 162 patients with daunorubicin-vincristine-prednisone. Eighty seven $\pm$ 4.6% of the former and 92.5 $\pm$ 4.3% of the latter,
achieved CR (P 0.04). Unfortunately, both studies were not properly randomized.

In relation to more intensive induction regimens, the Southwest Oncology Group has
shown, in randomized studies, that vincristine-prednisone achieved better induction remission rates and less toxicity that the combinations of vincristine-pred-
nisone-methotrexate-6 mercaptopurine (Berry and colleagues, 1975) or vincristine-

prednisone-cyclophosphamide-L-asparaginase (Komp and colleagues, 1976). Never—
theless, two different collaborative groups using another approach have shown
that the addition of L-asparaginase during (Ortega and colleagues, 1977) or
immediately after (Jones and colleagues, 1977) induction therapy with vincristine-
prednisone is useful to improve CR rate or prolong CR duration, respectively.

Intensification or consolidation phase. Information derived from animal studies
(Skipper and colleagues, 1964), several chemotherapy protocols have incorporated
a period of intensive therapy immediately after achieving CR, designed to reduce
leukemic cell numbers. The rationale of these studies was supported by the
observations of prolonged unmaintained remissions after multi-drug intensive
induction therapy (Freireich and colleagues, 1964; Hananian and colleagues, 1965;
Henderson and colleagues, 1970). However, at the time those induction regimens
were evaluated neither the importance of CNS prevention therapy was completely
appreciated nor the need of more aggresive maintenance regimens recognized.
Therefore, it is difficult at present to evaluate the effectiveness of this
intensification phase in prolonging the duration of CR.

In two recent protocols the importance of this phase was evaluated in a controlled
manner. Aur and colleagues studied the effect of one week course of high dosage
intravenous chemotherapy (cyclophosphamide-methotrexate-6 mercaptopurine). They
found no difference with the control group; however, it is necessary to emphasize
that the maintenance therapy employed in this study used the same drugs, though
at a lower dosage level. The GATLA's group used a short intensification period
with cytosine arabinoside-cyclophosphamide (Sackmann and colleagues, in press).

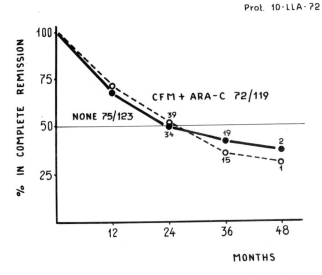

Fig. 3   Duration of complete remission in "standard risk" children
with ALL according to intensification (GATLA).

We did not find any difference between the duration of CR in the group so treated
or untreated. An explanation will be that current therapy protocols have mainte —
nance regimens which are designed to provide multi-drug exposure at maximally
tolerated dose level. Thus the maintenance period can be considered to be a
prolongation of the intensification phase. Actually, there is no definitive
demonstration that a period of intensification improves the overall results. How—
ever, Simone (1976) analysing the results of Total Therapy Studies have suggested

that adding a third drug (daunorubicin or L-asparaginase) to vincristine-prednisone for remission induction or giving an intensive phase of chemotherapy early
in remission is the wise therapy in ALL. Here we might mention that the Cancer
and Leukemia Group B has shown that use of 10-day L-asparaginase subsequent to
3-week course of vincristine-prednisone is superior to no L-asparaginase (Jones
and colleagues, 1977). However, we have used 5-day L-asparaginase after 4-week
course of daunorubicin-vincristine-prednisone and found no significant differences
with the control group (Sackmann and colleagues, 1974).

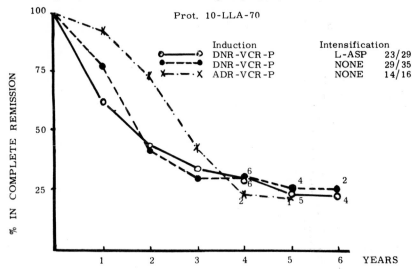

Fig. 4   Duration of complete remission in children with "standard
          risk" according to induction and intensification (GATLA).

In relation to the intensification phase, it is worth mentioning that with similar
rationality some studies add irradiation to thymus, liver, spleen, kidney and
testis (Fish and colleagues, 1966; Nesbit and colleagues, 1977; Sharp and
colleagues, 1967). So far, it is difficult to evaluate this form of therapy.

Prevention of CNS leukemia. Without any form of prevention the cumulative incidence of overt CNS disease during the first 3 years exceeds 50% (Evans and colleagues, 1970; West and colleagues, 1972). Though it is impossible to predict with
certainty which children are most likely to develop this complication, there are
some factors which predispose CNS leukemia: age and initial WBC count were, in
our experience (Pavlovsky and colleagues, 1973), the most significant indicators.
Therefore, CNS prevention treatment is nowadays mandatory in patients with ALL.
Price and Johnson (1973) have shown that CNS leukemic infiltration follows a
predictable anatomical pattern with the earliest lesions in the walls of the
veins of superficial arachnoid tissues. In this study it is clear that the leukemic infiltration is primarily an arachnoid disease. As the large mass of arach—
noid tissue is contained into cranium, it is logic to think that cranial irradiation may be succesful in the prevention of CNS disease.

At present, several regimens are available. The value of the combination of craniocervical irradiation (2400 rads) and a course of five intrathecal injections of
methotrexate was first established by Aur and colleagues (1971). In a controlled
study of the GATLA's group we corroborated that this regimen is highly effective
(Sackmann and colleagues, 1974).

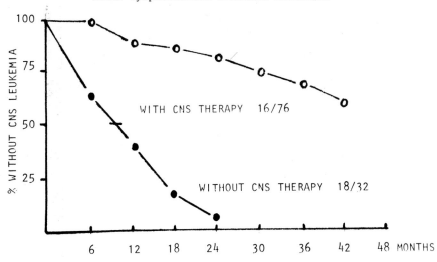

Fig. 5   Incidence of CNS leukemia in children with ALL in
          relation to CNS prevention therapy (GATLA).

Aur and colleagues (1973) have also shown, in a controlled study, that craniospi—
nal irradiation without intrathecal methotrexate was equally effective; however,
the latter is associated with more leukopenia and interruptions of chemotherapy.
Incidentally, some recent unpublished results show that 1800 rads of craniocervi—
cal irradiation seems to have the same preventive effects than 2400 rads.

In other studies the CNS prevention is given by periodic intrathecal injections of
methotrexate only (Haghbin and colleagues, 1972; Haghbin and colleagues, 1974;
Haghbin and colleagues, 1975). With this regimen the frequency of CNS leukemia
has been reduced from the expected rate. However, a longer follow-up is needed.

Another approach is being currently tested. The use of intermediate dose of intra—
venous methotrexate over 24 hours period followed by leucovorin rescue, produced
a significant cerebro-spinal-fluid level. Thus, this approach coupled simultaneous—
ly with intrathecal methotrexate can be used as CNS prevention and also as inten —
sification phase. The preliminary results indicate that this treatment program is
safe to administer and, at present, it appears effective in preventing CNS leuke —
mia (Wang and colleagues, 1976). Here also a longer follow-up is really needed.

In order to decrease the neurological toxicity of irradiation, another interesting
approach is the use of fractional radiotherapy (100 rads craniospinal irradiation
every 10 weeks) together with intrathecal methotrexate. The results thus far
obtained are comparable to those with more aggressive prevention (Yaddanapudi and
colleagues, 1978; Zuelzer and colleagues, 1976).

In the current GATLA protocol, we are administering three injections of intrathe—
cal methotrexate and dexamethasone during the induction period and another three
(six in total) during early in remission followed by one injection every three
months as prevention of CNS disease. Thus far the results, in comparison with
earlier protocols in which we used craniocervical irradiation coupled with five
doses of intrathecal methotrexate and dexamethasone, compares favourably in
standard and also in high risk children.

F. Sackmann-Muriel

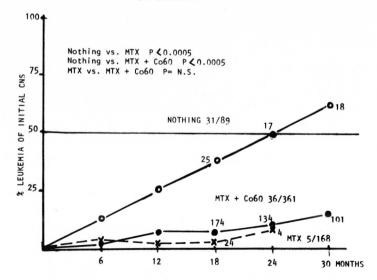

Fig. 6   Incidence of leukemic infiltration of the CNS in ALL with
         less than 50.000 WBC at diagnosis according to CNS prevention.

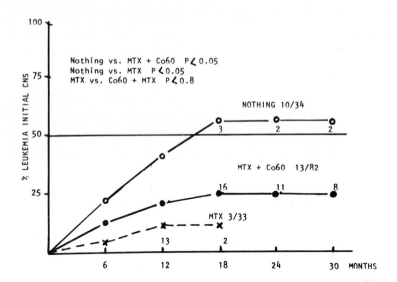

Fig. 7   Incidence of leukemic infiltration of the CNS in ALL with
         more than 50.000 WBC at diagnosis according to CNS prevention.

It is very difficult to evaluate, at present, which is the most effective and less
toxic CNS preventive therapy. Cranial irradiation with intrathecal methotrexate
and craniospinal irradiation are very effective but may be associated with higher
rate of hematological relapse (Medical Research Council, 1973). In addition, both
types of treatment leave the patients with highly significant reduction in lympho —
cyte counts for at least two years (Medical Research Council, 1975). Furthermore,

the degree of long-term lymphopenia was shown to be dependent upon the number of fractions into which the standard cranial dose of 2400 rads is divided (Medical Research Council, 1978).

Many complications of these prevention regimens have been described and recently reviewed (Pochedly, 1977). There is a wide range of incidence of neurological symptoms and may vary from mild to letal. Often unusual manifestations of CNS leukemia per se or bizarre CNS infections can be difficult to separate from neuro-toxicity due to CNS prevention therapy. Actually, there is much concern about the long-term consequences of radio and chemotherapy in children with ALL (Fishman and colleagues, 1976; McIntosh and colleagues, 1977; Pochedly, 1977). For instance, the significance of abnormal computed tomography scans are as yet unknown but very common in cases which received cranial irradiation and intrathecal chemotherapy (Peylan-Ramu and colleagues, 1978) but very uncommon in cases treated with CNS prevention without radiotherapy (Ochs and colleagues, 1978). Growth hormone deficiency has been described in children successfully treated with irradiation as CNS prevention (Shalet and colleagues, 1976), however, most girls aggresively treated have an excellent prognosis for normal hypothalamic pituitary-ovarian function (Fisher and Aur, 1978; Siris and colleagues, 1976). Soni and colleagues (1975) demonstrated that 2400 rads of cranial irradiation has no manifest adverse effect on the neuropsychological function. Recently, Verzosa and colleagues (1976) showed no prohibitive toxicity on physical growth and neuropsychological competen-ce 5 years after CNS irradiation in children with ALL and off therapy.

Continuation or maintenance therapy. It has become very clear that continuation or maintenance chemotherapy after initial remission and CNS prevention is a crucial part of the therapeutic regimen in determining disease control. To achieve this, it has become apparent that treatment must be continued for at least two or more years. Also there is a general agreement that this phase should include several drugs given simultaneously and/or sequentially in continouos or intermittent manners. It is remarkable that similar results are now being obtained by different groups using diverse treatment regimens during this period but after an effective induction of remission program and CNS prevention treatment (Haghbin and colleagues, 1975; Sackmann and colleagues, in press; Sallan and colleagues, 1978; Simone and colleagues, 1975b; Spiers and colleagues, 1975).

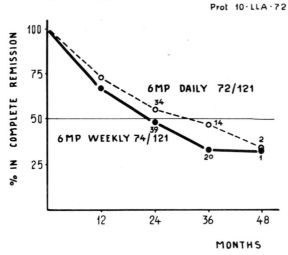

Fig. 8   Duration of complete remission in "standard risk" children with ALL according to maintenance treatment (GATLA).

However, many investigators will favour a schedule consisting of 6-mercaptopurine daily, methotrexate weekly and periodic reinforcement with vincristine and pred- nisone.

In addition, to evaluate the results in relation to remission duration it is very important to measure the degree of immunosuppresion and the frequency of infec — tions. A good example is a protocol which evaluates the effectiveness of using simultaneously one, two, three or four drugs during this phase. An early evalua — tion of this study shows no systematic association of efficacy with the numbers of drugs given (Simone and colleagues, 1975b). However, the three and four drug regimens are associated with much more toxicity, specially Pneumocystic Carinii pneumonitis (Hughes and colleagues, 1975). Another way to measure the effectiveness of therapy will be to determine by the number of cases that relapse when they are off therapy. For that reason, a longer follow-up is needed to assess the efficacy of any treatment regimen.

Experimental approaches. In 1969, Mathé and colleagues (1969) claimed that remissions induced by chemotherapy would be significantly prolonged by active immunotherapy with BCG and/or pooled irradiated leukemic cells. However, their data have not been supported but subsequent large controlled clinical trials (Heyn and colleagues, 1975; Medical Research Council, 1971). Nevertheless, very recently the same authors have insisted - again with few number of cases in uncontrolled studies - that their results are equal or superior to the best published outcome obtained with maintenance chemotherapy alone (Mathé and collea — gues, 1978)

Since 1975, in view that levamisole has proved useful to prolong disease-free survival in breast cancer, the GATLA's group is randomizing patients with ALL to receive or not this drug during continuation or maintenance phase, in a dosage of 120 mg/m2 daily orally. Preliminary results are very promising and they suggest that levamisole is effective to prolong the duration of CR (Pavlovsky and collea— gues, 1978).

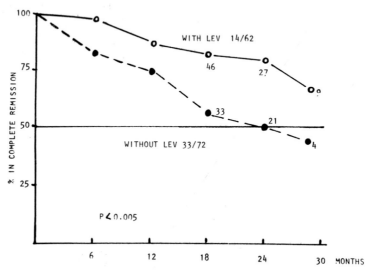

Fig. 9   Duration of hematological remission in ALL according to
         immunostimulation with levamisole (LEV) (Prot. 10-LLA-72)
         (GATLA).

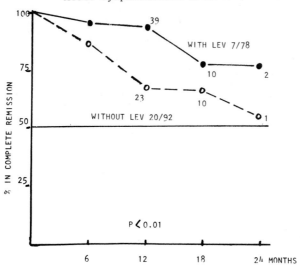

Fig. 10   Duration of complete remission in ALL according to
          immunostimulation with levamisole (LEV)(Prot. 1-LLA-76)
          (GATLA).

A recent report is noteworthy as far as the results obtained in terminal or end—
stage acute leukemia patients. One hundred of them were treated with chemotherapy,
total body irradiation and allogenic marrow transplantation. The long-term
remission of 13 endstage leukemia patients without any maintenance chemotherapy
after grafting, constitutes a unique achievement. However, this treatment was
possible because they were fortunate enough to have an HLA-matched sibling marrow
donour and the necessary facilities and expertise available (Thomas   and collea—
gues, 1977).

Cessation of therapy. Since all the chemotherapeutic regimens are also myelosuppre—
sive and immunosuppresive in addition to unknown potential late side effects, it
is important to determine when is it safe to stop it with very little risk of
leukemia relapse. There is much experience that a treatment for one year or less,
regardless how intensive was the previous chemotherapy, is insufficient to prevent
subsequent relapse in most cases.

St. Jude's group stops treatment after 2-3 years of CCR. An analysis of 132
patients removed from therapy showed a relapse rate of 16%. The likehood of
relapse after therapy is higher in the first year and no specific feature, other
than the abscence of CNS prevention, was found to predict whether relapse would
occur after stopping therapy (Aur and colleagues, 1974). Similar results were
obtained in a joint study between the Children's Cancer Group and the Southwest
Oncology Group with continued or discontinued chemotherapy after 3 years or more
of CCR. However, this study showed that boys are at high risk, specially if
discontinuing therapy, because the testis appears to be a significant site of
relapse (Baum and colleagues, 1977). Cancer and Leukemia Group B are randomizing
children to stop or continue chemotherapy after 5 years of CCR. No significant
differences have emerged yet. In the Medical Research Council's UKALL II trial
patients in CCR at 2 years have been randomized for either 2 or 3 years of chemo—
therapy: so far the results indicate no clear preference for either period
(Hardisty and Chessells, 1977). In the GATLA group we are stopping chemotherapy
in all patients after reaching 4 years of CCR. The last evaluation of this study

has shown that 37 patients were removed from therapy and 3 so far have relapsed.
We cannot make any conclusion yet but about 75% of the patients who live for 4
years from diagnosis without relapse can be expected to remain alive and without
evidence of disease indefinitely.(Pavlovsky and Sackmann, 1977).

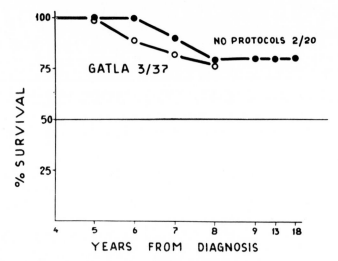

Fig. 11   Long-term survival in acute leukemia with more than
          four years in complete remission according to
          previous therapy (GATLA).

CONCLUSION

During the last decade a giant step has been made in the treatment of ALL.However,
despite modern therapy hematological relapse occurs in more than half of the
patients and long-term sequalae have emerged. This represents a real challenge for
all of us and our efforts must continue because every ALL patient should have the
opportunity of cure.

REFERENCES

Aur, R.J.A., Simone, J., Hustu, H.O., Walters, T., Borrela, L., Pratt, C., Pinkel,
D. (1971). Central nervous system therapy and combination chemotherapy of childhood acute lymphocytic leukemia. Blood, 37, 272-281.
Aur, R.J.A., Simone, J.V., Hustu, H.O., Verzosa, M.S. (1972). A comparative study
of central nervous system irradiation and intensive chemotherapy early in remissi-
on of childhood acute lymphocytic leukemia. Cancer, 29, 381-391.
Aur, R.J.A., Hustu, H.O., Verzosa, M.S., Wood, A., Simone, J.V. (1973). Comparison
of two methods of preventing central nervous system leukemia. Blood, 42, 349-357.
Aur, R.J.A., Simone, J.V., Hustu, H.O., Verzosa, M.S., Pinkel, D. (1974). Cessa-
tion of therapy during complete remission of childhood acute lymphocytic leukemia.
N. Engl. J. Med., 291, 1230-1234.
Baum, E., Land, V., Joo, P., Starling, K., Leikin, S., Miale, T., Krivit, W.,
Miller, D., Chard, R., Nesbit, M., Sather, H., Hammond, D. (1977). Cessation of
chemotherapy (Ch) during complete remission (CR) of childhood acute lymphocytic
leukemia (ALL). Proc. AACR-ASCO, 18, 290.
Bennett, J.M., Henderson, E.S. (1969). Lymphoblastic leukaemia. Brit. Med. J., 2,
513.
Bennett, J.M., Catovsky, D., Daniel, M.T., Flandrin, G., Galton, D.A.G., Gralnick,

H.R., Sultan, C. (1976). Proposals for the classification of acute leukaemias.
French-American-British (FAB) Co-operative Group. Brit. J. Haemat., 33, 451-458.
Bernard, J., Weil, M., Jacquillat, C.L. (1975). Prognostic factors in human acute
leukemia. In Advances in the Biosciences 14, Workshop on Prognostic Factors in
Human Acute Leukemia, Reisensburg, Germany, October 1-3, 1973; New York, Pergamon
Press, 97-121.
Berry, D.H., Pullen, J., George, S., Vietti, T.J., Sullivan, M.P., Fernbach, D.
(1975). Comparison of prednisolone, vincristine, methotrexate and 6-mercaptopurine
vs. vincristine and prednisone induction therapy in childhood acute leukemia.
Cancer, 36, 98-102.
Brouet, J.C., Valensi, F., Dariel, M.T., Flandrin, G., Preud'homme, J.L., Seligman,
M. (1976). Immunological classification of acute lymphoblastic leukaemias. Evalua—
tion of its clinical significance in a hundred patients. Brit. J. Haemat., 33,
319-328.
Campuzano Maya, G., Hayes, A., Pavlovsky, S., Sackmann Muriel, F. (1976). Valor
pronóstico del tamaño y de la coloración del PAS en el linfoblasto de la leucemia
linfoblástica aguda de la niñez. Sangre (Barcel.), 21, 441-450.
Catovsky, D. (1977). Cell markers in acute lymphoblastic leukaemia and lympho —
proliferative disorders. In Recent Advances in Haematology, edited by A.V. Hoff —
brand, M.C. Brain, J. Hirsh, number two, Churchill Livingstone, Edimburg, London,
New York, 201-217.
Dow, L.W., Borella, L., Sen, L., Aur, R.J.A., George, S.L., Mauer, A.M., Simone,
J.V. (1977). Initial prognostic factors and lymphoblast-erythrocyte rosette
formation in 109 children with acute lymphoblastic leukemia. Blood, 50, 671-682.
Evans, A.E., Gilbert, E.S., Zandstra, R. (1970). The increasing incidence of
central nervous system leukemia in children (Children's Cancer Study Group A).
Cancer, 26, 404-409.
Feldges, A.J., Aur, R.J.A., Verzosa, M.S., Daniel, S. (1974). Periodic Acid-Schiff
reaction, a useful index of duration of complete remission in acute lymphocytic
leukemia. Acta Hemat., 52, 8-13.
Fish, V.J., Winchell, H.S., Lawrence, J.H. (1966). Thymic and splenic irradiation
in treatment of acute lymphatic leukemia. Amer. J. Roentg., 97, 989-990.
Fisher, J.N., Aur, R.J.A.: Neuroendocrine assesment of children with acute lympho—
cytic leukemia (ALL) in continuous complete remission (CCR) on Total Therapy
Study VIII. Proc. AACR-ASCO, 19, 336, (1978).
Fishman, M.L., Bear, S.C., Cogan, D.G.: Opticatrophy following prophylactic chemo—
therapy and cranial radiation for acute lymphocytic leukemia. Amer. J. Opthal.,82,
571-576, (1976).
Freireich, E.J., Karon, M., Frei, E. III. (1964). Quadruple combination chemothe —
rapy (VAMP) for acute lymphocytic leukemia of childhood. Proc. AACR, 5, 20.
George, S.L., Fernbach, D.J., Vietti, T.J., Sullivan, M.P., Lane, D.M., Haggard,
M.E., Berry, D.H., Lonsdale, D., Komp, D. (1973). Factors influencing survival
in pediatric acute leukemia. The SWCCSG experience, 1958-1970. Cancer, 32, 1542-
1553.
Haghbin, M., Tan, C., Clarkson, B., Sykes, M., Murphy, M.L. (1972). Intensive
chemotherapy and prophylactic intrathecal methotrexate in acute lymphoblastic
leukemia (ALL). Proc. AACR, 13, 22.
Haghbin, M., Tan, C., Clarkson, B.D., Miké, V., Burchenal, J.H., Murphy, M.L.
(1974). Intensive chemotherapy in children with acute lymphoblastic leukemia
(L-2 protocol). Cancer, 33, 1491-1498.
Haghbin, M., Tan, C., Clarkson, B.D., Miké, V., Burchenal, J.H., Murphy, M.L.
(1975). Treatment of acute lymphoblastic leukemia in children with "prophylactic"
intrathecal methotrexate and intensive systemic chemotherapy. Cancer Res., 35,
807-811.
Hananian, J., Holland, J.F., Sheehe, P. (1965). Intensive chemotherapy of acute
lymphocytic leukemia in children. Proc. AACR, 6, 26.
Hardisty, R.M., Till, M.M. (1968). Acute leukaemia 1959-64. Factors affecting

46   F. Sackmann-Muriel

prognosis. Arch. Dis. Childh., 43, 107-115.
Hardisty, R.M., Chessells, J.M. (1977). Acute leukaemias in childhood: management
and prognosis. In Recent Advances in Haematology, edited by A.V. Hoffbrand, M.C.
Brain, J. Hirsh, number two, Churchill Livingstone, Edimburg, London, New York,
159-173.
Hayhoe, F.G.J., Quaglino, D., Doll, R. (1964). The cytology and cytochemistry of
acute leukaemias. A study of 140 cases. Medical Research Council Special Reports
Series, number 304, London, HMSO.
Henderson, E.S., Freireich, E.J., Karon, M., Rosse, W. (1970). High dose of combi-
nation chemotherapy in acute lymphocytic leukemia of childhood. Proc. AACR, 11,
38.
Heyn, R.N., Joo, P., Karon, M., Nesbit, M., Shore, N., Breslow, N., Weiner, J.,
Reed, A., Hammond, D. (1975). BCG in the treatment of acute lymphocytic leukemia.
Blood, 46, 431-442.
Holland, J.F. (1971). E Pluribus Unum: Presidential address. Cancer Res., 31,
1319-1329.
Hughes, W.T., Feldman, S., Aur, R.J.A., Verzosa, M.S., Hustu, H.O., Simone, J.V.
(1975). Intensity of immunosuppressive therapy and the incidence of pneumocystis
carinii pneumonitis. Cancer, 36, 2004-2009.
Jones, B., Holland, J.F., Glidewell, O., Jacquillat, C., Weil, M., Pochedly, C.,
Sinks, L., Chevalier, L., Maurer, H.M., Koch, K., Falkson, G., Patterson, R.,
Seligman, B., Sartorius, J., Kung, F., Haurani, F., Stuart, M., Burgert, E.O.,
Ruymann, F., Sawitsky, A., Forman, E., Pluess, H., Truman, J., and Hakami, N.
(1977). Optimal use of L-asparaginase (NSC-109229) in acute lymphocytic leukemia.
Med. Ped. Oncol., 3, 387-400.
Komp, D.M., George, S.L., Falletta, J., Land, V.J., Starling, K.A., Humprey, G.B.,
Lowman, J. (1976). Cyclophosphamide-asparaginase-vincristine-prednisone induction
therapy in childhood acute lymphocytic and non-lymphocytic leukemia. Cancer, 37,
1243-1247.
Laurie, H.C. (1968). Duration of remission in lymphoblastic leukemia in childhood.
Brit. Med. J., 2, 95-97.
Mathé, G., Amiel, J.L., Schwarzenberg, L., Schneider, M., Cattan, A., Schlumber-
ger, J.R., Hayat, M., DeVassal, F. (1969). Active immunotherapy for acute lympho-
blastic leukaemia. Lancet, 697-699.
Mathé, G., Pouilliart, P., Sterecu, M., Amiel, J.L., Schwarzenberg, L., Schneider,
M., Hayat, M., DeVassal, F., Jasmin, C., Lafleur, M. (1971). Subdivision of
classical varieties of acute leukemia. Correlation with prognosis and cure
expectancy. Europ. J. Clin. Biol. Res., 16, 554-560.
Mathé, G., DeVassal, F., Schwarzenberg, L., Delgado, M., Weiner, R., Gil, M.A.,
Pena-Angulo, J., Belpomme, D., Pouillart, P., Machover, D., Misset, J.L., Pico,
J.L., Jasmin, C., Hayat, M., Schneider, M., Cattan, A., Amiel, J.L., Musset, M.,
Rosenfeld, C. and Ribaud, P. (1978). Preliminary results of three protocols for
the treatment of acute lymphoid leukemia in children. Distinction of two groups
of patients according to predictable prognosis. Med. Ped. Oncol., 4, 17-27.
McIntosh, S., Fisher, D., Rothman, S.G., Rosenfeld, N., Lebel, J.F., O'Brien, R.T.
(1977). Intracranial calcifications in childhood leukemia. J. Pediat., 91, 909-913.
Medical Research Council (1971). Treatment of acute lymphoblastic leukaemia. Comparison of immunotherapy (BCG), intermittent methotrexate, and no therapy after
a five-month intensive cytotoxic regimen (Concord trial). Brit. Med. J., 4,
189-194.
Medical Research Council (1973). Working party on leukaemia in childhood. Treatment of acute lymphoblastic leukaemia: Effect of "prophylactic" therapy against
central nervous system leukaemia. Brit. Med. J., 2, 381-384.
Medical Research Council.(1975).Working party on leukaemia in childhood: Analysis
on treatment in childhood leukaemia: I. Prolonged predisposition to drug induced
neutropenia following craniospinal irradiation. Brit. Med. J., 3, 563-566.
Medical Research Council (1978). Working party on leukemia in childhood: Analysis
of treatment in childhood leukemia. IV. The critical association between dose

fractionation and immunosuppression induced by cranial irradiation. Cancer, 41, 108-111.
Murphy, S.B., Borella, L., Sen, L., Mauer, A.M. (1975). Lack of correlation of lymphoblast cell size with presence of T-cell markers or with outcome in child-hood acute lymphoblastic leukaemia. Brit. J. Haemat., 31, 95-102.
Nesbit, M., Ortega, J., Donaldson, M., Hittle, R., Hammond, D., Weiner, J. (1977). Prevention of testicular relapse by prophylactic radiation (XRT) in childhood acute lymphoblastic leukemia (ALL). Proc. AACR-ASCO, 18, 317.
Ochs, J., Berger, P., Brecher, M., Sinks, L.F., Freeman, A.I. (1978). Computed tomography (CT) scans in children with acute lymphocytic leukemia (ALL) following CNS prophylaxis without radiotherapy. Proc. AACR-ASCO, 19, 391.
Ortega, J.A., Nesbit, M.E., Donaldson, M.H., Hittle, R.E., Weiner, J., Karon, M., Hammond, D. (1977). L-asparaginase, vincristine and prednisone for induction of first remission in acute lymphocytic leukemia. Cancer Res., 37, 535-540.
Oster, M.W., Margileth, D.A., Simon, R., Leventhal, B.G. (1976).Lack of prognostic value of lymphoblast size in acute lymphoblastic leukemia. Brit. J. Haemat., 33, 131-135.
Pantazopoulos, N., Sinks, L.F. (1974). Morphological criteria for prognostication of acute lymphoblastic leukaemia. Brit. J. Haemat., 27, 25-30.
Pavlovsky, S., Eppinger-Helft, M., Sackmann Muriel, F. (1973). Factors that influence the appearance of central nervous system leukemia. Blood, 42, 935-938.
Pavlovsky, S., Sackmann, F., Eppinger, M., Svarch, E., Braier, J.L. (1975). Evaluation of intensification and maintenance combination in acute lymphoblastic leukemia. Proc. AACR-ASCO, 16, 7.
Pavlovsky, S., Sackmann, F. (1977). Long-term survival in acute leukemia in Argen-tina. A study of 78 cases. Cancer, 40, 1402-1409.
Pavlovsky, S., Garay, G., Giraudo, C., Sackmann, F., Hayes, A., Svarch, E. (1978). Chemoimmunotherapy with levamisole (LEV) in acute lymphocytic leukemia. Proc. AACR ASCO, 19, 204.
Peylan-Ramu, N., Poplack, D.G., Pizzo, P.A., Adornato, B.T., DiChero, G. (1978). Abnormal CT scans in asymptomatic children after prophylactic cranial irradiation and intrathecal chemotherapy. N. Engl. J. Med., 298, 815-819.
Pochedly, C. (1977). Neurotoxicity due to CNS therapy for leukemia. Med. Ped. Oncol 3, 101-115.
Price, R.A., Johnson, W.W. (1973). The central nervous system in childhood leuke-mia. I. The arachnoid. Cancer, 31, 520-533.
Sackmann Muriel, F., Pavlovsky, S., Peñalver, J.A., Hidalgo, G., Cebrian Bonesana, A., Eppinger Helft, M., Macchi, G., Pavlovsky, A. (1974). Evaluation of induction, intensification and central nervous system prophylactic treatment in acute lympho-blastic leukemia. Cancer, 34, 418-426.
Sackmann, F., Pavlovsky, S., Goldar, D. (1978). Prognostic factors in acute lympho-blastic leukemia (ALL). Proc. AACR-ASCO, 19, 403.
Sackmann, F., Svarch, E., Eppinger Helft, M., Braier, J.L., Pavlovsky, S., Guman, L., Vergara, B., Ponzinibbio, C., Failace, R., Garay, G., Bugnard, E., Ojeda, F., De Bellis, R., Sijvarger, S.R., Saslavsky, J. (in press). Evaluation of intensifi-cation and maintenance programs in the treatment of acute lymphoblastic leukemia. Cancer.
Sallan, S.E., Camitta, B.M., Cassady, J.R., Nathan, D.G., Frei, E.III (1978). Intermittent combination chemotherapy with adriamycin for childhood acute lympho-blastic leukemia: clinical results. Blood, 51, 425-433.
Sather, H.N., Coccia, P., Nesbit, M., Level, C., Hammond, D. (1978). Disappearance of the predictive value of prognostic factors for childhood acute lymphocytic leukemia (ALL). Proc. AACR-ASCO, 19, 330.
Sen, L., Borella, L. (1975). Clinical importance of lymphoblasts with T markers in childhood acute leukemia. N. Engl. J. Med., 292, 828-832.
Shalet, S.M., Beardwell, C.G., Morris Jones, P.H., Pearson, D. (1976).Growth hormone deficiency after treatment of acute leukemia in children. Arch. Dis. Childh

51, 489-493.

Sharp, H.L., Nesbit, M.E., D'Angio, G.J., Krivit, W. (1967). Addition of local radiation after bone marrow remission in acute leukemia in children. Cancer, 20, 1403-1404.

Simone, J.V., Aur, R.J.A., Hustu, H.O., Verzosa, M. (1975a). Acute lymphocytic leukemia in children. Cancer, 36, 770-774.

Simone, J.V., Aur, R.J.A., Hustu, H.O., Verzosa, M., Pinkel, D. (1975b). Combined modality therapy of acute lymphocytic leukemia. Cancer, 35, 25-35.

Simone, J.V., Verzosa, M.S., Rudy, J.A. (1975c). Initial features and prognosis in 363 children with acute lymphocytic leukemia. Cancer, 36, 2099-2108.

Simone, J.V. (1976). Factors that influence haematological remission duration in acute lymphocytic leukaemia. Brit. J. Haemat., 32, 465-472.

Siris, E.S., Leventhal, B.G., Vaitukaitis, J.L. (1976). Effects of childhood leukemia and chemotherapy on puberty and reproductive function in girls. N. Engl. J. Med., 294, 1143-1146.

Skipper, H.E., Schaber, F.M.Jr., Wilcox, W.S. (1964). Experimental evaluation of potential anticancer agents. XIII. On the criteria and kinetics associated with "curability" of experimental leukemia. Cancer Chemoth. Rep., 35, 1-111.

Soni, S., Marten, G.W., Pitner, S.E., Duenas, D.A., Powazek, M. (1975). Effects of central-nervous-system irradiation on neuropsychologic functioning of children with acute lymphocytic leukemia. N. Engl. J. Med., 293, 113-118.

Spiers, A.S.D., Roberts, P.D., Marsh, G.W., Parekh, S.J., Franklin, A.J., Galton, D.A.G., Szur, Z.L., Paul, E.A., Husband, P., Wiltshaw, E. (1975). Acute lympho-cytic leukaemia: Cyclical chemotherapy with three combinations of four drugs (COAP-POMP-CART regimen). Brit. Med. J., 4, 614-617.

Thomas, E.D., Buckner, C.D., Banaji, M., Clift, R.A., Fefer, A., Flournoy, N., Goodell, B.W., Hickman, R.O., Lerner, K.G., Neiman, P.E., Sale, G.E., Sanders, J.E., Singer, J., Stevens, M., Storb, R., Weiden, P.L. (1977). One hundred patients with acute leukemia treated by chemotherapy, total body irradiation and allogenic marrow transplantation. Blood, 49, 511-533.

Verzosa, M., Fite, A.: Efficacy and morbidity of daunomycin (NSC-82151) added to vincristine (NSC-67574) and prednisone (NSC-10023) for remission induction of childhood acute lymphocytic leukemia. Cancer Chemoth. Rep., 55, 79-81.

Verzosa, M.S., Aur, R.J.A., Simone, J.V., Hustu, H.O., Pinkel, D.P. (1976). Five years after central nervous system irradiation of children with leukemia. Int. J. Radiat. Oncol. Biol. Phys., 1, 209-215.

Wagner, V.M., Baehner, R.L. (1977). Lack of correlation between blast cell size and length of first remission in acute lymphocytic leukemia in childhood. Med.Ped. Oncol., 3, 373-377.

Wang, J.J., Freeman, A.I., Sinks, L.F. (1976). Treatment of acute lymphoblastic leukemia by high-dose intravenous methotrexate. Cancer Res., 36, 1441-1444.

West, R.J., Graham-Pole, J., Hardisty, R.M., Pike, M.C. (1972). Factors in patho-genesis of central nervous system leukaemia. Brit. Med. J., 3, 311-314.

Yaddanapudi, R., Lusher, J., Sarnaik, S., Considine, B., Zuelzer, W. (1978). Intermittent intrathecal (IT) methotrexate (MTX) and fractional radiation (IMFRA) plus chemotherapy in acute lymphoblastic leukemia (ALL). Proc. AACR-ASCO, 19,414.

Zuelzer, W.W., Ravindranath, Y., Lusher, J.M., Sarnaik, S., Considine, B. (1976). Infra (intermittent intrathecal methotre xate and fractional radiation) plus chemo-therapy in childhood leukemia. Amer. J. Hemat., 1, 191-199.

Treatment of Adult Acute Myeloblastic Leukemia

**K. B. McCredie*, K. A. Dicke*, G. P. Bodey*, J. P. Hester*,
T. Smith** and E. J. Freireich***

**Developmental Therapeutics, **Biomathematics
The University of Texas Cancer Center,
M.D. Anderson Hospital and Tumor Institute, Houston, Texas 77030, U.S.A.*

ABSTRACT

Combination chemotherapy for the management of adults with acute myeloblastic leukemia has significantly improved the response rate and duration of survival. The additional use of immunotherapeutic agents such as BCG has improved both the duration of response and survival rates compared to chemotherapy alone. The addition of late intensification therapy also prolongs disease and survival. For those patients that relapse, preliminary data suggests that autologous bone marrow transplantation may play a significant role in improving prognosis.

KEYWORDS

AML, anthracycline, Ara-C, Ad-OAP, rubidazone, late intensification, transplantation.

INTRODUCTION

The combination of cytosine arabinoside with an anthracycline antibiotic, either daunorubicin, adriamycin or rubidazone, has been responsible over the last decade for dramatic improvements in the response rates seen in patients with acute myeloblastic leukemia. The use of cytosine arabinoside alone or in combination with immunotherapeutic agents and/or 6-thioguanine for remission maintenance therapy has also prolonged the duration of remission and survival of these patients.

In a study at the M. D. Anderson Hospital in 1973, adriamycin and cytosine arabinoside were combined in a sequential fashion with vincristine and prednisone for remission induction therapy in acute myeloblastic leukemia. In addition, BCG was administered to these patients during the remission induction phase. Subsequent to the achievement of complete remission, patients had three further courses of the adriamycin-cytosine arabinoside regimen before being put on a maintenance program consisting of cytosine arabinoside, vincristine and prednisone for five days at approximately monthly intervals. Table 1 shows the results of the initial induction therapy, 58 adults with ages ranging between 15 and 71 were treated with this regimen for the diagnosis of acute myeloblastic leukemia. The median duration of survival in 58 patients was 58 weeks, 43 patients achieved a complete remission (74%) with 31 of 35 patients under the age of 50 achieving a complete remission (McCredie, 1975). Nine patients remain alive between four and five years from diagnosis. Of these nine, eight are in their original first complete remission, all of whom were under the age of 50 at the time of diagnosis and represents

49

26% of the patients under the age of 50 who achieved a complete remission or 23% of patients entered on the program under the age of 50.

TABLE 1   AD-OAP Acute Myeloblastic Leukemia

Entered	58	
Complete Remission	43 (74%)	
Complete Remission	< 50	31/35 (88.5%)
	≥ 50	12/23 (51%)

The initial success of this program led to the same combination of agents being utilized in the Southwest Oncology Group for remission induction therapy and maintenance. Four hundred and twenty patients with a diagnosis of myeloblastic disease were entered, 224 achieved a complete remission. The survival of all patients and the survival of those patients achieving a complete remission is shown in Fig. 1. Vertical lines on these survival curves represent patients still alive and can effect the overall curve. The median duration of survival for all patients is 50 weeks and the projected median duration of survival for those patients that achieve a complete remission is almost double this, approximately two years (McCredie, 1977). This study also has a randomization between BCG and no BCG during the remission maintenance phase. It is, however, too early to determine the role BCG will play in the study.

Acute Myeloblastic Leukemia
Survival From First Treatment

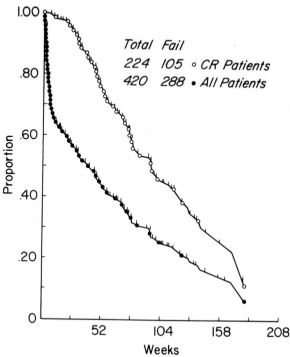

Total	Fail	
224	105	∘ CR Patients
420	288	• All Patients

Fig. 1

Rubidazone, a new anthracycline antibiotic related to daunorubicin, has been recently utilized in combination with cytosine arabinoside for the management of patients for remission induction therapy with patients over the age of fifty. In an attempt to improve the overall response in this poor prognostic group, results of this study is shown in Table 2 and are similar to the previous results using the combination of adriamycin and Ara-C (Keating, 1977).

TABLE 2   ROAP
Acute Myeloblastic Leukemia
> 50 Years of Age

Entered   57

Complete Remission   28 (49%)

Immunotherapy utilizing BCG by the scarification technique, originally described by Mathe, has been used in patients achieving a complete remission with a diagnosis of acute myeloblastic leukemia in conjunction with the Ara-C, vincristine and prednisone program. The BCG was administered weekly during the weeks that chemotherapy was not administered in doses of 6×10^8 viable units. Two groups of patients were studied and compared with 24 patients in a control group who received OAP alone and compared to 14 patients that received OAP plus BCG, Table 3. There was a significant improvement both in the duration of remission and in the survival of these patients. Six of 14 patients on OAP-BCG remain alive and in complete remission (43%) compared to 8 (33%) of the patients receiving OAP. Two additional patients, long term survivors in the OAP-BCG group, have relapsed and subsequently have been reinduced into complete remission (Gutterman, 1978).

TABLE 3   Chemoimmunotherapy of
Acute Myeloblastic Leukemia

	No. of Patients	Median Duration of Remission (Weeks)	Duration of Remission (Weeks)
OAP	24	52	96
OAP+BCG	14	85	165

(52/85 > 0.08)   (96/165 > 0.05)

Late intensification therapy utilizing drugs to which patients have not been previously exposed has been administered to a total of 62 patients. The majority of these patients received a combination of 6-mercaptopurine, methotrexate, vincristine and prednisone, administered 12 to 24 months after remission induction and maintenance therapy.

Table 4 shows that 29 or 47% of the patients remain in complete remission. The majority of the patients that relapsed, relapsed in the first 6 months and almost all of the patients that relapsed, relapsed within 24 months of discontinuation of chemotherapy.

K. B. McCredie *et al.*

TABLE 4   Late Intensification Therapy In Acute Leukemia

Patients Entered	62	
Patients Still In CR	29	(47%)
Relapsed By 6 Months	21	(64%)
Relapsed By 24 Months	31	(94%)

Table 5 shows the risk of relapse following late intensification and demonstrates that the risk of subsequent relapse after one year of continuous remission without chemotherapy is less than 10% and that these patients are potentially cured of their leukemia (Bodey, 1975).

TABLE 5   Duration Of Unmaintained Remission After Late Intensification Therapy

Duration of CR (Yrs from LI)	Number of Patients	Subsequent Relapses	
1	36	9	(25%)
2	25	2	(8%)
3	18	1	(6%)
4	12	0	

Although there is a potential cure rate in adults with myeloblastic leukemia, for those patients who relapse subsequent to achieving a complete remission, the survival is poor, Fig. 2, with median durations of survival being less than 20 weeks and only 5% of patients are projected to be alive one year after their initial relapse.

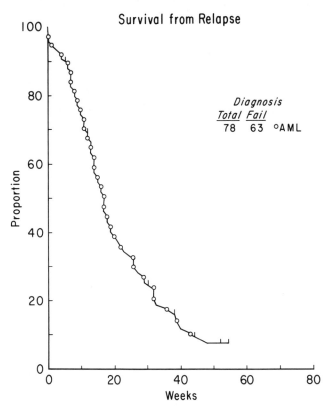

Fig. 2

Because of the poor results and the lack of available therapy subsequent to relapse, a program of autologous bone marrow transplantation has been introduced
utilizing marrow collected and stored from patients during periods of remission.
The combination of piperazinedione and total body irradiation has been utilized
to eradicate the leukemia prior to the thawing and administration of previously
stored bone marrow. This program has resulted in the clearing of leukemia and
evidence of engraftment with normal myeloid recovery in 5 of 11 patients (Dicke,
1977). Survival of these patients, duration of remission and duration of bone
marrow storage in months and interval between storage and relapse and the number of cells and the number of colony forming units reinfused is shown in Table
6.

TABLE 6 Autologous Bone Marrow Transplantation

Number of Evaluable Patients	11
Number Showing Evidence of Engraftment	9
Number Achieving Complete Remission Survival (days) 17 - 320+	5
Interval Between Remission and Storage (months)	2 - 5 Median 12
Interval Between Storage and Relapse (months)	10 - 30 Median 19
Cells Transfused/kg b.w.	$6.8x10^6 - 3.2x10^8$ Median $1.2x10^8$
CFT-C/10^5 Cells	0 - 15 Median 5

Effective remission induction therapy for acute myeloblastic leukemia, particularly under the age of 50, the use of aggressive maintenance chemotherapy, late intensification, immunotherapy, and a potential for bone marrow transplantation has improved substantially the outlook for patients with this disease with the potential of a cure in a percentage of patients. Better understanding the factors which predict for response in survival may allow us to individualize therapy for patients in these groups and improve the outlook for long term survival in the majority of patients.

REFERENCES

Bodey, G.P., E.J Freireich, K.B. McCredie, V. Rodriguez, J.U. Gutterman and M.A. Burgess (1976). Late intensification chemotherapy for patients with acute leukemia in remission. JAMA, 235:1021-1025.
Dicke, K.A., K.B. McCredie, E.E. Stevens, G. Spitzer and J.C. Bottino (1977). Autologous bone marrow transplantation in a case of acute adult leukemia. Transplantation Proceedings, 9:193-195.
Gutterman, J.U., V. Rodriguez, K.B. McCredie, J.P. Hester, G.P. Bodey, E.J Freireich, and E.M. Hersh (1978). Chemoimmunotherapy of acute myeloblastic leukemia: 4-year follow-up with BCG. In W.D. Terry and D. Windhorst (Ed.), Immunotherapy of Cancer: Present Status of Trials in Man, Vol.6, Raven Press, New York. pp.375-381.
Keating, M.J., R.S. Benjamin, K.B. McCredie, G.P. Bodey and E.J Freireich (1977). Remission induction therapy with a rubidazone containing combination (ROAP) in acute leukemia. Proceedings of the Sixty-Eight Annual Meeting of AACR/ASCO, #719:180.
McCredie, K.B. and E.J Freireich (1975). Acute Leukemia: Chemotherapy and Management. In E.M. Greenspan (Ed.), Clinical Cancer Chemotherapy, Raven Press, New York. pp. 71-109.
McCredie, K.B., J.S. Hewlett, E.A. Gehan and E.J Freireich (1977). Chemoimmunotherapy of adult acute leukemia (CIAL). Proceedings of the Sixty-Eight Annual Meeting of the AACR/ASCO, #506:127.

New Drugs against Human Acute Leukemia

Franco M. Muggia, Delia F. Chiuten, Daniel D. Von Hoff,
Marcel Rozencweig and Peter H. Wiernik

Division of Cancer Treatment, National Cancer Institute, Bethesda, Maryland,
U.S.A.

ABSTRACT

AMSA, maytansine, 3-deazauridine and chlorozotocin have recently demonstrated favorable features for future therapeutic trials in leukemia. This paper summarizes relevant preclinical and clinical data on these four potentially promising antileukemic agents.

KEYWORDS

Antineoplastic agents, AMSA, maytansine, 3-deazauridine, chlorozotocin, leukemia

INTRODUCTION

In the past, the median survival from the time of diagnosis of acute leukemia was 2.2 months for both children and adults (Tivey, 1954). With presently available chemotherapeutic agents and improved therapeutic approaches, considerable advances have been made in the treatment of acute leukemia, particularly in acute lymphocytic leukemia (ALL). Leukemic remissions have been induced in a majority of patients through the use of a number of well established sequences of single or combination chemotherapy regimens resulting in significant prolongation of survival. However, prolonged intensive cytostatic therapy may be complicated by the emergence of resistant leukemic cell lines pointing to the need for new anticancer agents.

Unfavorable prognostic factors, including chemo-resistance, poor drug tolerance from previous treatment, and complicating diseases, lead to difficulties in perceiving the true extent of activity of new agents being explored at a late stage of the disease. Nevertheless, several investigational drugs such as 5-azacytidine (Von Hoff, Slavik, and Muggia, 1976), VP-16-213 (Rozencweig and others, 1977), and neocarzinostatin (Legha and others, 1976) have demonstrated some reproducible efficacy against advanced leukemias. More recently, AMSA, maytansine, 3-deazauridine and chlorozotocin have shown promising potential in leukemia refractory to extensive prior chemotherapy.

AMSA

AMSA or 4'-(9-acridinylamino) methane sulfon-m-anisidide, is a synthetic acridine derivative (Cain, Seelye, and Atwell, 1974) having DNA binding properties (Gormley, Sethi, and Cysyk, 1978). Its antitumor activity has been established in various murine tumors, including the P388 and L1210 leukemia, the C3H/HeJ spontaneous mammary tumor and the B16 melanocarcinoma (Cain and Atwell, 1974). The drug seems to retain its antitumor activity when given orally (Shoemaker and others, 1977). AMSA also has antiviral activity (Byrd, 1977) and immunosuppressive properties (Baguley and others, 1974).

Pharmacologic disposition of AMSA in mice and rats seems related to an enzymatic conversion by glutathione-S-transferase and to a non-enzymatic nucleophilic attack on the 9-carbon atom of the acridine nucleus by endogenous thiols in the liver (Cysyk, Shoemaker, and Adamson, 1977). Following parenteral administration of 14C-AMSA in rodents, sustained concentrations of total radioactivity are noted in the liver and, within 2 hours, more than 50% of the administered dose is excreted in the bile with a bile to plasma ratio of > 400 : 1. Multiphasic plasma decay curves are observed with an early rapid component followed by a much more gradual decline. This pattern of disappearance is believed to be due to an interaction of AMSA with thiol groups of protein, thus forming stable protein-acridine complexes and causing prolonged retention of the acridine moiety in plasma and certain tissues.

Phase I clinical trials with i.v. AMSA have just been completed in the United States. Myelosuppression, especially transient leucopenia, was the dose-limiting toxicity (Van Echo and others, 1978; Von Hoff and others, 1978; Legha and others, 1978). In addition, nausea and vomiting, fever, skin rash, local irritation and phlebitis have been reported. In general, AMSA has tolerable, acceptable, and reversible toxicity. The recommended dosages are 70 mg/m^2 q 2 weeks (Van Echo and others, 1978), 120 mg/m^2 q 4 weeks (Von Hoff and others, 1978) for the single dose schedule and 40 mg/m^2 for the daily x 3 schedule (Legha and others, 1978).

An early evaluation of a Phase I-II trial of AMSA in heavily pretreated and refractory leukemic patients at the Baltimore Cancer Research Program, National Cancer Institute (BCRP-NCI) revealed some responses in both ALL and acute myelocytic leukemia (AML). One patient with ALL exhibited clearing of blasts in a hypocellular marrow with circulating WBC decreasing from 47,000 to 8,000 twelve hours after chemotherapy. Two patients with AML developed aplastic marrow and a third patient with AML had a decrease in peripheral blasts from 60% to 2% by day 4. All of the six patients treated so far had at least a 50% reduction in the total WBC. Further investigation is ongoing at BCRP-NCI and additional experience will also be forthcoming from studies at the M.D. Anderson Hospital.

MAYTANSINE

Maytansine (MYT), a plant product isolated from the East African shrubs, Maytenus seratta and Maytenus buchanii, is an ansa macrolide structurally related to the rifamycins. Preclinical and clinical information on this new agent is reviewed elsewhere in this volume (Douros and others, 1979). This agent exhibits significant cytotoxic antitumor activity against P388 leukemia, B16 melanocarcinoma, and Lewis lung carcinoma (Kupchan and others, 1972, 1974). MYT possesses stathmokinetic properties and induces metaphase arrest similar to the vinca alkaloids (Sieber and others, 1976). MYT and vincristine (VCR) appear to share common tubulin binding sites, but an additional site specific for MYT

seems to be present (Mandelbaum-Shavit, Wolpert-DeFilippes, and Johns, 1976).
Both drugs inhibit tubulin polymerization at similar concentration but MYT is
about 100 fold more potent than VCR in inhibiting mitosis in sea urchin eggs
(Remillard and others, 1975). However, investigation of the activity of MYT
against VCR-sensitive and resistant variants of P388 leukemia has revealed
cross-resistance with VCR (Sieber and others, 1976).

MYT blocks the fast axoplasmic transport of proteins at dosages that do not induce perceptible change in axonal ultrastructure as observed at electron microscopy (Donoso and others, 1977). Unlike with VCR, toxicologic studies in beagle
dogs and rhesus monkeys did not reveal any neurotoxicity with MYT (Helman,
Henney, and Slavik, 1976). However, hind limb paralysis was induced in 10%
of the mice given MYT by i.p. route (Sieber and others, 1976).

Clinical trials with MYT have been sponsored since 1975 by the Investigational
Drug Branch of the Cancer Therapy Evaluation Program, NCI. Recently completed studies have identified the drug-induced toxic effects in man (Eagan and
others, 1978; Chabner and others, 1978; Cabanillas and others, 1978; Blum and
Kahlert, 1978). Dose-related gastrointestinal toxicity, manifested by nausea,
vomiting and diarrhea, is the major dose-limiting factor. Hepatotoxicity, varying from subclinical transient elevation of liver enzymes to overt jaundice, has
been reported. Dose-related neurotoxicity is manifested as central and peripheral neuropathy. Impairment of the central nervous system is characterized by
lethargy, dysphoria, insomnia, agitated depression and lightheadedness. Peripheral neuropathy is less frequent and resembles vinca alkaloid neuropathy
with paresthesias, jaw pain, loss of deep tendon reflexes, muscle pain and weak-
ness. Hematologic toxicity is minimal and infrequent, and is usually manifested
by transient thrombocytopenia. Local phlebitis, alopecia, stomatitis, metallic
taste and constipation have also been occasionally encountered. Phase II studies
are ongoing using intermittent schedules (0.5 mg/m^2 daily x 3 or 2 mg/m^2 single dose every three weeks) or weekly administration (0.75 mg/m^2). Dose re-
ductions may be required in the presence of liver dysfunction.

In the initial Phase I-II clinical trials, antitumor activity was seen in 2 of 4 patients with ALL even though the patients had all received prior VCR (Chabner
and others, 1978). Because of its similarity to VCR, both in animal antitumor
spectrum and stathmokinetic properties, these very preliminary results should
encourage further trials in acute leukemia, where VCR has been particularly
effective.

3-DEAZAURIDINE

3-Deazauridine (DU), an analogue of the pyrimidine nucleoside uridine (Robins
and Currie, 1968) is a compound with antibacterial (Wang and Bloch, 1972) and
antiviral properties particularly against Gross leukemia virus (Shannon and
others, 1974). Interest as an antitumor compound was based on its activity
against murine L1210 leukemia especially since it is significantly more active
against a cytosine arabinoside (Ara-C)-resistant subline (L1210/Ara-C) than
against the parent Ara-C-sensitive line (L1210/0) (Brockman and others, 1975).
Ara-C is currently part of every primary combination for AML. Relapsing patients, therefore, may be considered for clinical validation of the observation
that L1210/Ara-C is significantly more sensitive to DU than the parent L1210/0
cell line.

The mechanism of action of DU is thought to be inhibition of cytidine triphosphate
(CTP) synthetase (McPartland and others, 1974). DU is phosphorylated to the
nucleoside triphosphate, (3-deaza UTP), and accumulates in the cell (Wang and

Bloch, 1972). At this metabolic stage, it prevents DNA synthesis through inhibition of CTP synthetase (Brockman and others, 1975; McPartland and others, 1974). DU is not incorporated into cellular RNA or DNA despite its extensive conversion to its major metabolite (3-deaza UTP) in tumor cells (Wang and Bloch, 1972).

DU is currently undergoing Phase I clinical trials in the United States (Minutes of Phase I Working Group, 1978). The main toxic effects are myelosuppression, manifested as mild leukopenia and thrombocytopenia, and gastrointestinal (i.e. nausea and vomiting); diarrhea and stomatitis are also reported. Occasional fever, skin rash, and transient elevation in SGOT are also observed. The maximum tolerated dose (MTD) is 1.2 gm/m^2 for solid tumors and 6 gm/m^2 for leukemic patients, at a daily x 5 schedule given by rapid i.v. infusion. When given as a continuous infusion, the MTD is 3 gm/m^2 for leukemic patients. It is of note that DU seems much better tolerated in leukemic patients where the MTD is six times higher than in solid tumors. Therapeutic results have not yet been published but there has been some evidence of antileukemic activity.

DU is a potent competitive inhibitor of cytidine deaminase (Hande, Lewis, and Chabner, 1978), the enzyme which degrades Ara-C. Synergistic antitumor activity has been observed in vitro when DU was given together with Ara-C (Lauzon, Paran, and Paterson, 1978; Mills-Yamamoto, Lauzon, and Paterson, 1978). This phenomenon, due to increased cellular uptake of Ara-C after pretreatment with DU and to enhancement of Ara-C anabolism by DU (Lauzon, Paran, and Paterson, 1978), provides a reasonable rationale for combining DU and Ara-C in the treatment of AML.

CHLOROZOTOCIN

Chlorozotocin (CLZ) is a water-soluble 2-chloro ethyl analog of the nitrosourea, streptozotocin (Johnston, McCaleb, and Montgomery, 1975). It is of particular interest because it exhibits low marrow toxicity and a high level of activity in L1210 leukemia (Anderson, McMenamin, and Schein, 1975). Based on structure-activity studies, the attachment of the cytotoxic nitrosourea moiety on the C2 of the glucose carrier may be responsible for the reduction of bone marrow toxicity (Heal and others, 1977; Schein, 1969; Schein, McMenamin, and Anderson, 1973). Schein and his coworkers (1978), using soft agar bone marrow cultures assays for colony-forming units committed to granulocyte-macrophage differentiation (CFU-c), have shown that CLZ produced less depression in mouse as well as in human bone marrow hematopoietic precursor cells relative to BCNU. Interestingly, CLZ had demonstrated selective sparing of normal murine bone marrow DNA synthesis but produced significant inhibition of L1210 DNA synthesis (Anderson, McMenamin, and Schein, 1975; Schein and others, 1976; Panasci, Green, and Schein, 1977). However, unlike STZ, a methylnitrosourea derivative, CLZ produces DNA damage in L1210 leukemia cells by cross-linking similar to other chloroethyl nitrosoureas (Ewig and Kohn, 1977; Erickson, 1978). Biochemical studies have shown that CLZ exerts its greatest activity on G1 arrested cells rather than on cells in exponential growth phase (Bhuyan, Fraser, and Day, 1977). As other chloroethyl nitrosoureas, it also prolongs S phase, causes cells to accumulate in G2 phase, and allows only a small fraction of the population to divide (Tobey and Crissman, 1975; Tobey, Oka, and Crissman, 1975). Of all clinically used chloroethyl nitrosoureas, with the exception of the Japanese ACNU, CLZ possesses the most alkylating activity relative to carbamoylating activity as judged by the ability of the isocyanate component to react with lysine (Heal and others, 1978; Panasci and others, 1977). Myelosuppression has been observed in clinical Phase I studies at doses higher than 120 mg/m^2. This has been manifested as thrombocytopenia, the nadir typically occurring four weeks after treatment (Hoth and others, 1978; Kovach and others, 1978). Leukopenia has not been prominent at doses as high as 220 mg/m^2, and there may be less cumulative toxicity on repeated dosing than with BCNU, CCNU or MeCCNU, as judged by experience in previously untreated patients. Gastrointestinal toxicity (i.e. nausea and vomiting) has been tolerable. Some hepatotoxicity (transient elevation of transaminases) has been reported (Hoth and others, 1978; Kovach and others, 1978), perhaps in relation to the hepatic metabolism of the drug partly by glutathione conjugation (Franza, Wang, and Woolley, 1977; Woolley and Wang, 1978). Hyperglycemia, which occurred in rats with CLZ (Tutwiler and others, 1976), was not observed in the clinic (Tan and others, 1978). No renal toxicity has been noted. Responses were noted in hematologic malignancies, i.e., lymphoma (Hoth and others, 1978; Tan and others, 1978) and leukemia (Hoth and others, 1978). A patient with ALL had a fall in bone marrow blasts from 90% to 25% (Hoth and others, 1978). Current dosages in Phase II studies are 30-40 mg/m^2 for the daily x 5 and 120 mg/m^2 to 180 mg/m^2 for the single dose q 6 week schedule.

CONCLUSION

In spite of the difficulties of assessing responses in very heavily pretreated patients, acute leukemia remains an important area for new drug testing. Advances in supportive care, coupled with enhanced selective cell killing of malignant cells through induction regimens, treatment of sanctuaries, and crossover to non-cross-resistant combinations, continue to give tangible proof of therapeutic benefits resulting from efforts at improving systemic chemotherapy.

REFERENCES

Anderson, T., M. G. McMenamin,, and P. S. Schein (1975). Chlorozotocin, 2-[3-(2-chlorethyl)-3-nitrosoureido]-D-glucopyranose, an antitumor agent with modified bone marrow toxicity. Cancer Res., 35, 761-765.

Baguley, B. C., E. M. Falkenhaug, J. M. Rastrick, and J. Marbrook (1974). An assessment of the immunosuppressive activity of the anti-tumour compound 4'-[(9-acridinyl) amino] methanesulphon-m-anisidide (m-AMSA). Eur. J. Cancer, 10, 169-176.

Bhuyan, B. K., T. J. Fraser, and K. J. Day (1977). Cell proliferation kinetics and drug sensitivity of exponential and stationary populations of cultured L1210 cells. Cancer Res., 37, 1057-1063.

Blum, R. H., and T. Kahlert (1978). Maytansine: A phase I study of an ansa macrolide with antitumor activity. Cancer Treat. Rep., 62, 435-438.

Brockman, R. W., S. C. Shaddix, M. Williams, J. A. Nelson, L. M. Rose, and F. M. Schabel, Jr. (1975). The mechanism of action of 3-deazauridine in tumor cells sensitive and resistant to arabinosylcytosine. Ann. N. Y. Acad. Sci., 255, 501-521.

Byrd, D. M. (1977). Antiviral activities of 4'-(9-acridinylamino)-methanesulfon-m-aniside (SN 11841). Ann. N. Y. Acad. Sci., 284, 463-471.

Cabanillas, F., V. Rodriguez, S. W. Hall, M. A. Burgess, G. P. Bodey, and E. J. Freireich (1978). Phase I study of maytansine using a 3-day schedule. Cancer Treat. Rep., 62, 425-428.

Cain, B. F. and G. J. Atwell (1974). The experimental antitumour properties of three congeners of the acridylmethanesulphonanilide (AMSA) series. Eur. J. Cancer, 10, 539-549.

Cain, B. F., R. N. Seelye, and G. J. Atwell (1974). Potential antitumour agents. 14'acridylmethanesulphonanilides. J. Med. Chem., 17, 922-930.

Chabner, B. A., A. S. Levine, B. L. Johnson, and R. C. Young (1978). Initial clinical trials of maytansine, an antitumor plant alkaloid. Cancer

Treat. Rep., 62, 429-433.

Cysyk, R. L., D. D. Shoemaker, and R. H. Adamson (1977). The pharmaco-
    logic disposition of 4'-(9-acridinylamino)-methanesulfon-m-anisidide in
    mice and rats. Drug Metab. Dispos., 5, 579-590.

Donoso, J. A., D. F. Watson, I. Bettinger, and F. E. Samson (1977). Effect
    of maytansine on fast axonal transport. Fed. Proc., 36, 560.

Douros, J. D., M. Suffness, D. F. Chiuten, and R. H. Adamson (1979). May-
    tansine. (This volume).

Eagan, R. T., J.N. Ingle, J. Rubin, S. Frytak, and C. G. Moertel (1978). Ear-
    ly clinical study of an intermittent schedule for maytansine (NSC-153858):
    Brief communication. J. Natl. Cancer Inst., 60, 93-96.

Erickson, L. C. (1978). Measurements of DNA damage in Chinese hamster
    cells treated with equi-toxic and equi-mutagenic doses of nitrosoureas.
    Proc. Am. Assoc. Cancer Res., 19, 210.

Ewig, R. A. G. and K. W. Kohn (1977). DNA damage and repair in mouse leu-
    kemia L1210 cells treated with nitrogen mustard, 1,3-bis(2-chloroethyl)-1-
    nitrosourea, and other nitrosoureas. Cancer Res., 37, 2114-2122.

Franza, R., A. Wang, and P. V. Woolley (1977). Alterations in murine hepatic
    glutathione levels by streptozotocin and chlorozotocin. Proc. Am. Assoc.
    Cancer Res., 18, 132.

Gormley, P. E., V. S. Sethi, and R. L. Cysyk (1978). Interaction of 4'-(9-acri-
    dinylamino) methanesulphon-m-anisidide with DNA and inhibition of oncorna-
    virus reverse transcriptase and cellular nucleic acid polymerases. Cancer
    Res., 38, 1300-1306.

Hande, K., B. Lewis, and B. Chabner (1978). Inhibition of cytosine arabinoside
    (AraC) deamination by uridine analogs. Proc. Am. Assoc. Cancer Res.,
    19, 149.

Heal, J.M., P. A. Fox, D. Doukas, and P. S. Schein (1978). Biological and
    biochemical properties of the 2-hydroxyl metabolites of 1-(2-chloroethyl)-3-
    cyclohexyl-1-nitrosourea. Cancer Res., 38, 1070-1074.

Heal, J., P. Fox, R. Nagourney, J. McDonald, and P. Schein (1978). Biolog-
    ical and biochemical properties of new water soluble nitrosoureas. Proc.
    Am. Assoc. Cancer Res., 18, 132.

Helman, L., J. Henney, and M. Slavik (1976). Clinical brochure on maytansine
    (NSC 153858). Investigational Drug Branch, CTEP, DCT, NCI.

Hoth, D., T. Butler, S. Winokur, A. Kales, P. Woolley, and P. Schein (1978).
    Phase II study of chlorozotocin. Proc. Am. Assoc. Cancer Res., 19, 381.

Hoth, D., P. Woolley, D. Green, J. MacDonald, and P. Schein (1978). Phase I
    studies on chlorozotocin. Clin. Pharmacol. Ther., 23, 712-722.

Johnston, T. P., G. S. McCaleb, and J. A. Montgomery (1975). Synthesis of
    chlorozotocin, the 2-chloroethyl analog of the anticancer antibiotic strepto-
    zotocin. J. Med. Chem., 18, 104-106.

Kovach, J., C. G. Moertel, A. J. Schutt, and M. J. O'Connell (1978). A
    phase I study of chlorozotocin (NSC 178248). Proc. Am. Assoc. Cancer
    Res., 19, 408.

Kupchan, S. M., Y. Komoda, A. R. Branfman, R. G. Dailey, Jr., and V. A.
    Zimmerly (1974) Novel maytansinoids. Structural interrelations and re-
    quirements for antileukemic activity. J. Am. Chem. Soc., 96, 3706-3708.

Kupchan, S. M., Y. Komoda, W. A. Court, G. J. Thomas, R. M. Smith, A.
    Karim, C. G. Gilmore, R. C. Haltiwanger, and R. F. Bryan (1972). May-
    tansine, a novel antileukemic ansa macrolide from Maytenus ovatus. J.
    Am. Chem. Soc., 94, 1354-1356.

Lauzon, G. J., J. H. Paran, and A. R. P. Paterson (1978) Formation of 1-β-D-
    arabinofuranosylcytosine diphosphate choline in cultured human leukemic
    RPMI 6410 cells. Cancer Res., 38, 1723-1729.

Legha, S. S., J. U. Gutterman, S. W. Hall, R. S. Benjamin, M. A. Burgess,
    M. Valdivieso, and G. P. Bodey (1978). Phase I clinical investigation of

4'-(9-acridinylamino) methanesulfon-m-anisidide (NSC 249992), a new acri-
    dine derivative. Cancer Res. (In press).
Legha, S. S., D. D. Von Hoff, M. Rozencweig, D. Abraham, M. Slavik, and
    F. M. Muggia (1976). Neocarzinostatin (NSC 157365): A new cancerostatic
    compound. Oncology, 33, 265-270.
Mandelbaum-Shavit, F., M. K. Wolpert-DeFilippes, and D. G. Johns (1976).
    Binding of maytansine to rat brain tubulin. Biochem. Biophys. Res. Com-
    mun., 72, 47-54.
McPartland, R. P., M. C. Wang, A. Bloch, and H. Weinfeld (1974). Cytidine
    5'-triphosphate synthetase as a target for inhibition by the antitumor agent
    3-deazauridine. Cancer Res., 34, 3107-3111.
Mills-Yamamoto, C., G. J. Lauzon, and A. R. P. Paterson (1978). Toxicity
    of combinations of arabinosylcytosine and 3-deazauridine toward neoplastic
    cells in culture. Biochem. Pharmacol., 27, 181-186.
Minutes of the Phase I Working Group Meeting, January 19-20, 1978. Investiga-
    tional Drug Branch, CTEP, DCT, NCI, Bethesda, Md.
Panasci, L. C., D. Green, R. Nagourney, P. Fox, and P. S. Schein (1977).
    A structure-activity analysis of chemical and biological parameters of
    chloroethylnitrosoureas in mice. Cancer Res., 37, 2615-2618.
Panasci, L., D. Green, and P. Schein (1977). Chlorozotocin (CLZ): Mecha-
    nism of reduced myelotoxicity for mice. Proc. Am. Assoc. Cancer Res.,
    18, 123.
Remillard, S., L. I. Rehbun, G. A. Howie, and S. M. Kupchan (1975). Anti-
    mitotic activity of the potent tumor inhibitor maytansine. Science, 189,
    1002-1005.
Robins, M. J. and B. L. Currie (1968). The synthesis of 3-deazauridine
    [4-hydroxy-1-(β-D-ribopentofuranosyl)-2-pyridone]. Chem. Commun., 2,
    1547-1548.
Rozencweig, M., D. D. Von Hoff, J. E. Henney, and F. M. Muggia (1977).
    VM-26 and VP-16-213: A comparative analysis. Cancer, 40, 334-342.
Schein, P. S. (1969). 1-methyl-1-nitrosourea and dialkyl-nitrosamine depression
    of nicotinamide adenine dinucleotide. Cancer Res., 29, 1226-1232.
Schein, P. S., J. M. Bull, D. Doukas, and D. Hoth (1978). Sensitivity of human
    and murine hematopoietic precursor cells to 2-[3-(2-chloroethyl)-3-nitro-
    soureido]-D-glucopyranose and 1,3-Bis (2-chloroethyl)-1-nitrosourea.
    Cancer Res., 38, 257-260.
Schein, P. S., M. McMenamin, and T. Anderson (1973). 3-(tetraacetyl gluco-
    pyranose-2-yl)-1-(2-chloroethyl)-1-nitrosourea, an antitumor agent with
    modified bone marrow toxicity. Cancer Res., 33, 2005-2009.
Schein, P. S., L. Panasci, P. V. Woolley, and T. Anderson (1976). Pharma-
    cology of chlorozotocin (NSC-178248), a new nitrosourea antitumor agent.
    Cancer Treat. Rep., 60, 801-805.
Shannon, W. M., R. W. Brockman, L. Westbrook, S. Shaddix, and F. M.
    Schabel, Jr. (1974). Inhibition of Gross leukemia virus-induced plaque
    formation in XC cells by 3-deazauridine. J. Natl. Cancer Inst., 52, 199-
    205.
Shoemaker, D. D., O. Ayers, M. E. D'Anna, and R. L. Cysyk (1977). Selec-
    tive toxic effect of 4'-(9-acridinylamino)-methanesulfon-m-anisidide (AMSA,
    NSC 141549) on liver metastases in mice. Proc. Am. Assoc. Cancer Res.,
    18, 166.
Sieber, S. M., M. K. Wolpert, R. H. Adamson, R. L. Cysyk, V. H. Bono, and
    D. G. Johns (1976). Experimental studies with maytansine - a new antitumor
    agent. Bibl. Haematol., 43, 495-500.
Tan, C., R. Gralla, P. Steinherz, and C. W. Young (1978). Phase I study of
    chlorozotocin. Proc. Am. Assoc. Cancer Res., 19, 126.
Tivey, H. (1954). The natural history of untreated acute leukemia. Ann. N. Y.
    Acad. Sci., 60, 322-358.
Tobey, R. A. and H. A. Crissman (1975). Unique techniques for cell cycle

analysis utilizing mithramycin and flow microfluorometry. <u>Exp. Cell Res.</u>, <u>93</u>, 235-239.

Tobey, R. A., M. S. Oka, and H. A. Crissman (1975). Differential effects of two chemotherapeutic agents, streptozotocin and chlorozotocin, on the mammalian cell cycle. <u>Eur. J. Cancer</u>, <u>11</u>, 433-441.

Tutwiler, G. F., G. J. Bridi, T. J. Kirsch, H. D. Burns, and N. D. Heindel. Hyperglycemic activity of some non-nitrosated streptozotocin analogs. <u>Proc. Soc. Exp. Biol. Med.</u>, <u>152</u>, 195-198.

Van Echo, D., D. F. Chiuten, M. Scoltack, and P. H. Wiernik (1978). A phase I study of m-AMSA (NSC 249992) employing an intermittent every other week schedule. (In preparation).

Von Hoff, D. D., D. Howser, P. E. Gormley, R. Bender, D. Glaubiger, A. Levine, and R. Young (1978). A phase I study of 4'(9-acridinylamino) methane-sulfon-m-anisidide (m-AMSA) using a single dose schedule. <u>Cancer Treat. Rep.</u> (In press).

Von Hoff, D. D., M. Slavik, and F. M. Muggia (1976). 5-Azacytidine, a new anticancer drug with effectiveness in acute myelogenous leukemia. <u>Ann. Intern. Med.</u>, 85, 237-245.

Wang, M. C. and A. Bloch (1972). Studies on the mode of action of 3-deazapyrimidines-1. Metabolism of 3-deazauridine and 3-deazacytidine in microbial and tumor cells. <u>Biochem. Pharmacol.</u>, <u>21</u>, 1063-1073.

Woolley, P. V and A. L. Wang (1978). Studies on the hepatic toxicity of chlorozotocin. <u>Proc. Am. Assoc. Cancer Res.</u>, <u>19</u>, 130.

Immunotherapy of Acute Myelocytic Leukemia with Neuraminidase treated Myeloblasts and MER

J. George Bekesi and James F. Holland

Department of Neoplastic Diseases, Mount Sinai School of Medicine and Hospital of the City University of New York, New York, N. Y. 10029, U.S.A.

Varying degrees of success have been demonstrated by immunization of experimental animals with x-irradiated syngeneic tumor cells in conjunction with or without BCG or MER, methanol extraction residue of BCG (1,2). Similarly, improved remission duration and survival of leukemic patients have been reported after immunization with x-irradiated ALL or AML blast cells in combination with or without BCG (3-6).

Neuraminidase of Vibrio Cholerae origin has been used successfully in increasing the immunogenicity of a variety of spontaneous and experimental tumors (7-12). The immunoprotection evoked by stimulation from the neuraminidase-modified tumor cells was found to be specific for the particular tumor and could be transferred by either the sera or splenic lymphocytes of immunized syngeneic mice (8,9,10).

The vertically transmitted Gross leukemia virus is the etiologic agent for lymphoma in AKR mice. In many respects this disease has similarities to acute lymphocytic leukemia in children. In our laboratory spontaneous leukemic AKR mice were treated with combination durg therapy plus immunization with neuraminidase modified syngeneic or allogeneic Gross virus induced E_2G leukemia cells (13). The success of this therapy indicated the existence of a cross-reacting common viral antigen and suggested that if a similar etiology existed for human acute leukemia it would not be essential to use autologous myeloblasts or lymphoblasts for immunization.

The work to be reported describes a successful chemoimmunotherapy study in AML patients in complete remission using neuraminidase modified allogeneic myeloblasts as immunogen.

Chemotherapy

The chemoimmunotherapy program has been predicated on the maximal chemotherapeutic reduction of leukemic body burden. The chemotherapy constituted 7 days of continuous infusion of cytosine arabinoside at 100 mg/m^2/day and 3 days of daunorubicin at 45 mg/m^2/day on days 1, 2 and 3. All patients were 15 to 70 years of age. The drugs led to remission in approximately 70% of the patients. Maintenance consisted of rotational cycles of cytosine arabinoside 100 mg/m^2 q.12.h. (k.v.) x 10 doses and thioguanine 100 mg/m^2 q.12.h.(p.o.) x 10, cytosine arabinoside and cyclophosphamide 1000 mg/m^2(i.v.) x 1 and cytosine arabinoside and

daunorubicin 45 mg/m^2 x 2. Later in the study, an additional maintenance cycle
of cytosine arabinoside for 5 days and CCNU were added. Beginning on day 8,
after the first sustaining course of chemotherapy and on day 15 of each cycle
thereafter, patients were randomly allocated to receive chemotherapy alone, or
chemotherapy plus neuraminidase treated allogeneic myeloblasts or chemotherapy
plus neuraminidase treated myeloblasts plus MER, the mentanol extraction residue
of BCG (see Fig. 1). This rotational cycle was continued till relapse.

Immunotherapy

Patients become eligible for collection of myeloblasts after satisfying the
following criteria: negative HA-A determined by radioimmunoassay, no previous
chemotherapy, total WBC higher than 35,000 per µl and 70% myeloblasts in the
peripheral blood. The separation of myeloblasts is achieved by leukophoresis.
In the last 3 years, 2.4 x 10^{13} myeloblasts were collected from 60 patients
between the ages of 14 and 72 years. None of the patients showed important side
effects from the procedure which was performed in 1 to 4 hours.

Myeloblasts were collected in transfer bags containing acid citrate-dextrose
solution. After cessation of the leukophoresis, the myeloblasts were separated
from contaminating red blood cells by sedimentation. Because of their cryosensi-
tivity, granulocytes were removed by passage through glass beads or nylon wool if
they constituted greater than 3 per cent of the cell population. The myeloblasts
were mixed with special freezing media containing 15 per cent autologous or AB
plasma and 10 per cent dimethylsulfoxide and were frozen in transfer bags by
programmed freezing at a temperature drop of 0.5 to 1°C per minute until 38°C was
reached, and then rapidly to -85°C. The frozen cells were immediately stored in
the vapor phase of liquid nitrogen.

In order to avoid using non-antigenic myeloblasts for immunotherapy, a battery of
tests designated to pretest their antigenicity was run. Fresh myeloblasts from
all donors were tested in mixed lymphocyte-tumor culture. In addition, delayed
type hypersensitivity response to neuraminidase treated myeloblasts in designated
AML patients in complete remission was measured.

Modification of Allogeneic Myeloblasts with Neuraminidase

Myeloblasts retrieved from liquid nitrogen storage prior to immunization were
layered over a 22 per cent human albumin gradient supported by 45 per cent
sucrose (1:3) to separate the viable from nonviable blast cells. After purifica-
tion, myeloblasts were incubated with Vibrio Cholerae neuraminidase. The neuraminidase for this study has been purified 2500 to 3000-fold and was free of
other enzymes and bacterial endotoxins. The incubation mixture contained 50 units
of enzyme per 5 x 10^7 cells per ml in sodium acetate buffer at pH 5.6 for 60
minutes at 37°C. The cells were washed and a total of 10^{10} modified myeloblasts
were used for immunotherapy.

Immunotherapy

Immunization with neuraminidase treated allogeneic myeloblasts was given in 48
intradermal sites. In order to get maximum exposure to the immunogen, sites were
widely spread in the supraclavicular, infraclavicular, arm, forearm, parasternal,
thoracic, suprainguinal and femoral regions draining into several node bearing
areas. Reaction to neuraminidase-treated cells at 48 hours as measured by the
induration at the injection sites was proportional to the number of cells injected per site and increased with the frequency of administration. (Table 1) The
injections of neuraminidase treated myeloblasts produced no local lesions other
than the delayed type hypersensitivity reaction and none of the patients developed

chill, fever, or adenopathy. The biopsies of the cutaneous reactions induced
by neuraminidase treated myeloblasts showed immunoblastic infiltration. For
patients randomized to receive MER too, ten intradermal sites of 100 µg/.1 ml
each totaling 1.0 mg of MER were used. The DCH reaction to cells was not altered
by intradermal injection of the nonspecific immunoadjuvant MER when compared to
the induration in patients immunized with neuraminidase-treated cells from the
same donor.

Immunotherapy with Neuraminidase-Treated Myeloblasts in Patients with Acute Mye-locytic Leukemia

Sixty-eight previously untreated patients with AML were induced into complete
remission by cytosine arabinoside and daunorubicin. The three way randomization
was accomplished on condition of the patient being in complete remission and
having received the first course of cytosine arabinoside and thioguanine. Figure
2 shows the remission duration of AML patients who were given chemotherapy alone,
versus those who received neuraminidase treated allogeneic myeloblasts with or
without MER. The median remission of the chemotherapy group is about 6 months
while that of patients immunized with neuraminidase modified myeloblasts is 22
months. The difference between the two groups is statistically significant.
While in laboratory studies the combination of specific and non-specific immunotherapy appeared to be more effective than either therapy alone, in this clinical
study MER impaired the immunotherapeutic value of neuraminidase modified myeloblasts.

Immunological Status of AML Patients in the Chemoimmunotherapy Study

The in vivo immunocompetence of AML patients in this study was measured by the
delayed cutaneous hypersensitivity (DCH) response to: PPD, mumps, candida, vari-
dase and dermatophytin. Interpretation of the skin tests was based on the indu-
rations as measured in diameter at 48 hours and were considered positive if the
diameter of induration exceeded 5 mm. Initially, there was considerable improvement in the DCH response in patients in both immunotherapy regimens (Figure 3).
While this improvement continued for patients who received neuraminidase modified
myeloblasts, the group of patients immunized with modified myeloblasts plus MER
showed a gradual decline and subsequent loss of DCH after 6 months. The decline
or loss in response to recall antigens often preceeded subsequent relapse of
those patients who have been receiving MER in addition to neuraminidase treated
myeloblasts.

Quantification of the E-rosette forming peripheral blood lymphocytes from patients
in the chemoimmunotherapy protocol was performed at 4°C. The median value for
normal donors of E-rosetting lymphocytes is 74.4%, with 1986 as the number of
absolute T-lymphocytes (Table 2). Patients at the time of randomization, still
in recovery from induction and consolidating chemotherapy, have shown significantly lower percentage (49.2 and 51.7) and absolute number (412 and 487) of
T-cells in both immunotherapy groups. Patients in both chemoimmunotherapy groups
showed a significant increase of T-lymphocytes as compared to values at the time
of randomization (Table 2).

Lymphocyte blastogenesis for the peripheral blood lymphocytes was determined by
selected mitogens: phytohemagglutinin (PHA) and pokeweed mitogen (PWM). Remission lymphocytes obtained from patients receiving chemotherapy alone showed considerably lower degree of stimulation to both mitogens all through the observation period (Figure 4). On the other hand patients treated with chemotherapy
plus modified myeloblasts showed progressively higher response to PHA and PWM,
and by the 12th cycle of immunotherapy the stimulation values were similar to

that of healthy donors. Of those patients who received modified myeloblasts plus MER there was a steady increase of lymphocyte function during the first six months. This was followed by a gradual decline (Figure 4).

This study clearly demonstrates the therapeutic advantage of combining neuraminidase modified allogeneic myeloblasts with a highly effective remission inducing and sustaining chemotherapeutic protocol in the treatment of acute myelocytic leukemia as compared to the use of neuraminidase-treated myeloblasts plus MER or chemotherapy alone.

REFERENCES

1. Revesz, L., (1960). Cancer Res., 20, 443.

2. Mathe, G., Pouillart, P., and Lapeyrague, F., (1969).Br. J. Cancer, 23, 814-824.

3. Mathe, G., Amiel, J. L., Schwarzenberg, L., Schneider, M., Schlumberger, J. R., Hayat, M., and DeVassal, F., (1969). Lancet, 1, 697-699.

4. Sokol, J.F., Aungst, C.W., and Grace, J.T., Jr., (1973). Natl. Cancer Inst. Monogr., 39, 195-198.

5. Powles, R. L., Growther, D., Bateman, C. J. T., Beard, M. E. J., McElwain, T. J., Russell, J., Lister, T. A., Whitehouse, J. M. A., Wrigley, P. F. M., Pike, M., Alexander, P., and Hamilton-Fairley, G., (1973). Cancer, 28, 365-376.

6. Gutterman, J. U., Hersh, E. M., Rodriguez, V., McCredie, K. G., Mavligit, G., Reed, R., Burgess, M. A., Smith, T., Gehan, E., and Bodey, G. P., Sr., (1974). Lancet, 2, 1405-1409.

7. Sanford, B. H., (1967). Transplantation, 5, 1273-1279.

8. Bekesi, J. G., St-Arneault, G., and Holland, J. F., (1971). Cancer Res., 31, 2130-2132.

9. Bekesi, J. G., St-Areault, G., Walter, L., and Holland, J. F., (1972). J. Natl. Cancer Inst., 49, 107-118.

10. Sethi, K, K., and Brandis, H., (1973). Br. J. Cancer, 27, 106-113.

11. Rios, A., Simmons, R. L., (1974). Intern J. Cancer, 13, 71-81.

12. Sedlacek, H. H., Meesmann, H., Seiler, F. R., (1975). Int. J. Cancer, 15, 409.

13. Bekesi, J. G., Roboz, J. P., Holland, J. F., (1976). N. Y. Acad. Sci., 277, 313-331.

ACKNOWLEDGEMENTS

This work was supported in part by grant and contracts CA-1-5936-02, CA-5834, NCI Cancer Virus Program No. 1-CB-43879, and NCI Immunotherapy Program No. 1-CP-43225.

We express our appreciation to the Behring Institute Behringwerke Ag. Marburg,

West Germany, for supplying the highly purified neuraminidase for this study.

We also thank Suzan Sattler-Gillman, RN, for the excellent assistance in performing the immunotherapeutic maniuplations, Robert Schechter for excellent
technical assistance and Rogena Brown for secretarial assistance.

TABLE 1

DELAYED HYPERSENSITIVITY RESPONSE TO X-IRRADIATED OR NEURAMINIDASE TREATED MYELOBLASTS

IMMUNIZATION CYCLES	INDURATION[1]						
	NUMBER OF N'ASE TREATED MYELOBLASTS INJECTED PER SITE x 10^8				NUMBER OF X-IRRADIATED MYELOBLASTS INJECTED PER SITE x 10^8		
	0.5	1.0	2.0	3.0	1	2	3
1	3.5±1.5	6.2±2	14±4	18±3	3.0±1	5.4±1.5	7.8±2
6	7.1±2	12.9±3	19.8±6.1	24±6	4.2±2.1	7.5±3	8.4±3.2
12	8.3±2.4	14.1±2.9	20.3±5	25.1±7	4.6±1.6	7.2±2.4	8.1±2.5

(1) MEAN INDURATION IN MM OBTAINED FROM AT LEAST 40 INJECTED SITES, MEASURED 48 HOURS
     AFTER THE INTRADERMAL INJECTION OF MYELOBLASTS.

*   STANDARD ERROR OF MEAN

TABLE 2   E-ROSETTING LYMPHOCYTE SUBPOPULATION IN AML PATIENTS IN THE IMMUNOTHERAPY STUDY

	At Randomization		After 12 Cycles		After 24 Cycles	
	% T-Cells	T-Lymphocytes*	% T-Cells	T-Lymphocytes	% T-Cells	T-Lymphocytes
Normal Subjects N=117	74.4	1,986 ± 251				
Immunotherapy with Neuraminidase Myeloblasts N=31	49.2	412 ± 35	69.3	889 ± 95 $p = .004$	70.1	1,122 ± 129 $p = .0001$
Immunotherapy with Neuraminidase Myeloblasts + MER N=21	51.7	487 ± 45	70.1	909 ± 101 $p = .009$		

+– Determined by the E-binding rosette technique at 4°C with SRBC.

* ± Standard error of mean

** Statistical significance between absolute E-rosetting lymphocytes at the time of randomization versus during therapy of AML patients.

CHEMOIMMUNOTHERAPY PROTOCOL IN AML

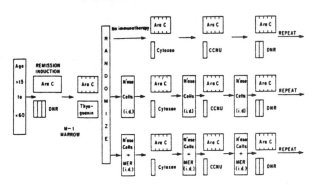

FIGURE 1 - CHEMOIMMUNOTHERAPY PROTOCOL FOR PATIENTS WITH ACUTE
MYELOCYTIC LEUKEMIA.

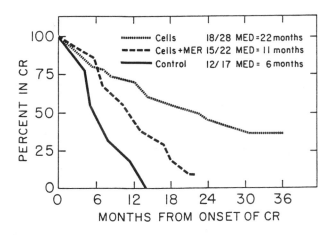

FIGURE 2 - REMISSION DURATION OF PATIENTS WITH ACUTE MYELOCYTIC
LEUKEMIA IMMUNIZED WITH NEURAMINIDASE MODIFIED ALLOGENEIC
MYELOBLASTS.

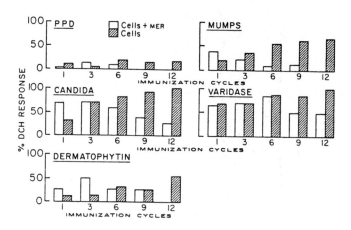

FIGURE 3 - CHANGE OF DELAYED HYPERSENSITIVITY RESPONSE TO RECALL
ANTIGENS DURING THE COURSE OF CHEMOIMMUNOTHERAPY.
SKIN TEST DIAMETER AT 48 HOURS >5MM.

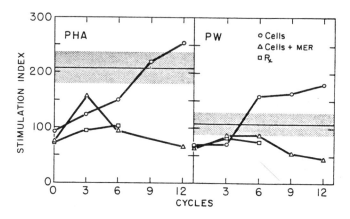

FIGURE 4 - KINETICS OF PHA AND PWM INDUCED BLASTOGENESIS OF PERIPHERIAL
LYMPHOCYTES FROM AML PATIENTS IMMUNIZED WITH NEURAMINIDASE
TREATED MYELOBLASTS.

The Use of Bone Marrow Grafting in the Treatment of Acute Leukemia

M. Territo, R. Gale, M. Cline, S. Feig, T. Gossett, P. Graze,
G. Sarna, R. Sparkes, A. Tesler, D. Winston and L. Young

Department of Medicine and Pediatrics, Center for Health Sciences,
University of California at Los Angeles, Los Angeles, California 90024, U.S.A.

With intensive combination chemotherapy and radiation programs definite progress
has been made in therapy of acute leukemia. Despite this progress, about half of
the patients with Acute Lymphoblastic Leukemia (ALL), and over 95% of those with
Acute Myelogenous Leukemia (AML) will eventually die of resistant leukemia. Studies at our institution and others have clearly demonstrated the feasibility of
transplantation of normal hematopoietic stem cells in man. In view of this and because of the disappointing results of conventional therapy in patients with acute
leukemia who relapse, the potential role of bone marrow transplantation in the therapy of resistant leukemia has gained increasing interest (Thomas, and Co-workers,
1977).

It is clearly possible to transplant hematopoietic stem cells in man. Requirements
for engraftment include histocompatibility matching between donor and recipient,
immunosuppression to prevent graft rejection and a minimal dose of marrow cells.
In the leukemic patient an additional problem is the permanent eradication of the
leukemic clone(s).

The human major histocompatibility complex, referred to as HLA, has been assigned
to chromosome 6 (Bach and Van Rood, 1976). The HLA locus has been further subdivided into the HLA - A,B,C, and D subloci. The first three are commonly defined by
serologic techniques, while the HLA-D region is conventionally studied in the mixed lymphocyte culture (MLC) test. While HLA is of prime importance in determining
graft outcome, other histocompatibility systems are undoubtedly involved. Little
is known regarding these non-HLA systems and no attempt has been made to match for
non-HLA antigens in clinical transplantation. This factor probably accounts for
the high incidence of graft rejection and graft versus host disease (GVHD). There
is a high degree of polymorphism in the HLA system. Since these antigens are inherited in a Mendelian fashion as co-alleles, there is a reasonable possibility
(25%) of finding an HLA-identical donor within a family. In the general population
the probability is in the range of one in 10,000. Because of this, most transplants
have been performed between the HLA-identical siblings.

The transplant procedure itself is relatively simple (Thomas et al, 1975). Approximately one liter of bone marrow is removed from the donor by multiple aspirations
from the posterior-iliac crest. A single cell suspension is prepared and infused
intravenously into the recipient. The infused cells home to the marrow after a
brief delay in the lungs and spleen. The usual dose is $1-15 \times 10^8$ nucleated marrow
cells per kg. In most instances discrete clusters of hematopoises are observed in

the marrow within the first 2 weeks following transplantation. Peripheral white
blood cells and platelets begin to rise within 2-3 weeks following transplantation
and may return to normal levels by 1-2 months. Cytogenetic marker studies clearly
indicate that red cells, granulocytes, lymphocytes, platelets, monocytes, and hepatic and alveolar macrophages are of donor origin (Gale, Sparkes, and Golde, 1977;
Thomas, and Co-workers, 1976; Sparkes, and Co-workers, 1977).

Following successful engraftment, the recipient is at risk to develop several immune-
related problems including graft-versus-host disease, post transplant immunodeficiency, interstitial pneumonitis and infectious complications. Graft rejection which
is a significant problem in transplantation for aplastic anemia, is rare in acute
leukemia, however, leukemic recurrence is an additional potential complication in
leukemic recipients.

Graft-versus-host disease results from the introduction of immunocompetent donor
cells into the immunosuppressed recipient. Principle target organs of GVHD include
the lymphoid system, skin, liver, and gastrointestinal tract (Thomas, and Co-workers,
1975). While GVHD initially results from immune stimulation, the end result is
immunodeficiency. The incidence of GVHD following HLA-identical marrow transplantation is 70%, and over one-half of these cases are fatal. The prevention and
treatment of GVHD are problematic. Methotrexate is routinely given prophylactically
to modify GVHD but this is not completely effective. Attempts to prevent GVHD with
antithymocyte globulin (ATG) or to treat active GVHD with ATG, corticosteroids, and
other immunosuppressive drugs have been largely unsuccessful. The complete prevention of GVHD is not necessarily desirable since GVHD may have antileukemic effects.

Approximately 60-70% of marrow graft recipients develop interstitial pneumonitis
(Neiman, and Colleagues, 1977). One-half of the cases are related to cytomegalovirus (CMV), 10% to pneumocystis, and 10% to other viruses or fungi. No etiology
is identified in the remaining cases. It is likely that immunologic factors including immunodeficiency and GVHD play a critical role in the development of interstitial pneumonia.

Bacterial and fungal infections are an important complication of bone marrow transplantation. These usually occur during the period of granulocytopenia immediately
following the transplant and their magnitude is related to the intensity of the
pre-transplant conditioning regimen. Most patients receive oral non-absorbable
antibiotics and granulocyte transfusions. The value of prophylactic granulocyte
transfusions and laminar air flow environments is controversial but recent data
suggest they may decrease the incidence of infection without a substantial effect
on survival.

Using conventional therapy programs, the survival of patients with resistant acute
leukemia is poor, with a median survival of less than 6 months in several large
series. Because of this, we and others have studied the potential role of allogeneic bone marrow transplantation in patients with resistant disease (Gale, 1977;
Santos, and Colleagues, 1976; Sarna, and Colleagues, 1977; and Thomas, and Colleagues, 1977).

Transplantation in acute leukemia is difficult. In addition the the previously described immunologic problems, it is necessary to permanently eradicate the leukemic
clone(s). A variety of chemotherapy-radiation therapy regimens have been developed
to achieve this goal. These regimens serve as pre-transplantation conditioning
programs both for immunologic suppression of the host to prevent graft rejection
and for the eradication of the leukemia. Three representative regimens are indicated in Figure 1 and remission and survival data in Figures 2 & 3.

Fig. 1   The treatment sche-
         dule in days pre-
         transplantation for
         three chemoradio-
         therapy condition-
         ing regimens CY =
         cytoxan, TBI = total
         body irradiation,
         BM = Donor marrow
         infusion, Ara-C =
         cytosine arabinoside,
         TG = 6-thioguanine,
         DNR = Daunorubicin,
         FTBI = fractionated
         total body irradia-
         tion.

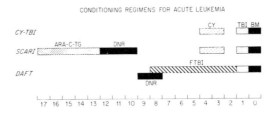

Fig. 2   Actuarial remission
         following bone mar-
         row transplantation.
         CY = cytoxan (Santos
         197**6**), TBI = Total
         body irradiation
         (Thomas et al 1975),
         CY-TBI (Thomas et al
         1977), SCARI (Sarna
         et al 1977), DAFT
         (see text). Number
         in parenthesis re-
         fers to number of
         patients initially
         in each study.

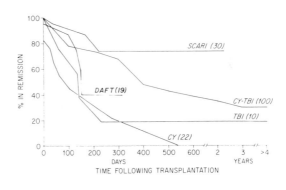

Fig. 3   Cumulative survival
         of leukemic patients
         treated with three
         different condition-
         ing regimens.

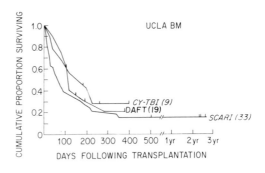

Several important points emerge from these studies: 1) leukemic relapse is common despite the use of supralethal levels of drug and radiation; 2) the risk of relapse is high during the first 2 years, but lower thereafter; 3) that with the possible exception of SCARI (Fig. 1), more intensive conditioning has not been associated with a lower relapse rate; and 4) 15-20% of patients with resistant leukemia may become long-term disease-free survivors. While this survival rate is not a satisfactory end result, it is probably superior to chemotherapy alone. It is noteworthy that immunologic problems rather than resistant leukemia are the major cause of death in some series. These problems may ultimately prove more soluable than resistant leukemia.

TABLE 1   Leukemic Recurrence Following Bone Marrow Transplantation

Indefinite time at risk
Predominantly in recipient cells
Maintains genetic markers of original disease
Residual normal hematopoiesis of donor origin

TABLE 2   Approaches to Decreasing Leukemic Relapse
Following Bone Marrow Transplantation

More effective Radiotherapy
Intensive chemoradiotherapy with optimal support facilities
Treat leukemic "Sanctuaries"
Transplant before "Resistance" develops
Combination of approaches

Major features of leukemic relapse in bone marrow transplantation are reviewed in Table 1. It should be emphasized that 98% of relapses occur in recipient cells so that progress is dependent upon development of more effective conditioning regimens. Potential approaches to this problem are indicated in Table 2. Perhaps the most promising are the development of more effective regimens, and transplantation in remission. Preliminary data from Thomas and Co-workers has indicated a low relapse rate in AML patients transplanted in remission. Unfortunately, ALL patients have not fared as well, probably because most are in second or later remission. Finally, the introduction of new myelosuppressive drugs or innovative uses of radiation may improve the results of transplantation in acute leukemia.

Our institution has recently been investigating a new conditioning regimen utilizing fractionated total body irradiation (TBI). This approach was considered because of the known anti-leukemia effect of radiotherapy. Single dose escalation beyond 1000 rads in man is thought to be limited by irreversible gastrointestinal toxicity. When X-irradiation is fractionated at lower doses, however, tissue tolerance can be considerably increased. The DAFT regimen consisted of fractionated TBI 20 rads/day given for 7 consecutive days (day -8 to -2) and followed by a single high dose TBI (1000 rads, 5-7 rads/min) on day -1 (Fig. 1). Daunorubicin, a potent antileukemic and radiosensitizing drug, was given at a dose of 60 mg/m^2 on day -9 and -8. Patients who had received high doses of anthracyclines ($\geq$ 550 mg/m^2) received reduced doses of daunorubicin (30-45 mg/m^2/day). Donor bone marrow was infused intravenously on day 0. Nineteen patients with resistant acute leukemia (14 with AML, 5 with ALL) ranging in age from 6 to 44 years, were transplanted. The conditioning regimen was well tolerated by all patients. There was no evidence of cardiotoxicity, hepatotoxicity or nephrotoxicity. Actuarial remission data are indicated in Figure 2. One patient never achieved a remission. The remaining 18 patients showed prompt evidence of hematologic engraftment within 7-14 days. Six patients relapsed. Median remission duration was 361 days (range 0-405+days). In all instances the relapse occurred in the recipient cells. There was no evidence of graft rejection. GVHD occurred in 12 of 17 (70%) patients at risk. Nine of 12 died of GVHD and its related infectious complications. One additional patient developed chronic cutaneous GVHD. Interstitial pneumonia occurred in 6 of 18 (33%) patients at risk. Four cases occurred in association with GVHD. All six patients died. Cytomegalovirus was documented in 2 cases. In 4 cases the etiology was not defined. Three patients are currently alive 180-440 days following transplantation, including 1 identical twin. Median survival was 104 days (range 40-440^{+} days) Fig. 3. Reasons for failure include: recurrent or resistant leukemia in 6, GVHD in 6, interstitial pneumonia in 1, and GVHD with interstitial pneumonia in 3.

Overall, these results were disappointing, clearly the anti-leukemic effect was inadequate with an actuarial relapse rate exceeding 50% at one year. Relapses occurred in recipient cells indicating that the addition of fractionated TBI and daunorubicin in these doses was insufficient to eradicate resistant disease. Several points, are however, of interest. This regimen was extremely well tolerated and there were no early deaths due to toxicity or infection. A substantial reduction in the resistant leukemia cell burden was observed with these relatively low doses of fractionated TBI such that some patients had hypocellular bone marrow biopsies before they received the high single dose TBI. The incidence of interstitial pneumonitis and GVHD was comparable to other trials using lower doses of radiation. These observations have led us to consider escalation of the dose of fractionated TBI and additional chemotherapeutic agents in our future trials.

Future research in the field of marrow grafting in the treatment of acute leukemia must concentrate on two critical problems: 1) more effective leukemia eradication, and 2) solutions to immunologic problems including GVHD, infection, immunodeficiency, and interstitial pneumonitis.

A recent area of considerable interest is autotransplantation using cryopreserved remission bone marrow. Preliminary studies have clearly indicated that cryopreserved autologous marrow can reconstitute a lethally irradiated recipient but leukemic relapse has been a major obstacle (Graze, and Gale, 1978). Whether this relates to residual leukemia in the patient, or in the cryopreserved marrow is as yet uncertain. The concept of autotransplantation is of considerable theoretical interest since these patients would not be at risk to develop many of the immunologic problems associated with allogeneic transplantation such as GVHD. Autotransplantation could expand the applicability of marrow transplantation since most patients with leukemia lack an HLA identical sibling donor. Leukemic relapse remains the major problem in autotransplantation and attempts to deplete clinically undetectable leukemic cells from remission marrow using either physical or immunologic techniques needs to be critically evaluated.

IN SUMMARY: Bone marrow transplantation is an experimental approach to the treatment of patients with acute leukemia. To date, long-term disease-free survival has been achieved in a small proportion of carefully selected patients with resistant acute leukemia. While results are far from optimal, they are at least encouraging in late stage patients where there are no effective alternatives. Major problems in marrow transplantation for leukemia include resistant tumor and spectrum of immunologic complications including GVHD, immunodeficiency, and interstitial pneumonia. Progress in any one area would have a substantial impact on improving survival and extended the applicability of marrow transplantation to patients at an earlier stage of their disease.

REFERENCES

1. Bach, F.H., and Van Rood, J.J. (1976). The Major Histocompatibility Complex. New Engl. J. Med., 295, 806-812; 872-878; 927-935.

2. Gale, R.P. (for the UCLA Bone Marrow Transplant Team), (1977). Bone Marrow Transplantation in Acute Leukemia. Lancet, 2:1197-1200.

3. Gale, R.P., Sparkes, R.S., and Golde, D.W. (1978). Bone Marrow Origin of Hepatic Macrophages (Kupffer Cells) in Man. Science 201:937-938.

4. Graze, P.R., and Gale, R.P. (1978). Autotransplantation for Leukemia and Solid Tumors. Transplant. Proc. 10:177-186.

5. Sarna, G., Feig, S., Opelz, G., Young, L., Langdon, E., Julliard, G., Farawarz, N., Sparkes, R., Golde, D., Territo, M., Haskell, C., Smith, G., Fawzi, F., Falk, P., Fahey, J., Cline, M., and Gale, R. (1977). Bone Marrow Transplantation with Intensive Combination Chemotherapy/Radiation Therapy (SCARI) in Acute Leukemia. Ann. Int. Med. 86:155-161.

6. Santos, G.W., Sensenbrenner, L.K., Anderson, P.M., Burke, P.J., Klein, D.L, Slavin, R.E., Schauer, B., Borganhan, D.S. (1976). HLA-Identical Marrow Transplants in Aplastic Anemia, Acute Leukemia, and Lymphosarcoma Employing Cyclophosphamide. Transplant. Proc. 8:607-612.

7. Thomas, E.D., Buchner, C.D., Banaji, M., Clift, R.A., Fefer, A., Flournoy, N., Goodell, B.W., Hickman, R.O., Lerner, K.G., Neiman, P.E., Sale, G.E., Sanders, J.E., Singer, J., Stevens, M., Storb, R., and Weiden, P.L. (1977). One-hundred Patients with Acute Leukemia Treated by Chemotherapy, Total Body Irradiation, and Allogeneic Bone Marrow Transplantation. Blood 49:511-533.

8. Thomas, E.D., Ramberg, R.E., Sale, G.E., Sparkes, R.S., and Golde, D.W. (1976). Direct Evidence for Bone Marrow Origin of the Alveolar Macrophage in Man. Science 2:1016-1018.

9. Thomas, E.D., Storb, R., Clift, R.A., Fefer, A., Johnson, F.L., Neiman, P.E., Lerner, K.G., Glucksberg, H., and Buchner, C.D. (1975). Bone Marrow Transplantation. New Engl. J. Med. 292, 832-843; 895-902.

Non-Hodgkin's Lymphomas

Non-Hodgkin Lymphoma: Etiology and Epidemiology

F. P. Li and C. D. Atkins

Clinical Studies Section, Clinical Epidemiology Branch,
National Cancer Institute, Boston, Massachusetts, 02115, U.S.A.

ABSTRACT

Epidemiologic studies have implicated diverse factors in the etiology of non-Hodgkin lymphomas (NHL) in man. Host susceptibility is indicated by predisposing constitutional immunodeficiency diseases, and by family aggregates of NHL. Environmental agents associated with the development of NHL include ionizing radiation, industrial chemicals, and immunosupressive drugs administered to organ transplant recipients. In addition, Epstein-Barr virus may be a causal agent in African Burkitt's lymphoma, as suggested by epidemiologic and laboratory studies. Reported variations in NHL rates with nationality, race, age, and sex cannot be fully explained by these factors, and may result from other host and environmental influences. Further classification of NHL through immunological, chromosomal and other markers may help to identify more homogeneous groups of patients with etiologic factors in common.

Keywords: non-Hodgkin lymphoma/Burkitt's lymphoma/epidemiology/immunodeficiency/viral oncogenesis

INTRODUCTION

Studies of the epidemiologic characteristics of non-Hodgkin lymphoma (NHL) in man have been hindered by difficulties in diagnosis and disease classification. NHL must be differentiated from benign diseases and from other cancers, e.g., Hodgkin's disease, lymphocytic leukemia, malignant reticulosis, and anaplastic carcinoma. Furthermore, the clinical and histological diversity of NHL has prompted proposals for multiple classification schemes based on morphology, anatomic site, and immunologic markers (Dorfman, 1977), and for new diagnostic categories, such as immunoblastic sarcoma (Lukes and Tindle, 1975) and Lennert lymphoma (Burke and Butler, 1976).

RATES AND PATTERNS OF DISEASE

The validity of international comparisons of NHL incidence is limited by potential inaccuracies in the data, but some observations can be made. Reported figures show that most countries have annual NHL incidence rates that range from 1 to 8

per 100,000 persons (Waterhouse and others, 1976). NHL incidence generally increases logarithmically with age (Basa, Hirayama and Cruz-Basa, 1977; Besuschio
and Ghinelli, 1973; Edington and Hendrickse, 1973; Misad, Brandon and Albujar,
1973; Nasr, Tawfik and El-Einen, 1973; Waterhouse and others, 1976); data from the
Third National Cancer Survey of the U.S. are typical (Fig. 1) (Cutler and Young,
1975). Rates are usually about 50% higher among men than among women (Waterhouse

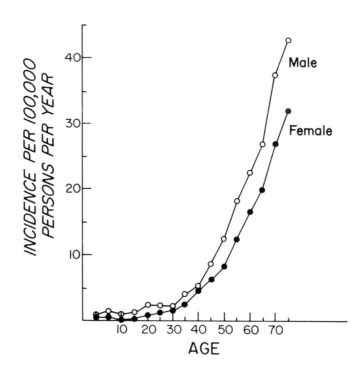

Fig. 1. Annual age-specific incidence of non-Hodgkin
         lymphoma, U. S. white males and females. Data
         from the Third National Cancer Survey, 1969-1971.

and others, 1976). Racial and ethnic groups within one geographic area can show
different rates: the incidence of NHL is higher in whites than in blacks in the
U. S. (Fig. 2), and higher in Jews than in non-Jews in Israel (Waterhouse and
others, 1976). The relative frequencies of histologic subtypes vary among different countries (Correa and O'Conor, 1973), but data using modern classification
schemes are lacking.

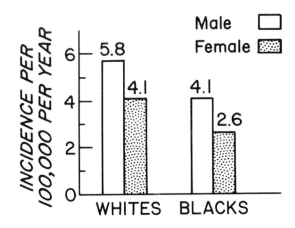

Fig. 2.   Age-standardized U. S. incidence of non-Hodgkin
          lymphoma, by race and sex. Data from the Third
          National Cancer Survey, 1969-1971.

Burkitt's lymphoma (BL) rates show striking international variations. The
incidence is many-fold higher in tropical Africa (Burkitt, 1964) and Papua,
New Guinea (Booth and others, 1967) than in other parts of the world where BL
is extremely rare. African BL predominates in males and develops infrequently
after 15 years of age (Booth and others, 1967). The mean age at diagnosis of BL
is reported to be 9.1 years in Africa and 12.2 years in the U. S., where a higher
proportion of affected are adults (Levine and others, 1975). Immigrants to high-
rate areas in Africa have also been reported to develop BL at older ages than
the indigenous population (Burkitt and Wright, 1966). However, differences in
age structure of these disparate populations can, in part, explain the findings,
and appropriate age adjustment of the data is needed.

Primary intestinal lymphoma also shows considerable geographic variation in
incidence. This lymphoma typically affects the small intestine of adolescents
and young adults and, in some cases, is associated with abnormal IgA heavy chains
in the serum (Tabbane and others, 1976). The disease is common in Mediterranean
populations, particularly in Israel, North Africa, Spain, and Italy (Ramot and
Many, 1972). In Israel, rates are lower among Jews of European origin than among
Arabs and other Jews (Abramson, Avitzour and Peritz, 1975). This pattern may be
due to differences in inherited susceptibilities, or to culturally determined
environmental influences (Modan and others, 1969; Royston and Modan, 1968).

An association between social class and mortality from NHL has been reported in
Great Britain. Persons in the highest social class have a 50% greater NHL mortality than those in the lowest stratum (MacMahon, 1966). This may reflect differences in disease incidence or in diagnostic practices.

CONSTITUTIONAL STATES OF IMMUNODEFICIENCY

The incidence of NHL is increased in patients with diverse constitutional immunologic deficiency diseases. The excess risk is well demonstrated for several autosomal recessive diseases (ataxia-telangiectasia and severe combined-system immuno-

deficiency) and X-linked diseases (Wiskott-Aldrich syndrome, congenital X-linked agammaglobulinemia, and X-linked recessive lymphoproliferative syndrome) (Kersey, Spector and Good, 1973; Purtilo and others, 1975). Patients with severe immuno-deficiency usually die of infection in childhood, but during the markedly shor-tened lifespan of these children the overall risk of fatal malignancy is 7%, more than 100 times the risk for children in the general population (Kersey and Spector, 1975). Nearly one-third of these cancers are NHL (i.e., lymphomas ex-cluding Hodgkin's disease and malignant reticuloses) (Gatti and Good, 1971), which normally represent less than 10% of childhood malignancies. NHL has also been reported in patients with common variable immunodeficiency and selective immunoglobulin deficiencies. However, the risk of NHL is more difficult to estimate for these heterogeneous disorders.

NHL may aggregate in families. Some of the family pedigrees suggest autosomal dominant or recessive inheritance, but a genetic basis for these aggregates is not proven. Clinically healthy relatives in some of these families have subtle immunologic abnormalities (Buehler and others, 1975; Fraumeni and others, 1975; Freeman, Sinks and Cohen, 1970; Potolsky and others, 1971). Further study of affected families may help identify immunological and other factors that induce NHL.

An associated finding in ataxia-telangiectasia, one of the predisposing immuno-deficiency states, is the monoclonal proliferation of peripheral lympho-cytes which have rearrangements of the long arm of chromosome 14. Some fibroblast lines of ataxia-telangiectasia patients show a similar change (McCaw and others, 1975; Oxford and others, 1975). The development of CLL from the aberrant clone has been observed in one ataxia-telangiectasia patient (McCaw and others, 1975). Translocations involving chromosome 14 have also been found in tumor cells from a high proportion of Burkitt's lymphomas (8q-; 14q+) (Manolov and Manolova, 1975; McCaw and others, 1977; Zech and others, 1976), and in malignant cell lines of other lymphomas (Fleischman and Prigogina,1977; Fukuhara, Shirakawa and Uschino, 1976). These findings suggest that abnormalities of chromosome 14 may have an etiologic role in diverse types of NHL.

ACQUIRED STATES OF ALTERED IMMUNITY

Renal transplant recipients have an approximately 50-fold increase in the risk of NHL (Hoover and Fraumeni, 1973; Penn and Starzl, 1972). The immunologic status of these patients is complex and the relative importance of the foreign antigens of the renal allografts and the drug-induced immunosuppression in the development of NHL is not known. Histiocytic lymphomas account for most of the excess NHL in this group and over 50% are localized to the brain, normally a rare site for this tumor (Hoover and Fraumeni, 1973). In one large study, the risk of NHL reached a maximum within a few months after transplantation, and 40% of the lymphomas developed within the first year (Hoover and Fraumeni, 1973). This interval is a very short latency period for cancer induction in humans. Preliminary data on cardiac transplant recipients suggest a similar trend. Three of 124 patients developed NHL within 2 years of cardiac transplantation (4.5, 7.6 and 20.8 months). There were 2 histiocytic lymphomas, and one of these was localized to the brain (Krikorian and others, 1978).

Isolated studies have suggested a small excess of NHL in patients with auto-immune diseases and other acquired states of altered immunity (Table 1). An excess risk of NHL in Sjogren's syndrome (Kassan and Gardy, 1978), and excess gastrointestinal NHL in longstanding celiac sprue (Harris and others, 1967) have been reported. Follow-up series on patients with sarcoidosis (Brincker and Wilbek, 1974) or leprosy (Purtilo and Pangi, 1975) have found NHL in a few

TABLE 1   Estimates of Risk of Non-Hodgkin Lymphoma in States of Altered Immunity

Disease	No. with NHL	Estimated No. with the Immune Disorder	Relative Risk*	Reference
Inborn Immunodeficiency	98	1800	100	Kersey, Spector & Good, 1973
Renal Transplant Recipients	25	6297	50	Fraumeni & Hoover, 1973
Celiac Sprue	10	202	10	Harris & others, 1967
Sjogren's Syndrome	7	136	7	Kassan & Gardy, 1978
Cardiac Transplant Recipients	3	124	–	Krikorian & others, 1978
Leprosy	3	185	–	Purtilo & Pangi, 1975
Sarcoidosis	2	2544	–	Brincker & Wilbeck, 1974

*Risk of NHL in study group as compared with normal population.

individuals. In addition, case reports have noted an association of NHL with systemic lupus erythematosis, rheumatoid arthritis, and inflammatory bowel diseases
(Lee, Smith and Seal, 1977; Oleinick, 1967; Vieta and Delgado, 1976), but the
risk of the neoplasm was not determined.

The immunostimulatory effects of Bacillus Calmett-Guerin (BCG) have prompted
several studies of the incidence of cancer in BCG vaccinees. Both increased and
decreased risks for some lymphoreticular malignancies have been reported, but the
overall evidence shows no substantial effect of BCG on the risk of cancer in
general, or NHL in particular (Hoover, 1976; Skegg, 1978; Snider and others, 1978).

The pathogenesis of NHL in these states of altered immunity is unclear. Proposed
mechanisms include reduced host immunosurveillance, stimulation of clonal proliferation of abnormal lymphocytes, and activation of oncogenic viruses (Stutman,
1977).

ENVIRONMENTAL FACTORS

Exposures to radiation and certain chemicals have been implicated in some cases
of NHL. An increased mortality from NHL has been reported for several groups of
chemical workers or handlers, namely, professional chemists, anesthesiologists,
electrical workers, and rubber workers (Table 2). However, the findings of excess
risk of NHL should be viewed as preliminary because of such methodological considerations as small sample size and potential ascertainment bias. Specific
chemical carcinogens involved were not identified, since these workers are usually
exposed to multiple toxic agents.

The anticonvulsant, phenytoin (Dilantin), can induce a pseudolymphoma which
resolves upon discontinuation of the drug. In addition, cases of NHL after
chronic ingestion of phenytoin have been reported (Editorial, 1971). However,
the excess risk for NHL after long-term therapy with this drug is small (Li and
others, 1975).

TABLE 2 Occupational Groups Found at Excess Risk of Mortality from Lympho-
         reticular Malignancies

	Deaths from Lymphoreticular Malignancies		
	No. Observed	No. Expected	Reference
Chemists[1]	78	42	Li & others, 1969
Anesthesiologists[1]	17	9	Bruce & others, 1968
Electrical Workers[2]	28	18	Goldsmith & Guidotti, 1977
Rubber Workers[2]	9	6	McMichael & others, 1975

[1]Non-Hodgkin lymphoma, Hodgkin's disease, multiple myeloma, and malignant
reticuloses.

[2]Non-Hodgkin lymphoma only.

A two-fold increase in the incidence of lymphoreticular neoplasms (NHL was not
evaluated separately) has been noted in patients irradiated for ankylosing spondylitis (Court-Brown and Doll, 1965) and in atomic-bomb survivors in Hiroshima
(Nishayama and others, 1973). The data from Hiroshima reveal an average latency
period of at least 12 years from the time of exposure to development of lymphoma
(Nishayama and others, 1973). No increase has been seen in other radiation-
exposed populations, e.g., radiologists (Matanoski and others, 1975; Lewis, 1963)
and survivors of the Nagasaki atomic bomb (Nishayama and others, 1973). The
discordant findings may be due to differences in radiation dose received by these
groups (Anderson and others, 1972).

VIRUSES

The incidence of BL in Uganda is increased in the hot lowlands with high rainfall.
This geographic distribution has suggested the hypothesis that BL is caused by an
oncogenic virus transmitted by an endemic arthropod vector (Burkitt and Wright,
1966). Time-space clustering of an BL, which might further support an infectious
origin of the disease, has been observed in some parts of Uganda (Baikie, Kinlen
and Pike, 1972), but not in others (Morrow, Pike and Smith, 1977).

The evidence favoring Epstein-Barr virus (EBV) as the cause of African BL has
been recently reviewed (zur Hausen, 1975). Relevant data include uniformly high
EBV-antibody titers in BL patients and the presence of EBV antigens in fresh
biopsy cells. High concentrations of EBV-specific deoxyribonucleic acid (DNA)
have been demonstrated in 97% of biopsy specimens of African BL. EBV-specific
DNA is found infrequently in non-African BL (Goldblum and others, 1977; Koliais
and others, 1978). Laboratory studies have also shown that EBV can transform
human lymphocytes in vitro, and that certain primates may develop lymphoma
after inoculation with EBV (Miller and others, 1977).

EBV is a common organism worldwide, whereas BL is rare and has a distinct geographic pattern. Several explanations to reconcile this discrepancy with an etiologic hypothesis have been suggested: (1) Strains of EBV may differ in oncogenic
potential (Gerber and others, 1976). (2) Oncogenicity may be determined by the

mode or timing of exposure to EBV, e.g., infection in infancy (de-The, 1977).
(3) Carcinogenesis may require cofactors which are present in specific geographic
areas, e.g., malaria (Burkitt, 1969).

Evidence for a viral etiology of NHL other than BL is weak. The hypothesis that
some human cancers may be caused by transmission of oncogenic viruses from pets
and other animals to man has been recently reviewed (Essex and Francis, 1976).
Feline leukemia and sarcoma viruses induce neoplasia in cats and grow readily in
human cell cultures. Feline sarcoma virus can also transform human lymphocytes
in vitro and induce lymphomas in inoculated monkeys. However, one study found
no serological evidence of infection by these agents among 1300 humans, including
patients with NHL (Krakower and Aaronson, 1978). Additionally, epidemiologic
studies of the association between human malignancy and pet exposure have
generally been negative, and highly exposed individuals, i.e., veterinarians,
have shown no increased incidence of cancer (Essex and Francis, 1976).

The action of an oncogenic virus may be difficult to demonstrate with the methods
of classical infectious disease epidemiology. This approach most easily detects
the effects of infectious agents with short, constant incubation periods and high
attack rates-- characteristics which are probably absent in malignant disease.
The paucity of putative oncogenic viruses in man further limits epidemiologic
studies that employ serological or other laboratory measures of exposure.

If NHL does have a viral etiology, interpersonal contact might play a role in
spreading the disease. Studies of this question have produced conflicting
results (Gunz, Gunz, and Leigh, 1978; Schimpff and others, 1976; Zack and others,
1977). The methodology used in these studies is complex, and caution is needed
to avoid faulty study design which would bias the outcome of the investigation.

HOST-ENVIRONMENT INTERACTIONS

Host and environmental factors may interact to induce NHL. Genes, immunodeficiency and viruses have been considered individually in this report as potential etiologic factors. The X-linked recessive lymphoproliferative syndrome has
been proposed as a model for interaction among these three factors (Purtilo and
others, 1975; 1978). Affected boys appear to inherit an intrinsic defect in
immune response, particularly to EBV. After infection with the virus, these
patients may develop fatal infectious mononucleosis, American BL, immunoblastic
sarcoma, or a non-cancerous immunologic disorder (Purtilo, 1976; Purtilo and
others, 1977). Impairment of the immune response to EBV infection by a host
lesion may be a pathogenetic mechanism in the development of BL and other B-cell
diseases.

REFERENCES

Abramson, J. H., M. Avitzour, and E. Peritz (1975). Mortality from lymphomas in
    Israel, 1950-71: the possible role of environmental factors. Int. J.
    Epidemiol., 4, 321-329.

Anderson, R. E., H. Nishiyama, Y. Ii, K. Ishida, and N. Okabe (1972). Patho-
    genesis of radiation-related leukaemia and lymphoma: speculations based
    primarily on experience of Hiroshima and Nagasaki. Lancet, 1, 1060-1062.

Baikie, A. G., L. J. Kinlen, and M. C. Pike (1972). Detection and assessment of
    case clustering in Burkitt's lymphoma and Hodgkin's disease. In E. Grundmann
    and H. Tulinius (Eds.), Current Problems in the Epidemiology of Cancer and
    Lymphomas, Springer-Verlag, New York. pp. 201-209.

Basa, G. F., T. Kirayama, and A. G. Cruz-Basa (1977). Cancer epidemiology in the Philippines. Natl. Cancer Inst. Monogr., 47, 45-56.

Besuschio, S. and C. Ghinelli (1973). Lymphoreticular tumors in Argentina. J. Natl. Cancer Inst., 50, 1639-1643.

Booth, K., D. P. Burkitt, D. J. Bassett, R. A. Cooke, and J. Biddulph (1967). Burkitt lymphoma in Papua, New Guinea. Br. J. Cancer, 21, 657-664.

Brincker, H., and E. Wilbek (1974). The incidence of malignant tumours in patients with respiratory sarcoidosis. Br. J. Cancer, 29, 247-251.

Bruce, D. L., K. A. Eide, H. W. Linde, and J. E. Eckenhoff (1968). Causes of death among anesthesiologists: a 20-year survey. Anesthesiology, 29, 565-569.

Buehler, S. K., F. Firme, G. Fodor, G. R. Fraser, W. H. Marchall, and P. Vaze (1975). Common variable immunodeficiency, Hodgkin's disease, and other malignancies in a Newfoundland family. Lancet, 1, 195-197.

Burke, J. S., and J. J. Butler (1976). Malignant lymphoma with a high content of epithelioid histiocytes (Lennert's lymphoma). Am. J. of Clin. Pathol., 66, 1-9.

Burkitt, D. (1964). A lymphoma syndrome dependent on environment. In F. C. Roulet (Ed.), Symp. Lymph. Tumours in Africa, Paris, 1963, S. Karger, New York, pp. 119-136.

Burkitt, D. P. (1969). Etiology of Burkitt's lymphoma--an alternative hypothesis to a vectored virus. J. Natl. Cancer Inst., 42, 19-28.

Burkitt, D., and D. Wright (1966). Geographical and tribal distribution of the African lymphoma in Uganda. Br. Med. J., 1, 569-573.

Correa, P., and G. T. O'Conor (1973). Geographic pathology of lymphoreticular tumors: summary of survey from the Geographic Pathology Committee of the International Union Against Cancer. J. Natl. Cancer Inst., 50, 1609-1617.

Court-Brown, W. M., and R. Doll (1965). Mortality from cancer and other causes after radiotherapy for ankylosing spondylitis. Br. Med. J., 2, 1327-1332.

Cutler, S. J., and J. L. Young, Jr. (Eds.), (1975). Third National Cancer Survey: Incidence Data. Natl. Cancer Inst. Monogr., 41.

de-The, G. (1977). Is Burkitt's lymphoma related to perinatal infection by Epstein-Barr virus? Lancet, 1, 335-337.

Dorfman, R. F. (1977). Pathology of the non-Hodgkin's lymphomas: new classifications. Cancer Treat. Rep., 61, 945-951.

Edington, G. M., and M. Hendrickse (1973). Incidence and frequency of lymphoreticular tumors in Ibadan and the Western State of Nigeria. J. Natl. Cancer Inst., 50, 1623-1631.

Editorial (1971). Is Phenytoin carcinogenic? Lancet, 2, 1071-1072.

Essex, M., and D. P. Francis (1976). The risk to humans from malignant diseases of their pets: an unsettled issue. J. Am. Animal Hosp. Assoc., 12, 386-390.

Fleischman, E. W., and E. L. Prigogina (1977). Karyotype peculiarities of malignant lymphomas. Hum. Genet., 35, 269-279.

Fraumeni, J. F., Jr., W. Wertelecki, W. A. Blattner, R. D. Jensen, and B. G. Leventhal (1975). Varied manifestations of a familial lymphoproliferative disorder. Am. J. Med., 59, 145-151.

Freeman, A. I., L. F. Sinks, and M. M. Cohen (1970). Lymphosarcoma in siblings, associated with cytogenetic abnormalities, immune deficiency, and abnormal erythropoiesis. J. Pediatr., 77, 996-1003.

Fukuhara, S., S. Shirakawa, and H. Uchino (1976). Specific marker chromosome 14 in malignant lymphomas. Nature, 259, 210-211.

Gatti, R. A., and R. A. Good (1971). Occurrence of malignancy in immunodeficiency diseases: a literature review. Cancer, 28, 89-98.

Gerber, P., F. K. Nkrumah, R. Pritchett, and E. Kieff (1976). Comparative studies of Epstein-Barr virus strains from Ghana and the United States. Int. J. Cancer, 17, 71-81.

Goldblum, H., H. Ben-Bassat, S. Mitrani, M. Andersson-Anvret, T. Goldblum, E. Aghal, B. Ramot, and G. Klein (1977). A case of an Epstein-Barr virus (EBV) genome-carrying lymphoma in an Israeli Arab child. Europ. J. Cancer, 13, 693-698.

Goldsmith, J. R., and T. L. Guidotti (1977). Environmental factors in the epidemiology of lymphosarcoma. Pathol. Annu., 12 (Pt. 2), 411-425.

Gunz, F. W., J. P. Gunz, and J. Leigh (1978). Contacts among patients with hematological malignancies. Cancer, 41, 2379, 2387.

Harris, O. D., W. T. Cooke, H. Thompson, and J. A. H. Waterhouse (1967). Malignancy in adult coeliac disease and idiopathic steatorrhoea. Am. J. Med., 42, 899-912.

Hoover, R. N. (1976). Bacillus Calmette-Guerin vaccination and cancer prevention: a critical review of the human experience. Cancer Res., 36, 652-654.

Hoover, R., and J. F. Fraumeni, Jr. (1973). Risk of cancer in renal-transplant recipients. Lancet, 2, 55-57.

Kassan, S. S., and M. Gardy (1978). Sjogren's syndrome: an update and overview. Am. J. Med., 64, 1037-1046.

Kersey, J. H., and B. D. Spector (1975). Immune deficiency diseases. In J. F. Fraumeni, Jr. (Ed.), Persons at High Risk of Cancer: An Approach to Cancer Etiology and Control, Academic Press, New York. pp. 55-67.

Kersey, J. H., B. D. Spector, and R. A. Good (1973). Primary immunodeficiency diseases and cancer: the immunodeficiency-cancer registry. Int. J. Cancer, 12, 333-347.

Koliais, S., G. Gjursell, A. Adams, T. Lindahl, and G. Klein (1978). State of Epstein-Barr virus DNA in an American Burkitt's lymphoma line: brief communication. J. Natl. Cancer Inst., 60, 991-994.

Krakower, J. M., and S. A. Aaaronson (1978). Seroepidemiologic assessment of feline leukemia virus infection risk for man. Nature, 273, 463-464.

Krikorian, J. G., J. L. Anderson, C. P. Bieber, I. Penn, and E. B. Stinson (1978). Malignant neoplasms following cardiac transplantation. J. Am. Med. Assoc., 240, 639-643.

Lee, G. B., P. M. Smith, and R. M. E. Seal (1977). Lymphosarcoma in Crohn's disease: report of a case. Dis. Colon Rectum, 20, 351-354.

Levine, P. H., B. R. Cho, R. R. Connelly, C. W. Berard, G. T. O'Conor, R. F. Dorfman, J. M. Easton, and V. T. DeVita (1975). The American Burkitt lymphoma registry: a progress report. Ann. Intern. Med., 83, 31-36.

Lewis, E. B. (1963). Leukemia, multiple myeloma, and aplastic anemia in American radiologists. Science, 142, 1492-1494.

Li, F. P., J. F. Fraumeni, Jr., N. Mantel, and R. W. Miller (1969). Cancer mortality among chemists. J. Natl. Cancer Inst., 43, 1159-1164.

Li, F. P., D. R. Willard, R. Goodman, and G. Vawter (1975). Malignant lymphoma after diphenylhydantoin (Dilantin) therapy. Cancer, 36, 1359-1362.

Lukes, R. J., and B. H. Tindle (1975). Immunoblastic lymphadenopathy: a hyperimmune entity resembling Hodgkin's disease. N. Engl. J. Med., 292, 1-8.

MacMahon, B. (1966). Epidemiology of Hodgkin's disease. Cancer Res., 26, (Pt. 1), 1189-1200.

Manolov, G., and Manolova (1972). Marker band in one chromosome 14 from Burkitt lymphomas. Nature, 237, 33-34.

Matanoski, G. M., Seltser, P. Sartwell, E. L. Diamond, and E. A. Elliott (1975). The current mortality rates of radiologists and other physician specialists: specific causes of death. Am. J. Epidemiol., 101, 199-210.

McCaw, B. J., A. L. Epstein, H. S. Kaplan, and F. Hecht (1977). Chromosome 14 translocation in African and North American Burkitt's lymphoma. Int. J. Cancer, 19, 482-486.

McCaw, B. K., F. Hecht, D. G. Harnden, and R. L. Teplitz (1975). Somatic rearrangement of chromosome 14 in human lymphocytes. Proc. Natl. Acad. Sci. USA, 72, 2071-2075.

McMichael, A. J., R. Spirtas, L. L. Kupper, and J. F. Gamble (1975). Solvent exposure and leukemia among rubber workers: an epidemiologic study. J. Occup. Med., 17, 234-239.

Miller, G., T. Shope, D. Coope, L. Waters, J. Pagano, G. W. Bornkamm, and W. Henle (1977). Lymphoma in cotton-top marmosets after inoculation with Epstein-Barr virus: tumor incidence, histologic spectrum antibody responses, demonstration of viral DNA, and characterization of viruses. J. Exper. Med., 145, 948-988.

Misad, O., J. G. Brandon, and P. Albujar (1973). Lymphoreticular tumors in Peru. J. Natl. Cancer Inst., 50, 1663-1668.

Modan, B., B. Goldman, M. Shani, D. Meytes, and B. S. Mitchell (1969). Epidemiological aspects of neoplastic disorders in Israeli migrant population.

Non-Hodgkin's Lymphomas: a Search for Prognostic Factors

D. E. Bergsagel, M. Gospodarowicz, R. Bush and T. C. Brown

Ontario Cancer Institute, Toronto, Canada

ABSTRACT

We have assessed the influence of nine prognostic factors on the survival of 981 Non-Hodgkin's Lymphoma patients. Sex and the presentation of the lymphoma in nodal or extranodal sites did not influence prognosis. Pathology, age, B-symptoms, an ESR of $\geqslant 40$ mm/hr, an initial hemoglobin of <12.0 g/dl and Stage IV disease were found to be important prognostic factors. Patients with liver involvement have a worse prognosis than Stage IV patients with other organs involved.

NON-HODGKIN'S LYMPHOMAS, PROGNOSTIC FACTORS

INTRODUCTION

The Non-Hodgkin's Lymphomas are a heterogeneous group. The pathologic and clinical staging systems which we now use do not separate patients into definite risk categories. With accurate surgical staging about 65% of patients prove to have Stage IV disease (Chabner and others, 1975). The Rappaport pathologic classification separates patients into those with a relatively good prognosis (the well- and intermediately-differentiated lymphocytic and the nodular lymphomas), and those with a poor prognosis (diffuse poorly-differentiated lymphocytic and diffuse histiocytic lymphomas). In addition, some patients with histiocytic lymphomas appear to be cured with both x-irradiation for localized disease (Bush and others, 1977), and intensive combination chemotherapy for advanced disease (DeVita and others, 1975; Schein and others, 1976).

The survival curves for Non-Hodgkin's Lymphomas treated at the Ontario Cancer Institute have two components. Initially the survival curve falls rapidly for about two years, then bends and follows a slower exponential slope (Fig. 1). We have analysed the course of 981 patients with Non-Hodgkin's Lymphomas treated at the Ontario Cancer Institute between 1967-75, and assessed the significance of several prognostic factors. We identified seven important prognostic factors. Most of the factors exert their influence primarily on the steep portion of the curve during the first two years after diagnosis. We hope that further analysis of these patients will enable us to separate more accurately the poor prognosis group, which dies rapidly during the first two years, from the group with a relatively good prognosis which dies at a lower rate thereafter.

89

D. E. Bergsagel *et al.*

CLINICAL MATERIAL AND METHODS

All previously untreated patients with Non-Hodgkin's Lymphomas who were treated at the Ontario Cancer Institute between 1967 and 1975 are included. The diagnostic biopsies on all but 18 of these patients were reviewed by one of us (TCB) and classified (Table 1) by the Rappaport criteria (Rappaport, 1966). In our analysis we have combined the histiocytic and mixed cell categories.

TABLE 1   PMH NON-HODGKIN'S LYMPHOMAS 1967-75
RAPPAPORT PATHOLOGY CLASSIFICATION

Pathology	Nodal		Extranodal		Total	
	No.	%	No.	%	No.	%
Nodular						
LWD + ID	79	25	19	24	98	25
LPD	99	31	22	28	121	31
Histiocytic	88	28	30	38	118	30
Mixed	46	15	4	5	50	13
Stem cell	5	2	3	4	8	2
TOTALS	317	100	78	100	395	100
Diffuse						
LWD + ID	46	14	20	8	66	12
LPD	94	29	60	25	154	27
Histiocytic	130	41	149	61	279	50
Mixed	31	10	4	2	35	6
Stem cell	6	2	8	3	14	2
Non-Burkitt	12	4	2	1	14	2
TOTALS	319	100	243	100	562	100
Unclassified	4		2		6	0.6
Not reviewed	12		6		18	1.8
TOTAL	652		329		981	100

2243G

The staging procedures employed are shown in Table 2.

TABLE 2   PMH NON-HODGKIN'S LYMPHOMAS 1967-75
STAGING PROCEDURES

	Number	%
Total	981	100
Chest X-ray	953	97
Mediastinal tomograms	338	34
LAG	574	59
IVP	517	53
IVC	226	23
Liver/Spleen scan	550	56
Bone marrow : aspiration	498 ⎫ 680	51 ⎫ 70
biopsy	182 ⎭	19 ⎭
Serum alkaline phosphatase	855	87
BSP retention	470	48
ESR	563	57
B symptoms present	189	19
Laparotomy	55	6

2204G

The Ann Arbour Staging Classification (Carbone and others, 1971), and the initial form of treatment, are shown in Table 3. It will be noted that 46% of these patients were thought to have Stage IA or IIA disease. This proportion is much higher than has been reported in surgically staged groups (Chabner and others, 1975).

TABLE 3 PMH NON-HODGKIN'S LYMPHOMAS 1967-75

INITIAL TREATMENT BY STAGE

Stage	No.	% of pts. in each stage treated with :			
		XRT	CT	XRT + CT	NT
I̲ A	225	85.8	1.3	4.9	8.0
I̲I̲ A	225	80.4	4.9	10.2	4.4
I̲I̲I̲ A	184	34.8	34.2	13.6	17.4
I̲V̲ A	153	26.1	47.7	13.9	10.5
B	189	33.9	38.6	23.3	4.2
Not staged	5	80.0	-	-	20.0
Total	981	55.7	22.7	13.0	8.7

2244G

Actuarial survival curves were prepared using the method of Kaplan and Meier (1958). The significance of differences in survival was tested by the generalized Wilcoxan test, using the method of Gehan (1965).

PROGNOSTIC FACTORS

We tested the significance of nine possible prognostic factors. Sex, and the origin of the lymphoma in nodal or extranodal sites did not influence survival.

The other seven factors, described below, were found to be very important prognostic variables.

1. Pathologic Classification

It is well known that nodular lymphomas have a better survival prognosis than those with a diffuse pattern (Fig. 1). It will be noted, however, that the adverse effect of the diffuse pattern is exerted during the first two years; thereafter, the slopes for the nodular and diffuse lymphomas become parallel.

D. E. Bergsagel *et al.*

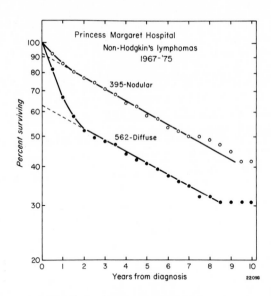

Fig. 1. Survival of Non-Hodgkin's Lymphomas with
nodular and diffuse patterns.

It is also well known that the survival of patients with well- and intermediately-differentiated lymphocytic lymphomas is better than for other lymphomas (Fig. 2). It is of interest that the major difference in these two survival curves occurs during the steeper first part of the curve. The initial slope of the survival curve for the well- and intermediately-differentiated lymphomas falls more slowly than for the other lymphomas, and does not bend until the fifth year. The steep initial slope for the other lymphomas bends at two years. Extrapolation of the slow part of the survival curve back to zero time suggests that about 70% of the patients in both groups belong to a better prognosis group.

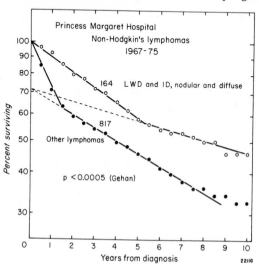

Fig. 2. Survival of lymphocytic,
well- and intermediately-
differentiated lymphomas
(LWD + ID) compared to
the survival of other
lymphomas.

The survival curve for the histiocytic lymphomas is distinctly different from that
of the lymphocytic group in that the slow portion parallels the expected survival
of age- and sex-matched controls (Bush and others, 1977). These patients appear
to be cured by radiation therapy for localized disease (Bush and others, 1977)
and combination chemotherapy for advanced disease (DeVita and others, 1975; Schein
and others, 1976).

2. Age

To assess the influence of age on the survival of lymphoma patients, we calculated
the relative survival of patients with lymphocytic (Fig. 3) and histiocytic (Fig. 4)
lymphomas. Each point on the relative curves is determined by dividing the
surviving lymphoma fraction by the expected survival fraction of an age- and sex-
matched group of normals. It will be noted that the relative survival of lymphocytic lymphomas decreases progressively with advancing age (Fig. 3).

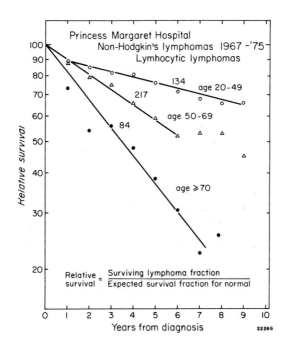

Fig. 3. Influence of age on the relative survival of
        lymphocytic lymphomas.

The influence of age on the histiocytic lymphomas is quite different. The relative
survival curve of patients between the ages of 20-59 years becomes horizontal at
50% after the fifth year, indicating that the survival of this group parallels
that of normals (Fig. 4). This suggests that this group is cured. For those over
60, a definite plateau phase has not been demonstrated, for the survival pattern
beyond seven years is not clearly established. However, if a plateau becomes
evident with further updating of the survival curve, it will probably occur at a
lower level than for the 20-59 year age group.

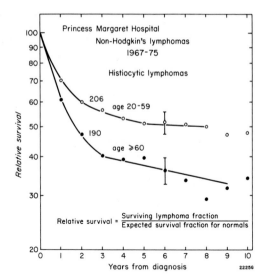

Fig. 4. Influence of age on the relative survival of
the histiocytic lymphomas.

Thus, age is a very important prognostic factor for the lymphocytic lymphomas, and
also appears to be important for the histiocytic group.

3. B-symptoms

B-symptoms are not recognized as important factors in determining survival prognosis
for Non-Hodgkin's Lymphoma patients by investigators at some centres (Fisher and
others, 1977). However, we have found that a history of B-symptoms (unexplained
fever, night sweats or weight loss of more than 10% body weight within three
months) influences survival adversely (Bergsagel and others, 1975; Peters and
others, 1975; Bush and others, 1977). The influence of B-symptoms on the survival
of our patients is shown in Fig. 5. Once again the occurrence of B-symptoms
influences survival during the first two years; thereafter the slower part of the
curve appears to be parallel to the slow part of the survival curve for A-patients.

4. Stage

The Ann Arbour staging system (Carbone and others, 1971) based on clinical, as
opposed to surgical staging, does not separate the survival curves of Stage IA and
IIA disease (Fig. 6). Indeed, IIIA does not separate from I and IIA until after
the third year. However, patients with extralymphatic involvement of organs
(Stage IVA) and those with B-symptoms, clearly have a poorer survival prognosis
than those with Stage I-IIIA disease.

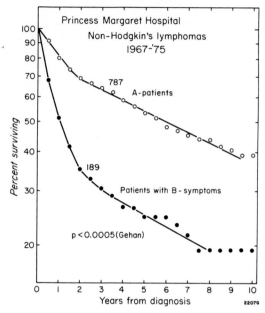

Fig. 5. Influence of B-symptoms on survival.

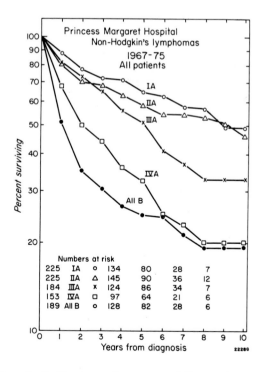

Fig. 6. Influence of stage and B-symptoms on
survival.

5. Erythrocyte Sedimentation Rate (ESR)

Peters and others (1975) noted that the survival prognosis for Non-Hodgkin's
Lymphoma patients becomes progressively worse with increasing ESR's. We have
found that the ESR is elevated above 40 mm/hour more frequently in patients with
B-symptoms (62/107, 58%) than in A-patients without B-symptoms (133/455, 29%).
In addition, an elevated ESR of 40 mm/hour, or more, identifies a group of both
A and B patients with a poor survival prognosis (Fig. 7). Thus, an elevated ESR
is a prognostic factor which acts independently of B-symptoms.

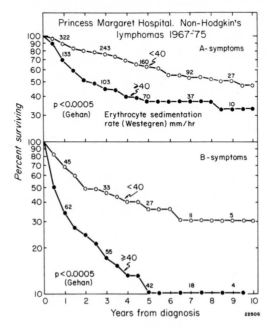

Fig. 7. The influence of ESR on the survival of A-patients
and those with B-symptoms.

6. Anemia

Patients who present with a hemoglobin concentration of less than 12.0 g/dl have a
significantly poorer survival prognosis than those who have higher initial
hemoglobin concentrations (Fig. 8). Again, the unfavorable influence of the lower
hemoglobin occurs during the first two years.

7. Influence of Organ Involvement on Survival in Stage IV

We wondered whether involvement of any particular extranodal site implied an
especially poor prognosis. We compared the survival of patients with multiple bony
lesions, lung lesions, splenomegaly, multiple skin lesions and liver involvement,
with Stage IV patients who did not have this organ involvement. For this study we
classified patients with an unexplained elevation of serum alkaline phosphatase
and a bromosulphalene retention of more than 6% at 45 minutes, a grossly enlarged
liver (> 8 cm below the right costal margin in the mid-clavicular line) and an
abnormal alkaline phosphatase and/or BSP retention, and those with positive liver
biopsies, as having involved livers. The significance of marrow and central nervous
system lesions are important (Fisher and others, 1977), but have not been assessed
yet in our group of patients.

The results are shown in Table 4. The prognosis for patients with bone, lung, spleen and skin involvement have a survival prognosis which is similar to that of other Stage IV patients. Liver involvement, however, identifies a group with a survival prognosis that is significantly poorer than other Stage IV disease.

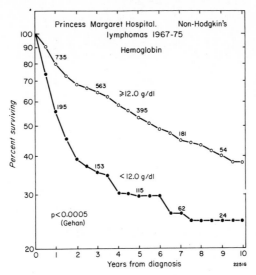

Fig. 8. The influence of anemia on the survival of lymphoma patients.

We are hopeful that further analysis of the prognostic factors in Non-Hodgkin's Lymphoma patients will allow us to identify the poor prognosis group which dies at a rapid rate during the first two years after diagnosis. This identification of important prognostic variables will lead to an improved staging system for these patients.

TABLE 4 PMH NON-HODGKIN'S LYMPHOMAS 1967-75

INFLUENCE OF ORGAN INVOLVEMENT
ON SURVIVAL IN STAGE IV

Organ	Involved	Number	p (Gehan)
Bone	No	227	0.328
	Yes	34	
Lung	No	223	0.839
	Yes	37	
Spleen	No	181	0.849
	Yes	80	
Skin	No	243	0.567
	Yes	17	
Liver	No	148	< 0.0005
	Yes	113	

2252G

REFERENCES

Bergsagel, D.E., T.C. Brown, and J. Reid (1975). The influence of chemotherapy on the management of Non-Hodgkin's Lymphomata at the Princess Margaret Hospital. Brit. J. Cancer, 31, Suppl. II, 489-496.

Bush, R.S., M. Gospodarowicz, J. Sturgeon, and R. Alison (1977). Radiation therapy of localized Non-Hodgkin's lymphoma. Cancer Chemother. Rep., 61, 1129-1136.

Carbone, P.P., H.S. Kaplan, K. Musshoff, D.W. Smithers, and M. Tubiana (1971). Report of the Committee on Hodgkin's Disease staging classification. Cancer Res., 31, 1860-1861.

Chabner, B.A., R.E. Johnson, P.B. Chretien, P.S. Schein, R.C. Young, G.P. Canellos, S.H. Hubbard, T. Anderson, S.H. Rosenoff, and V.T. DeVita, Jr. (1975). Percutaneous liver biopsy, peritoneoscopy and laparotomy: An assessment of relative merits in the lymphomata. Brit. J. Cancer, 31, Suppl. II, 242-247.

DeVita, V.T., Jr., G.P. Canellos, B. Chabner, P. Schein, S.P. Hubbard, and R.C. Young (1975). Advanced diffuse histiocytic lymphoma, a potentially curable disease. Results with combination chemotherapy. Lancet, i, 248-250.

Fisher, R.I., V.T. DeVita, Jr., B.L. Johnson, R. Simon, and R.C. Young (1977). Prognostic factors for advanced diffuse histiocytic lymphoma following treatment with combination chemotherapy. Am. J. Med., 63, 177-182.

Gehan, E.A. (1965). A generalized Wilcoxan test for comparing arbitrarily singly-censored samples. Biometrika, 52, 203.

Kaplan, E.L., and P. Meier (1958). Nonparametric estimation from incomplete observation. J. Am. Stat. Assoc., 53, 457-481.

Peters, M.V., R.S. Bush, T.C. Brown, and J. Reid (1975). The place of radiotherapy in the control of Non-Hodgkin's Lymphomata. Brit. J. Cancer, 31, Suppl. II, 386-401.

Rappaport, H. (1966). Tumors of the hemopoietic system. In Atlas of Tumor Pathology, Section 3, fascicle 8, Washington, D.C., U.S. Armed Forces Institute of Pathology.

Schein, P.S., V.T. DeVita, Jr., S. Hubbard, B.A. Chabner, G.P. Canellos, C. Berard, and R.C. Young (1976). Bleomycin, adriamycin, cyclophosphamide, vincristine and prednisone (BACOP) combination chemotherapy in the treatment of advanced, diffuse histiocytic lymphoma. Ann. Intern. Med., 85, 417-422.

Patterns of Presentation and Relapse in Childhood Non-Hodgkin's Lymphoma

S. B. Murphy, R. J. A. Aur and H. O. Hustu

*Hematology-Oncology Division, St. Jude Children's Research Hospital,
Memphis, Tennessee*

ABSTRACT

Childhood non-Hodgkin's lymphoma (NHL) is a heterogenous disease entity characterized by a variety of differing anatomic sites of involvement, extensions of
disease, blast-cell phenotypes, and prognoses in response to intensive combined
modality therapy. The presentation of disease is best assessed by adopting a
simplified clinical staging system, other than the Ann Arbor classification. The
most favorable prognosis (Stage I or II disease) is associated with a presentation of completely resectable gastrointestinal-tract lesions or strictly localized
or regional primary tumors in the peripheral nodes or the head and neck. A worse
prognosis (Stage III and IV disease) is carried by all other presentations,
particularly primary mediastinal masses or advanced unresectable intra-abdominal
disease, with or without initial involvement of the bone marrow and central nervous system. The hazard of relapse is limited largely to the first 2 years
following diagnosis; survival remains essentially unchanged thereafter. Relapse
in the bone marrow or central nervous system or both is the usual pattern of
recurrent disease. Patterns of presentation and relapse in childhood NHL are
illustrated from the authors' experience with 91 patients who were treated uniformly with multi-agent chemotherapy and involved-field irradiation.

Keywords: Childhood non-Hodgkin's lymphoma   staging   presenting features
           prognosis   relapse

PATTERNS OF PRESENTATION

Childhood non-Hodgkin's lymphoma (NHL) has a variable pattern of presentation
which takes into account a spectrum of clinical and biological factors, including
primary site of involvement, stage and classification of disease, and tumor cell
markers. Of these factors, stage of disease appears most important. Ideally,
a staging classification should (i) reflect the natural history of the cancer,
(ii) correlate with prognosis, (iii) provide helpful information in the assignment of treatment regimens, and (iv) promote a uniform description in scientific
communication, thus facilitating the interpretation of the end results of treatment. A staging system for childhood NHL that satisfies the above criteria is
shown in Table 1.

The assignment of stage is based on a clinical evaluation consisting of a careful history and physical examination, chest and skeletal roentgenography,
intravenous pyelography, tests of renal and hepatic function, and examination of
bone marrow and spinal fluid. In selected patients, additional noninvasive
studies - such as scans of bone, liver and spleen, whole-body ^{67}Ga scanning,
abdominal ultrasonography, and computerized axial tomography - may prove useful.
A pretreatment staging laparotomy is not indicated for children with NHL, but is
usually necessary for diagnosis or relief of obstruction or intussusception in
children with abdominal disease.

The staging classification in Table 1 retains the conventional distinction between lymphoma and leukemia. NHL with marrow involvement is defined by a normal
hemogram and less than 25% replacement of the marrow by tumor cells. This cri-
terion allows Stage IV NHL with marrow involvement to be distinguished from acute
leukemia with bulky extramedullary disease and complete replacement of marrow
with blasts. While this distinction may appear arbitrary, it is nevertheless of
prognostic importance.

TABLE 1   A Staging Classification for Childhood NHL

Stage I
    A single tumor (extranodal) or single anatomic site
(nodal), excluding the mediastinum or abdomen.

Stage II
    A single tumor (extranodal) with regional node
involvement.
    Two or more nodal sites on the same side of the
diaphragm.
    Two single (extranodal) tumors with or without re-
gional node involvement on the same side of the diaphragm.
    A resectable primary gastrointestinal tract tumor,
usually in the ileocecal area, with or without involvement of associated mesenteric nodes only.

Stage III
    Two single tumors (extranodal) on opposite sides of
the diaphragm.
    Two or more nodal areas above and below the diaphragm.
    All the primary intrathoracic tumors (mediastinal,
pleural, thymic).
    All extensive primary unresectable intra-abdominal
disease.
    All paraspinal or epidural tumors, regardless of other
tumor site(s).

Stage IV
    Any of the above with initial CNS or bone marrow
involvement or both.

The stage of disease and location of primary tumor in 66 consecutive untreated
children with NHL, admitted to St. Jude Children's Research Hospital from March
1975 to July 1978, are shown in Table 2. In our experience primary intra-abdominal disease is the most common presentation of childhood NHL, accounting for 25
(37.8%) of 66 cases in the current series. This figure is similar to reported
frequencies in other large series of childhood NHL patients (Jenkins, 1973;

Lemerle and others, 1975; Cebrian-Bonesana, Schwartzman, and Roca-Garcia, 1978). Next in frequency is mediastinal NHL, which was present in 17 (25%) of 66 patients.

TABLE 2   Relationship of Primary Site to Clinical Stage of Disease

Primary Site	Stage				
	I	II	III	IV	Total
Abdomen	--	8	14	3	25
Mediastinum	--	--	14	3	17
Head-Neck*	4	2	1	5	12
Peripheral Nodes	4	1	1	--	6
Other	--	--	2	4	6
Total	8	11	32	15	66

*Includes Waldeyer's ring with or without unilateral or bilateral cervical nodes.

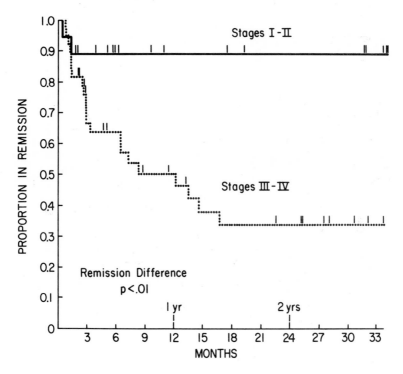

Fig. 1.   Influence of stage (Table 1) on the actuarial estimate of the proportion of children with NHL remaining in continuous complete remission.   The study group consisted of a consecutive series of 66 previously untreated children (Table 2) managed according to a protocol outlined elsewhere (Murphy, 1977; Murphy and Hustu, 1978).   The complete remission frequency for the group of patients assessable for induction therapy was 91.8% (56/61).   The 2-year estimate of disease-free survival for Stages I-II is 89%, compared to 37.5% for Stages III-IV (p < 0.01, log-rank test).

Stage of disease is clearly related to prognosis in NHL: comparison of the clinical course of children with localized vs. disseminated tumor has demonstrated a
significantly increased frequency and duration of complete remission and a significantly longer survival time for the former group (Murphy, 1977).   This relationship is illustrated in Fig. 1 by an actuarial estimate of remission duration for
the 66 patients included in Table 2, who were managed according to a previously
described treatment plan (Murphy, 1977; Murphy and Hustu, 1978).   The Ann Arbor
staging classification for Hodgkin's disease has also been applied to a series of
children with NHL and correlates with the outcome of therapy (Lemerle and others,
1975; Murphy, Frizzera,and Evans, 1975; Glatstein and others, 1974; Pinkel,
Johnson, and Aur, 1975).   For a variety of reasons, however, this system is poorly
suited to the staging of children with NHL (Murphy, 1978).

PATTERNS OF RELAPSE

Relapse patterns in childhood NHL are of three main types: central-nervous-system
(CNS) involvement, leukemic evolution, and lymphomatous recurrence - appearing
singly, in sequence, or in combination.   The frequency of reported relapse in
childhood NHL varies greatly depending upon the composition of the patient population and, of course, upon the type and intensity of treatment given.   Since 1968,
91 children in two consecutive series have been uniformly treated at this center
by modern intensive combined modality regimens.   The first series (Total V-III-C)
consisted of 25 patients with local or regional disease (Stages I-III, according
to the classification outlined in Table 1) who were treated during the period
1968-1975.   The second series (NHL-75) consists of the 66 children described
earlier in the review.   Preliminary results of treatment for the first group have
been published (Aur and others, 1971).

In the overall study population, the most common pattern of disease progression or
recurrence was dissemination to the bone marrow or to the CNS - or both, either
in combination or in sequence.   The cumulative frequency of patients exhibiting
leukemic evolution or CNS involvement (or both) is given in Table 3.   Bone marrow
and CNS disease occur more often in association than in isolation, as noted by
others as well (Watanabe, Sullivan, and Sutow, 1973; Gendelman, Rizzo, and Mones,
1969).   The cumulative frequencies shown in Table 3 may be regarded as minimal

TABLE 3   Central-Nervous-System and Leukemic Progression
of Childhood NHL

Series	Cumulative Frequency* with:		
	Leukemic Evolution[+]	Both Leukemic Evolution and CNS Disease	CNS Disease[§]
Total V-III-C	3/25	4/25	1/25
NHL-75	6/66	15/66	7/66
Total	9/91 (10%)	19/91 (21%)	8/91 (9%)
	28/91 (31%)		27/91 (30%)

*The proportion of patients with documented involvement at any
 time from diagnosis to death.
[+]Defined as greater than 25% replacement by blasts.
[§]Determined from autopsy evidence or by documented malignant
 cerebrospinal fluid pleocytosis.

estimates, since 27 of the 66 children registered in the NHL-75 protocol are still less than a year from diagnosis, the period of greatest risk for relapse. The likelihood of relapse in the bone marrow or CNS is clearly related to both the primary site and stage of disease; children with Stage I or II disease rarely relapse when managed by currently accepted methods.

Other patterns of progressive disease do occur in children with NHL, but less commonly. Gonadal involvement, for example, was found at the time of relapse in 6 (6.5%) of these 91 children. Tumor recurrence in nodal or extranodal sites, usually associated with malignant intracavitary effusions, rarely proved to be the initial evidence of recurrent or progressive disease in children who achieved a complete remission in response to induction therapy. In only 5 (6%) of the 82 children attaining an initial complete remission did bulky tumor recurrence represent the first evidence of disease progression.

From these observations it is clear that failure to control local tumor seldom constitutes an obstacle to cure. More typically, complete remissions are ended by the spread of tumor cells to the bone marrow and the CNS, indicating a need for more effective antileukemic regimens and improved prophylactic treatment of the CNS.

REFERENCES

Aur, R.J.A., H.O. Hustu, J.V. Simone, C.B. Pratt, and D. Pinkel (1971). Therapy of localized and regional lymphosarcoma of childhood. Cancer, 27, 1328-1331.

Cebrian-Bonesana, A., E. Schwartzman, C. Roca-Garcia, C. Pependieck, F. Sackmann-Muriel, F. Ojeda, R. Kvicala, S. Pavlovsky, J. Lein, and L. Penchansky (1978). Non-Hodgkin's lymphoma in children. An analysis of 122 cases from Argentina. Cancer, 41, 2372-2378.

Gendelman, S., F. Rizzo, and R.J. Mones (1969). Central nervous system complications of leukemic conversion of the lymphomas. Cancer, 24, 676-682.

Glatstein, E., H. Kim, S. Donaldson, R. Dorfman, T. Gribble, J. Wilbur, S. Rosenberg, and H. Kaplan (1974). Non-Hodgkin's lymphomas. VI. Results of treatment in childhood. Cancer, 34, 204-211.

Jenkins, R.D.T. (1973). The management of malignant lymphoma in childhood. In T.J. Deeley (Ed.) Modern Radiotherapy-Malignant Diseases in Children. Butterworths, London. pp. 341-359.

Lemerle, M., R. Gerard-Marchant, H. Sancho, and O. Scheweisguth (1975). Natural history of non-Hodgkin's malignant lymphomata in children. A retrospective study of 190 cases. Br. J. Cancer, 31, Suppl. II, 324-331.

Murphy, S.B. (1977). Management of childhood non-Hodgkin's lymphoma. Cancer Treat. Rep., 61, 1161-1173.

Murphy, S.B. (1977). Prognostic factors and obstacles to cure of childhood non-Hodgkin's lymphoma. Semin. Oncol., 4, 265-271.

Murphy, S.B., G. Frizzera, and A.E. Evans (1975). A study of childhood non-Hodgkin's lymphoma. Cancer, 36, 2121-2131.

Murphy, S.B., and H.O. Hustu (1978). A randomized trial of combined modality therapy in childhood non-Hodgkin's lymphoma. Proc. Amer. Soc. Clin. Oncol., 19, 365. (Abstract)

Pinkel, D., W. Johnson, and R.J.A. Aur (1975). Non-Hodgkin's lymphoma in children. Br. J. Cancer, 31, Suppl. II, 298-323.

Watanabe, A., M.P. Sullivan, and W. Sutow (1973). Undifferentiated lymphoma, non-Burkitt's type. Meningeal and bone marrow involvement in children. Am. J. Dis. Child., 125, 57-61.

Pathology of Non-Hodgkin's Malignant Lymphomas: Morphologic Classification in Adults and Children

M. Barcos

Roswell Park Memorial Institute, Buffalo, N.Y., U.S.A.

ABSTRACT

Recent reports on the histopathologic classification of malignant lymphomas and their clinical significance have been reviewed. Nodular poorly differentiated lymphocytic (centrocytic-centroblastic, cleaved cell) lymphomas in adults, and diffuse convoluted lymphocytic (lymphoblastic) lymphomas in children, share a predilection for presentation in peripheral nodes or mediastinum and for involvement of the marrow (Ann Arbor Stage IV): with modern therapeutic regimens these lymphomas may be associated with long term survivals. In contrast, diffuse histiocytic (immunoblastic, large non-cleaved cell) lymphomas in adults, as well as undifferentiated (Burkitt's, small non-cleaved cell) lymphomas in children, all share a tendency for presentation in extra nodal sites, mainly of the gastrointestinal tract, gonads, skin and bone. These lymphomas have a comparatively low incidence of leukemic dissemination but as a group are associated with relatively low median survival. Patients with abdominal lymphoma in Stages I-II fare significantly better than those in Stages III-IV.

The relative importance of nodular and diffuse patterns of lymph node involvement, compared to cytologic types, in determining the degree of malignancy of lymphomas in adults is not fully resolved. It appears that in poorly differentiated lymphocytic (cleaved cell) lymphomas a nodular or follicular pattern predetermines a longer median survival of 6-7.5 years, whereas in the histiocytic (immunoblastic, non-cleaved cell) lymphomas, nodular and diffuse patterns show equivocal differences in survival around a median period of about one year.

Keywords: Poorly differentiated lymphocytic lymphoma
Histiocytic lymphoma
Convoluted lymphocytic (lymphoblastic) lymphoma
Undifferentiated (Burkitt's) lymphoma
Nodular (follicular) lymphoma

HISTOPATHOLOGIC AND CLINICAL SPECIFICITY OF THE RAPPAPORT CLASSIFICATION

Traditionally, lymphomas were classified as giant follicle lymphomas, lymphosarcomas, or reticulum sarcomas (Jackson, Parker, 1947)(Table 1). In a retrospective study at Stanford University (Jones and colleagues, 1973), it was found that only half of 98 cases of lymphoma in the nodular class of Rappaport (1956) were previously

M. Barcos

classified as giant follicle lymphomas by the traditional criteria. Conversely, of 119 cases previously classified as reticulum cell sarcomas by the traditional criteria, almost half were reclassified among the Rappaport subclasses of non-histiocytic lymphomas, namely poorly differentiated lymphocytic and mixed cell lymphomas. Thus the traditional criteria often failed to distinguish nodular lymphomas and to separate from reticulum cell sarcoma histologic types with a more favorable prognosis.

TABLE 1   Distribution of Anatomic Sites and Clinical Responses in Poorly Differentiated Lymphocytic and Histiocytic Lymphomas

CLASSIFICATION	(NODULAR)	(DIFFUSE)
Rappaport	PDL-Mixed	Histiocytic
Kiel	Centrocytic-Blastic	Immunoblastic
Lukes-Collins	Cleaved FCC	Non-Cleaved FCC
Traditional	GFL – Lymphosarcoma – RCS	
Degree of Malignancy	**Low Grade**	**High Grade**
Median Survival (Yr) (1)	7.5	1.1
Cell Mediated Immunity (1)	Normal	Deficient
PROBABILITY OF DISTRIBUTION ANATOMIC SITES	%	%
Pattern (2, 3)	70 Nodular	84 Diffuse
Extranodal (2)	14	47
Mesenteric Nodes (2)	71 (47)*	27 (9)*
Spleen (2)	56 (41)*	21 (10)*
Liver (2)	16	11
Marrow (3, 4)	40-85	7-15
FIRST STAGING		
Stages III-IV (2, 3)	84-96	40-70
Complete Remission (CR) (1)	50-75	20-55
RE-STAGING IN CR		
False CR (5)	17	19
Newly Detected Sites (5)	18	40

REFERENCES
1. Jones (1975)
2. Goffinet (1977)
3. Chabner (1977)
4. Rosenberg (1975)
5. Herman (1977)

LEGEND
PDL – Poorly Differentiated Lymphocytic Lymphoma
FCC – Follicular Center Cell Lymphoma
GFL – Giant Follicle Lymphoma
RCS – Reticulum Cell Sarcoma
(*) – Positive with normal lymphangiogram (%)

The Rappaport classification defines two major histologic groups of lymphomas that have characteristic distributions of organ involvement and clinical stage, immunologic status, response to therapy and survival (Table 1). Poorly differentiated lymphocytic and mixed cell types of lymphomas share many clinical features and may be considered as a single group for the purpose of comparison with histiocytic lymphomas (Ultmann, 1977). The median age of presentation for these lymphomas is 50 years (Jones, 1975). The data shown on Table 1 is abstracted from prospective findings on a total of 693 cases of lymphoma reported by Stanford University (423 cases)(Jones & colleagues, 1973,   Rosenberg, 1975; Jones, 1975; Goffinet & colleagues, 1977; Rosenberg, 1977), the National Institute of Health (NIH) in USA (170 cases; Chabner & colleagues, 1977; Hande & colleagues, 1977), and the Southwest Oncology Group (100 cases; Herman & Jones, 1977).

Seventy percent of poorly differentiated lymphocytic lymphomas have a nodular pattern of lymph node involvement (Goffinet & colleagues, 1977; Chabner & colleagues, 1977). They characteristically tend to present with multicentric dissemination, only one in 10 cases remaining in Ann Arbor stages I and II after careful assessment with conventional and lymphangiographic radiologic studies, biopsies of liver and bone marrow, and abdominal laparotomy (Goffinet & colleagues, 1977; Chabner & colleagues, 1977), (Table 1). In recent reports (Rosenberg, 1975), the incidence of marrow involvement with improved biopsy techniques was so high (85%), as to suggest that additional sampling might prove involvement of the marrow in all patients with nodular poorly differentiated lymphocytic lymphoma. Nodular lymphomas also have a high tendency for involvement of at least one subdiaphragmatic site which can be predicted in over 75% of the patients presenting with supraclavicular lymph node involvement or with a positive lymphangiogram (Goffinet & colleagues, 1977; Chabner & colleagues, 1977). The value of a negative lymphangiogram in predicting absence of abdominal disease by nodular lymphomas is poor, however, since in over 40% of such cases, unsuspected involvement of mesenteric lymph nodes or spleen is found (Goffinet & colleagues, 1977)(Table 1).

Nodular lymphomas are rarely associated with cell mediated immune deficiency and up to 75% of affected patients appear to achieve clinical complete remission (CR) following chemotherapy (Jones, 1975). Ten of 58 patients (17%) with nodular lymphomas in CR, however, were noted by the Southwest Oncology Group (Herman & Jones, 1977) to have residual disease upon systematic re-staging, and of these 18% had newly found sites of involvement (Table 1). The median survival of patients with nodular poorly differentiated lymphocytic lymphoma in the Stanford series was 7.5 years.

Over 80% of histiocytic lymphomas show a diffuse pattern of tissue involvement (Goffinet & colleagues, 1977; Chabner & colleagues, 1977), and almost half of the cases present with extranodal involvement, mainly of the gastrointestinal tract, pleura and lung, and skin and bone (Goffinet & colleagues, 1977; Table 1). Patients with extra-nodal histiocytic lymphoma have the same incidence of dissemination to para-aortic lymph nodes, liver and marrow as patients with diffuse histiocytic lymphoma arising in lymph nodes (Hande & colleagues, 1977). In contrast to lymphocytic lymphomas, histiocytic lymphomas show a wider distribution of Ann Arbor stages, pathologic stages II and IV being the most common, and 30-60% of patients remaining in stages I-II (Goffinet & colleagues, 1977; Chabner & colleagues, 1977). The increased proportion in the series from NIH (Hande & colleagues, 1977) of stage IV cases with extranodal primaries (81%) as compared with nodal primaries (27%) is attributed mainly to the high incidence of positive lymphangiograms in the gastrointestinal lymphomas (which is considered by these authors to represent Stage IV disease) and not to differences in biologic behavior of the tumors. Extension beyond the primary site and draining lymph nodes was found in 81% of extranodal diffuse histiocytic lymphomas (Hande & colleagues, 1977), a finding which emphasizes the need for careful pathologic staging for radiotherapeutic management with curative intent. Problems with the application of the Ann Arbor staging classification to extranodal non-Hodgkin's lymphomas has led to revised staging criteria (Musshoff, 1977).

Patients with diffuse histiocytic lymphoma often have cellular immune deficiency and an unpredictable clinical course, only 20-55%, achieving apparent CR after chemotherapy (Jones, 1975; Table 1). Eight of 42 patients (19%) from the Southwest Oncology Group (Herman & Jones, 1977) with diffuse lymphoma in apparent CR were found to have residual disease during systematic re-staging and, of these, 40% had newly detected sites of disease. This latter figure is twice that reported for nodular lymphoma (Table 1). Although the overall median survival for histiocytic lymphomas is 1.1 years (Jones, 1975), results from NIH (Schein & colleagues, 1976), indicate significant prolongation of survival of patients with well-documented CR compared to those with residual disease on re-staging.

THE PLACE OF POORLY DIFFERENTIATED LYMPHOCYTIC AND HISTIOCYTIC LYMPHOMAS IN THE KIEL AND LUKES-COLLINS CLASSIFICATIONS

The remarkable activity in the field of non-Hodgkin's lymphomas during the present decade is reflected by the convergence, during a recent two-year period, of at least five new classifications (Bennett & colleagues, 1974; Gerard-Marchant & colleagues, 1974; Lukes & Collins, 1974; Dorfman, 1974; Mathe & colleagues, 1976). The historical background and immunologic advances that formed the basis of this conceptual revision of the lymphomas has been succintly reviewed by Dorfman (1977) and Taylor (1976,1977), who presented an appraisal of the theoretical and practical merits of each classification. The Kiel and Lukes-Collins classifications (Gerard-Marchant & colleagues, 1974; Lukes & Collins, 1974) are gaining increasing recognition. Implicit in these classifications is the hypothesis that cytologic type predetermines the biologic behavior of lymphomas, irrespective of their nodular or diffuse pattern. The Lukes-Collins classification also makes provision for their division into thymic-independent and thymic-dependent cell classes which is based on cytologic characteristics and on the topographic dominance of the lesions in follicular and para-cortical nodal areas, respectively. In this presentation only a brief reference will be made to the Kiel and Lukes-Collins classifications which also emphasize the differences in biologic behavior of those lymphomas termed as poorly differentiated lymphocytic and histiocytic lymphomas by the Rappaport nomenclature. Corresponding terms in the three classifications are listed in Table 1.

In a retrospective study of 405 cases reviewed by Stein in Kiel (Brittinger & colleagues, 1977), centrocytic-centroblastic lymphomas (129 cases) had a high survival of 75% at 72 months (6.0 years). In contrast, immunoblastic lymphomas (55 cases) had a median survival of only 9 months (0.8 years). These results are consistent with those reported in Table 1 for poorly differentiated lymphocytic-mixed cell lymphomas, and histiocytic lymphomas, respectively. The finding by the Kiel group (Brittinger & colleagues, 1977), of an intermediate median survival of 48 months (4.0 years) for "pure" centrocytic lymphomas (45 cases) is surprising, however, since this term corresponds closely to the highly favorable poorly differentiated lymphocytic lymphoma of the Rappaport classification. The "pure" centroblastic lymphoma, of high grade malignancy, is said to be of low frequency and was not represented in the study. The survivals among each of the remaining Kiel groups of lymphomas was not significantly different in Stage IV cases when compared to those in all (I to IV) stages. Among 19 cases of lymphomas with a median survival of 2.5 years that were classified as nodular with the Rappaport nomenclature, Mandard and colleagues, (1977) identified five cases (four centroblastic and one immunoblastic) of high grade malignancy with a median survival of six months. Duhmke and Quack (1977) report that the statistical difference in survival between centrocytic-centroblastic and immunoblastic lymphomas disappeared when the actuarial analysis was extended to 10 years, the corresponding plots merging near the 35% survival point.

A retrospective study of 202 cases of lymphoma from the City of Hope Medical Center (Nathwani & colleagues, 1978) compared the predictive value of the Rappaport and Lukes-Collins classifications and the relative importance of pattern and cell class in determining survival. In poorly differentiated lymphocytic or cleaved follicular center cell lymphomas, a nodular or follicular pattern predetermined a longer median survival of six years. In the histiocytic or large non-cleaved cell lymphomas, however, nodular and diffuse patterns showed equivocal differences in survival around a median period of about one year. Of 61 histiocytic lymphomas, seven (12%) were entered into the prognostically more favorable Lukes-Collins class of large-cleaved follicular center cell lymphomas. Only six nodular mixed cell lymphomas and no diffuse mixed cell lymphomas were reported. The low incidence of nodular mixed cell lymphomas (5%) contrasts with higher values of 35-41% reported in previous series (Rappaport & colleagues, 1956; Jones & colleagues, 1973) and suggests use of stringent new criteria for the diagnosis of this Rappaport class of lymphoma.

It has been reported that diffuse areas of infiltration impart a worse prognosis to nodular (follicular) poorly differentiated lymphocytic lymphomas (Patchefsky & colleagues, 1974), but other studies (Butler & colleagues, 1975; Warnke & colleagues, 1977; Barcos & colleagues, 1978), appear to be at variance with these findings and emphasize the need for recognition of a focal or even vague residual

*nodularity for assignment of a lesion to this prognostically favorable group. Be-
cause of high differences in responsiveness and survival reported in the literature and in its own studies between nodular and diffuse variants of poorly differentiated lymphocytic lymphomas, the Eastern Cooperative Oncology Group (Edzinli,
1976) urges the invalidation of chemotherapy protocols that fail to separate these
lesions histologically. A direct correlation between the number of small lymphocytes in the parafollicular thymic-dependent lymphoid tissue and survival has been
reported (Ree & Leone, 1978). This correlation was independent of the cytologic
type or clinical stage of the follicular lymphoma.*

Lymphomas of the First Two Decades

*The traditional terms lymphosarcoma and reticulum cell sarcoma are used in earlier
series of childhood and adolescent lymphomas of the past two decades (Rosenberg &
colleagues, 1958; Webster, 1961; Bailey & colleagues, 1961; Jones & Klinberg, 1963;
Jenkin & Sonley, 1969; Lemerle & colleagues, 1975; D'Angio & colleagues, 1965;
Olumide & colleagues, 1971; Fitzpatrick & colleagues, 1974)(Table 2A). The lack
of histopathologic specificity of these terms was noted above. The clinical specificity of the Rappaport classification (Rappaport & colleagues, 1956) in childhood lymphomas (Sullivan & colleagues, 1973; Watanabe & colleagues, 1973; Glatstein & colleagues, 1974; Pinkel & colleagues, 1975; Murphy & colleagues, 1975;
Hutter & colleagues, 1975; Hausner & colleagues, 1977) is not as clearly established as with adult disease. The remarkable improvements in staging and management of children with lymphoma reported in several recent series (Wollner & colleagues, 1975; Wollner & colleagues, 1976; Jaffe & colleagues, 1977; Murphy, 1977;
Ziegler, 1977; Brecher & colleagues, 1978)(Table 2B) point to unexpected, if not
surprising, trends in life expectancy which resemble, to some extent, those seen
in adults with lymphomas and which make assessment of the pathologic-clinical specificity of any classification premature. For example, in a retrospective study
of 38 children at Memorial Sloan Kettering Cancer Center (Wollner & colleagues,
1975), two-year survivals of 0% and 21% were reported for mediastinal and bowel
childhood lymphomas, respectively. These figures increased to 100% and 48%
respectively, in a prospective series beginning in 1971 (Table 2B), and these
latter values remained unchanged during a third year of follow-up. Independently
of cytologic class, also, lymphomas of the first decade of life show longer survivals than those in the second decade (Ziegler, 1978; Barcos & colleagues, 1978);
the reason for this difference is not known. Moreover, the clinical behavior of
childhood lymphomas is strongly dependent on the primary anatomic site of involvement, advanced clinical stage being prognostically more ominous in abdominal than
in mediastinal lymphomas (Wollner & colleagues, 1975; Sullivan, 1975; Nkrumah &
Perkins, 1976; Jaffe & colleagues, 1977, Murphy, 1977).*

*Mediastinal lymphomas in children show a male preponderance (Barcos & Lukes, 1975;
Hausner & colleagues, 1977), and in some smaller series all patients are male.
Most mediastinal lymphomas in children are now classified as convoluted lymphocytic lymphomas (Table 2B). The dominant population of the lesion consists of
small and intermediate size non-cohesive lymphocytes with finely dispersed nuclear
chromatin and scanty cytoplasm. The smaller cells have unconvoluted round nucleus.
The principal variable noted from one case to another is the number of large cells
with convoluted nuclei; this is proportional to the number of mitoses on section,
so that convoluted cells are associated with proliferative activity (Barcos &
Lukes, 1975). In the past these lesions were included with other hemopoietic malignancies under the traditional terms Sternberg sarcoma, lymphoblastic lymphosarcoma, lymphoblastoma, and reticulum cell sarcoma (Sternberg, 1916; Jackson & Parker, 1947; Rosenberg and colleagues, 1958). In the Rappaport nomenclature, these
lesions were previously classified as either poorly differentiated lymphocytic
lymphomas, or mixed cell lymphomas or undifferentiated (non-Burkitt) lymphomas
(Rappaport & colleagues, 1956; Sullivan & colleagues, 1973; Watanabe & colleagues,*

TABLE 2A *Distribution of Histologic Classes in Lymphomas of the First Two Decades*

CLASSIFICATION			TRADITIONAL			RAPPAPORT						RECENT	
REFERENCES	YEAR	NO.	LS	RCS	UNL	BL	UL	PDL	ML	HL	NOD	CL/NCL	SNCL/IL
Barcos	1953-62a	456	253	74	129								
	1949-72	23										23	
Lemerle	1950-72	190	126	64									
Glatstein	1961-73	32					4	11	3	14	1		
Pinkel	1962-73	64				2	41	2		19	2		
Murphy	1960-70	31			5		9	5		12	2		
	(Modified)				5								
Hutter	1958-73	26			4	2	3	2	16	4	2	5	11
Watanabe	1951-67	30					30						
Sullivan	1960-74	63				13b	30			8		12	
Banks	1958-73	30				30c							
Ziegler	1972-77	54				54							
Wright (AF)	1950-65	557				557d							
Nkrumah (AF)	1968-72	110				110e							
Hausner	1964-76	30				10	6			4		9/1	
Nathwani	1956-76	20										13/7	
Schneider	———	114			12							56	46
Brecker	1971-77	31											
Jaffee	1947-68	227				3	19	1		9			
	1973-76	30			2	7	9	2		10			
Woolner	1964-	38				10	16			7	5		
	1971-74	43				4	17	6			4		
TOTAL		2199	379	138	157	778	147	97	16	88	14	118/8	57

a. Review from: Rosenberg (1958), Webster (1961), Bailey (1961), Jones (1963), D'Angio (1965), Jenkin (1969), Olumide (1971) and Fitzpatrick (1974).
b, c, d, e. Facial bone tumors noted in 0 (0%), 5 (17%), 306 (55%), and 84 (76%) cases, respectively.

Abbreviations for lymphomas: LS — lymphosarcoma; RCS — reticulum cell sarcoma; UNL — unclassified or other types; BL — Burkitt's; UL — undifferentiated; PDL — poorly differentiated lymphocytic; ML — mixed cell; HL — histiocytic; NOD — nodular; CL — convoluted; NCL — non-convoluted; SNCL — small non-cleaved; IL — immunoblastic; AF — Africa.

TABLE 2B *Distribution of Anatomic Sites and Survival in Lymphomas of the First Two Decades*

REFERENCES	YEAR	MEDIASTINUM NO. HISTOL	% BM	% CNS	ABDOMEN NO. HISTOL	% BM	% CNS	SURVIVAL % I&II	SURVIVAL % III&IV	SURVIVAL % ALL STAGES	YRS
Barcos	1953-62a	LS-RCS	46-100		LS-RCS	5-30				50	<1
	1949-72	CL 23	75	20						50	<1
Lemerle	1950-72							58-25	9 (IV)	25	5
Glatstein	1961-73	PDL 6/11	81	36	PDL 3/6	17	17	55-38	0 (IV)	40	2
Pinkel	1962-73									50	<1
Murphy	1960-70 (Modified)										
Hutter	1958-73	PDL 8/12	50	50	PDL+ML 8/9	11	0	50	8	32	3
										NS	
Watanabe	1951-67	UL 11	91	45	UL 10	10	10			50	<1
Sullivan	1960-74	CL 7	54	46	BL 13	15				50CL	2.5
Banks	1958-73				BL 22	31	33				
Ziegler	1972-77				BL 47			60 (7YR)	50 (<1YR)		
Wright (AF)	1950-65				BL 139	8	18	82	41	54	2
Nkrumah (AF)	1968-72				BL 32		53	45-55	30-20	NS	4
Hausner	1964-76	CL 9	33	55	UL4+BL5	17-40				NS	
Nathwani	1956-76	CL-NCL	92							50	<1
Schneider	———	CL 29	72		SNCL 33					NS	
Brecker	1971-77							92CR	44CR	63CR	1-5
Jaffee	1947-68	85			14					50	<1
	1973-76									75CR	3
Woolner	1964-	0			21			58-0	0-3		3
	1971-74	100			48			100	85-75		3

(% SURVIVAL (3 YR) — Woolner, under Mediastinum and Abdomen columns)

a. Review from: Rosenberg (1958), Webster (1961), Bailey (1961), Jones (1963), D'Angio (1965), Jenkin (1969), Olumide (1971) and Fitzpatrick (1974).

Abbreviations for lymphomas: LS — lymphosarcoma; RCS — reticulum cell sarcoma; BL — Burkitt's; UL — undifferentiated; PDL — poorly differentiated lymphocytic; ML — mixed cell; CL — convoluted; NCL — non-convoluted; SNCL — small non-cleaved; CR — complete remission; BM — bone marrow; CNS — central nervous system; AF — Africa; NS — not stated.

1973). The Kiel study group (Gerard-Marchant & colleagues, 1974; Brittinger & colleagues, 1977) and Rappaport and colleagues (Nathwani & colleagues, 1976; Nathwani & colleagues, 1978) have introduced the traditional term lymphoblastic lymphoma into their respective classifications, and have incorporated the convoluted lymphocytic lymphoma within this class. Rappaport and his colleagues use the term lymphoblast in a conventional sense to correspond to the most immature-appearing cells of acute lymphocytic leukemia without necessarily implying that the lymphoblasts are precursor cells of the more mature-appearing cells (Nathwani & colleagues, 1976). They indicate that nuclear convolutions are helpful but not essential for the recognition of this type of lymphoma, which they believe is morphologically indistinguishable from lymphoblastic leukemia in tissue sections. If its intended histopathologic specificity is to be preserved, the term lymphoblastic lymphoma should be distinguished from the term lymphoblastic lymphosarcoma, which is still widely used by physicians and is endorsed also by the WHO classification (Mathe & colleagues, 1976).

Clinically, convoluted lymphocytic or lymphoblastic lymphomas often present with peripheral node or mediastinal involvement, respiratory and/or vena cava obstructive symptoms or pleural effusion (Barcos & Lukes, 1975; Sullivan, 1975; Nathwani, 1976; Hausner & colleagues, 1977; Lukes & colleagues, 1978; Williams & colleagues, 1978) and 20% of 56 cases reviewed recently (Schneider & colleagues) had lytic bone lesions. It is of interest that of ten lymphoblastic lymphomas reported by Hausner and colleagues (1977), nine (90%) had convoluted cells and a mediastinal mass. The incidence of marrow and central nervous system (CNS) dissemination is generally higher than is seen with undifferentiated and Burkitt lymphomas of the abdomen (Table 2B). Data supporting a thymic-dependent cell origin for these lesions has been reviewed (Nathwani & colleagues, 1976; Taylor, 1977; Lukes & colleagues, 1978; Williams & colleagues, 1978). Enzymic markers that are helpful in their diagnosis are terminal deoxynucleotidyl transferase, acid phosphatase and beta-glucoronidase (Donlon & colleagues, 1977; Stein & colleagues, 1976; Jaffe & colleagues, 1977). In their respective retrospective series, the Kiel group (Brittinger & colleagues, 1977) and Rappaport (Nathwani & colleagues, 1978) report that individuals with convoluted lymphocytic lymphoma have significantly lower survivals (median 7-9 months) than those with centrocytic-centroblastic lymphoma (85% at 72 months) or poorly differentiated lymphocytic lymphoma (median 72 months). The remarkable finding, with recent therapeutic regimens, of long term survivals and apparent cures of lymphomas with predilection for marrow and CNS involvement (Watanabe & colleagues, 1973; Wollner & colleagues, 1975; Sullivan, 1975; Jaffe & colleagues, 1977, Murphy, 1977; Brecher & colleagues, 1978)(Table 2B), would suggest that convoluted lymphocytic lymphomas may come to be regarded as a prognostically relatively favorable entity in the future.

Abdominal lymphomas generally can be classified as histiocytic or undifferentiated lymphomas in the nomenclature of Rappaport; the latter category includes Burkitt's lymphoma (Watanabe & colleagues, 1973; Glatstein & colleagues, 1974; Pinkel & colleagues, 1975; Murphy & colleagues, 1975; Hutter & colleagues, 1975; Hausner & colleagues, 1977; Wollner & colleagues, 1975). Lukes and his associates believe that these forms of childhood abdominal disease represent lymphomas of transformed B lymphocytes and classify most of these lesions as small non-cleaved follicular center cell lymphomas (SNCL) (Williams & colleagues, 1978). Thus, among 114 children with lymphoma, 46 (40%) had this type of lymphoma and, of these, 33 (72%) had an abdominal mass as main presenting sign (Schneider & colleagues)(Table 2B). Other authors classify these lesions as basophilic cell or immunoblastic lymphomas (Gerard-Marchant & colleagues, 1974; Brittinger & colleagues, 1977; Brouet & colleagues, 1975; Murphy & colleagues, 1975). Thus, of 21 lymphomas (nine undifferentiated and twelve histiocytic) reported by Murphy (1975), eleven (52%) were reclassified as basophilic cell (immunoblastic) lymphomas, and two (9%) as undifferentiated Burkitt lymphomas (Table 2A). Selective involvement of germinal centers by Burkitt's lymphoma has been shown (Mann & colleagues, 1976), supporting their inclusion among the group of follicular center cell lymphomas.

Undifferentiated Burkitt and non-Burkitt lymphomas share many clinical features, including their aggressive spread by contiguity from a primary extranodal site, and a decreased incidence of involvement of the marrow and meninges as compared to convoluted lymphocytic lymphomas (Sullivan, 1975; Levine & colleagues, 1975; Arsenau & colleagues, 1975; Banks & colleagues, 1975; Nkrumah & Perkins, 1976; Murphy, 1977; Hausner & colleagues, 1977)(Table 2B). The predominant abdominal sites of involvement in children with these types of lymphoma are the terminal ileum and ascending colon, ovaries and retroperitoneal soft tissues. Younger patients in the first decade of life survive significantly longer than older patients in the second decade (Ziegler, 1977; Barcos & colleagues, 1978). When considering both age groups together, patients with resectable localized abdominal disease in Stages I-II have long survivals compared to those with more extensive unresectable disease in Stages III-IV, (Wollner & colleagues, 1975; Murphy, 1977; Banks & colleagues, 1975; Levine & colleagues, 1975; Ziegler & colleagues, 1977)(Table 2B). In spite of these apparent clinical similarities, Burkitt's lymphomas should be separated by the pathologist from other undifferentiated forms of lymphoma according to the criteria of the World Health Organization (Berard & colleagues, 1969), because of their anatomic and biological peculiarities that have important bearing on patient management. The distinction is made primarily on the basis of the striking uniformity of cell size and of nuclear and cytoplasmic features in Burkitt's lymphoma.

Endemic (African) and non-endemic Burkitt lymphomas are similar in morphology and response to therapy (Nkrumah & Perkins, 1976; Ziegler, 1977), and share other biologic properties. Thus, they usually lack hydrolytic enzymes as detected by conventional cytochemical tests (Mann & colleagues, 1976), often contain surface-bound IgM of a single light chain class specificity, and may contain Epstein-Barr virus genomes (Bornkamm & colleagues, 1976; Anderson & colleagues, 1976; Gravell & colleagues, 1976) or an extra band in chromosome 14 (Zech & colleagues, 1976; Kakati, 1978). In contrast to most other forms of lymphoma, Burkitt lymphomas as reported in a recent series from NIH (Banks & colleagues, 1975) have little predilection for involvement of lymph nodes and spleen, even though they often form bulky cohesive tumor masses about the capsular surface of these organs[1]. Conversely, organs that are often spared by other lymphomas are frequently involved by Burkitt lymphomas; these include musculo-skeletal (jaw), integumentary, cardiovascular and endocrine systems (Banks & colleagues, 1975). The incidence of involvement of facial bones is higher in endemic Burkitt lymphoma (55-76%) than in non-endemic forms (0-17%). (Wright, 1971; Nkrumah & Perkins, 1976; Sullivan, 1973; Banks & colleagues, 1975)(Table 2A). In Africa, the incidence of CNS involvement is higher with abdominal than facial bone lymphomas (53% vs 26%) (Nkrumah & Perkins, 1976). The immediate response of endemic and non-endemic Burkitt's lymphoma to cyclophosphamide is striking, and its long-range therapeutic value of this single drug was found to be as effective as combination chemotherapy in a recent series of 54 American patients (Ziegler, 1977). CNS involvement by Burkitt's lymphoma is a preventable complication and the disease is potentially curable by chemotherapy alone (Nkrumah & Perkins, 1976; Ziegler, 1977; Murphy, 1977). Massive tumor regression may ensue within 24-48 hours of chemotherapy; this sensitivity of the tumor cells is attributed to their high proliferative rate and may be accompanied by severe

---

[1] A larger series of American Burkitt's culled from the literature from various institutions showed a higher incidence of hemopoietic and lymphoreticular involvement as compared with endemic Burkitt's lymphoma in Africa (Levine & colleagues, 1975). A prospective review indicated possible over-diagnosis of marrow involvement in some cases which continued to show lymphoid nodules in the marrow during states of clinical remission (Banks & colleagues, 1975).

metabolic disturbances such as hyperkalemia, hypocalcemia, hyperphosphatemia and lactic acidosis (Arsenau & colleagues, 1975).

A major report 19 years ago (Rosenberg & colleagues, 1958) succintly reviewed the disorderly state of studies on childhood lymphomas at that time: "pathologists have largely come to realize that histologic appearance does not define with much certainty the clinical course, extent of involvement and prognosis of these diseases". The recent improvements in classification, staging and management of children with lymphoma which have been reviewed here hopefully permit a more optimistic attitude. As is the case with lymphomas in adults, lymphomas in children can now be classified with more discrimination, which is predictive of anatomic site of presentation, marrow and central nervous system dissemination, and response to therapy. Convoluted lymphocytic lymphomas in children and poorly differentiated lymphocytic lymphomas in adults share a tendency for presentation in peripheral nodes and mediastinum and for leukemic dissemination. Paradoxically, these lymphomas may be associated with relatively long term survivals (Tables 1 and 2B). In contrast, undifferentiated or small non-cleaved lymphomas in children, and histiocytic or large non-cleaved lymphomas in adults, share a predilection for presentation in extranodal sites. They have a relatively low incidence of marrow involvement but may follow an aggressive course with decreased life expectancy unless arrested at an early stage of dissemination (Tables 1 and 2B).

Acknowledgement: I wish to thank the members of the Departments of Medicine B, Pediatrics and Pathology at Roswell Park Memorial Institute who kindly reviewed the manuscript. Dr. Richard Herrmann translated the literature in German.

114   M. Barcos

Andersson, M., G. Klein, J. L. Ziegler and W. Henle (1976). Association of Epstein-
   Barr Viral genomes with American Burkitt lymphoma. *Nature, 260*, 357.
Arsenau, J. C., G. P. Canellos, P. M. Banks, C. W. Berard, H. R. Gralnick, V. T.
   DeVita (1975). American Burkitt's lymphoma: a clinicopathologic study of 30
   cases. I. Clinical factors relating to prolonged survival. *Am. J. Med., 58*,
   314-321.
Bailey, R. J., E. O. Burgert, Jr., D. Dahlin (1961). Malignant lymphoma in children.
   Ped., 28, 985.
Banks, P. M., J. C. Arsenau, H. R. Gralnick, G. P. Canellos, V. T. DeVita and C. W.
   Berard (1975). American Burkitt lymphoma: a clinicopathologic study of 30 cases.
   II. Pathologic correlations. *Am. J. Med., 58*, 322-329.
Barcos, M. P. and R. J. Lukes (1975). Malignant lymphoma of convoluted lymphocytes:
   a new entity of possible T-cell type. In L. F. Sinks and J. O. Godden (Eds),
   Conflicts in Childhood Cancer: an evaluation of current management, Vol. 4.
   Alan Liss, Inc., New York. pp. 147-177.
Barcos, M., U. Kim, J. Pickren, P. Reese, A. Freeman and L. Stutzman (1978). Sur-
   vival of non-Hodgkin's malignant lymphomas according to two histopathologic
   classifications. Proceedings, XII International Cancer Congress, Buenos Aires.
Bennett, M. H., G. Farrer-Brown, K. Henry and A. M. Jeliffe (1974). Classification
   of non-Hodgkin's lymphomas. *Lancet, 2*, 405-406.
Berard, C. W., G. T. O'Conor, L. B. Thomas and H. Torloni (Eds)(1969). Histopathologic definition of Burkitt's tumor. *Bulletin of the World Health Organization,
   40*, 601-607.
Bornkamm, G. W., H. Stein, K. Lennert, F. Ruggeberg, H. Bartels and H. Zur Hausen
   (1976). Attempts to demonstrate virus-specific sequences in human tumors. IV.
   EB viral DNA in European Burkitt lymphoma and immunoblastic lymphadenopathy with
   excessive plasmacytosis. *Int. J. Cancer, 17*, 177.
Brecher, M. L., L. F. Sinks, R. R. M. Thomas and A. I. Freeman (1978). Non-Hodgkin's
   lymphoma in children. *Cancer, 41*, 1997-2001.
Brittinger, G., H. Bartels, K. Bremer, A. Burger, E. Duhmke, U. Gunzer, E. Konig, A.
   Stacher, H. Stein, H. Theml and R. Waldner (1975). Retrospective analysis of the
   clinical relevance of the Kiel classification of malignant non-Hodgkin's lymphomas.
   Strahlentherapie, 153, 222-228.
Brouet, J. C., S. Labaume and M. Seligmann (1975). Evaluation of T- and B-lymphocyte
   surface markers in human non-Hodgkin's malignant lymphoma. *Br. J. Cancer, 31*,
   (Suppl.).
Butler, J. J., J. A. Stryker and C. C. Schullenberger (1975). A clinicopathological
   study of stages I and II non-Hodgkin's malignant lymphomata using the Lukes-Collins
   classification. *Br. J. Cancer (Suppl.), 31*, 208-216.
Chabner, B. A., R. E. Johnson, V. T. DeVita, G. P. Canellos, S. P. Hubbard and R. C.
   Young (1977). Sequential staging in non-Hodgkin's lymphomas. *Can. Treat. Rep.,
   61*, 993-997.
D'Angio, A. Mitus and A. Evans (1965). The superior mediastinal syndrome in children
   with cancer. *Am. J. Roent., 93*, 537-544.
Donlon, J. A., E. S. Jaffe and R. C. Braylan (1977). Terminal deoxynucleotidyl trans-
   ferase activity in malignant lymphomas. *N. Eng. J. Med., 297*, 461-464.
Dorfman, R. F. (1974). Classification of non-Hodgkin's lymphoma. *Lancet, 1*, 1295.
Dorfman, R. F. (1977). Pathology of the non-Hodgkin's lymphomas: new classifications.
   Can. Treat. Rep., 61, 945-951.
Duhmke, E. and j. Quack (1977). A retrospective analysis of cases with non-Hodgkin's
   lymphomas treated in the Radiologic Clinic of the Kiel University between 1969
   and 1975. *Strahlentherapie, 153*, 229-231.
Ezdinli, E., S. Pocock, C. W. Berard, C. W. Aungst, M. Silverstein, J. Horton, J.
   Bennett, R. Bakemeier, L. Stolbach, C. Perlia, S. F. Brunk, R. E. Lenhard, D. J.
   Klaassen, P. Richter and P. Carbone (1976). Comparison of intensive versus
   moderate chemotherapy of lymphocytic lymphomas. *Cancer, 38*, 1060-1068.

Fitzpatrick, J., N. Lieberman and L. F. Sinks (1974). Staging of acute leukemia and
the relationship to central nervous system involvement. Cancer, 33, 1376-1381.

Gerard-Marchant, R., I. Hamlin, K. Lennert, F. Rilke, A. G. Stansfeld and J. A. M.
VanUnnik (1974). Classification of non-Hodgkin's lymphomas. Lancet, 2, 406-408.

Glatstein, E., H. Kim, S. S. Donaldson, R. F. Dorfman, J. J. Gribble, J. R. Wilbur,
S. A. Rosenberg and H. S. Kaplan (1974). Non-Hodgkin's lymphomas. VI. Results
of treatment in childhood. Cancer, 34, 204-211.

Goffinet, R. Warnke, N. R. Dunninck, R. Castellino, E. Glatstein, T. C. Nelsen, R.
F. Dorfman, S. A. Rosenberg and H. S. Kaplan (1977). Clinical and surgical (laparotomy) evaluation of patients with non-Hodgkin's lymphomas. Cancer Treat. Rep.,
61, 981-992.

Gravell, M., P. H. Levine, R. F. McIntyre, V. J. Land and J. S. Pagano (1976). Epstein-Barr virus in an American patient with Burkitt's lymphoma: detection of
viral genome in tumor tissue and establishment of a tumor-derived cell line (NAB).
J. Natl. Cancer Inst., 56, 701.

Hande, K. R., R. R. Reimer and R. I. Fisher. Comparison of nodal versus extranodal
primary histiocytic lymphoma. Can. Treat. Rep., 61, 999-1000.

Hausner, R. J., A. Rosas-Uribe, D. A. Wickstrum and P. C. Smith (1977). Non-Hodgkin's
lymphoma in the first two decades of life. A pathologic study of 30 cases. Cancer,
40, 1533-1547.

Herman, T. S. and S. E. Jones (1977). Systematic re-staging in the management of non-
Hodgkin's lymphomas. Cancer Treat. Rep., 61, 1009-1015.

Hutter, J. J., B. E. Favara, M. Nelson and C. P. Holton (1975). Non-Hodgkin's lymphoma
in children. Correlation of central nervous system disease with initial presentation. Cancer, 36, 2132-2137.

Jackson, H. and F. Parker (1947). Hodgkin's disease and allied disorders. New York,
Oxford University Press, Inc.

Jaffe, E. S., R. C. Braylan, K. Namba, M. M. Frank and C. W. Berard (1977). Functional
markers: A new perspective on malignant lymphomas. Cancer Treat. Rep., 61, 953-962.

Jaffe, N., D. Buell, J. R. Cassady, D. Traggis and H. Weinstein (1977). Role of staging
in childhood non-Hodgkin's lymphoma. Cancer Treat. Rep., 61, 1001-1007.

Jenkin, R. D. T. and M. J. Sonley (1969). The management of malignant lymphoma in
children. In neoplasia in childhood. Chicago, Yearbook Publishers, Inc., pp. 305-
319.

Jones, B. and W. G. Klinberg (1963). Lymphosarcoma in children. J. Ped., 63, 11-20.

Jones, S. E., Z. Fuks, M. Bull, M. D. Kadin, R. F. Dorfman, H. S. Kaplan, S. A. Rosenberg and H. Kim (1973). Non-Hodgkin's lymphomas. IV. Clinicopathologic correlation
in 405 cases. Cancer, 31, 806-823.

Jones, S. E. (1975). Non-Hodgkin's lymphomas. J. Am. Med. Assoc., 234, 633-638.

Kakati, S., A. Freeman, M. Barcos and A. A. Sandberg (1978). Chromosomes and causa-
tions of human cancer and leukemia. XXXV. 14q+ in an American Burkitt lymphoma
and the value of this chromosome anomaly in the definition of lymphoproliferative
disorders (Submitted for publication).

Lemerle, M., R. Gerard-Marchant, H. Sancho and O. Schweisguth (1975). Natural history
of non-Hodgkin's malignant lymphomata in children. A retrospective study of 190
cases. Br. J. Cancer (Suppl. II), 31, 324-331.

Lukes, R. J. and R. D. Collins (1974). Immunologic characterization of human malignant
lymphomas. Cancer, 34, 1488-1503.

Lukes, R. J., C. R. Taylor, J. W. Parker, T. L. Lincoln, P. K. Pattengale and B. H.
Tindle (1978). A morphologic and immunologic surface marker study of 299 cases
of non-Hodgkin's lymphomas and related leukemia. Am. J. Path., 90, 461-485.

Levine, P. H., R. R. Connelly, C. W. Berard, G. T. O'Conor, R. F. Dorfman, M. Easton
and V. T. DeVita (1975). The American Burkitt lymphoma registry: A progress
report. Ann. Int. Med., 83, 31-36.

Mann, R. B., E. S. Jaffe, R. C. Braylan, K. Namba, M. M. Frank, J. L. Ziegler and C. W. Berard (1976). Non-edemic Burkitt's lymphoma. A B-cell tumor related to germinal centers. N. Eng. J. Med., 295, 685-691.

Mandard, A. M., A. Tangoy, J. C. Vernhes, J. S. Arbatucci and J. C. Mandard (1977). Non-Hodgkin's malignant lymphomas. Retrospective study in terms of Kiel's and Rappaport's classifications. Bull. Cancer, 64, 347-364.

Mathe, G., H. Rappaport, G. T. O'Connor (1976). Histological and cytological typing of neoplastic diseases of hematcpcietic and lymphoid tissues. In WHO International Histological Classification of Tumors, No. 14. Geneva, World Health Organization.

Murphy, S. B., G. Frizzera and A. E. Evans (1975). A study of childhood non-Hodgkin's lymphoma. Cancer, 36, 2121-2131.

Murphy, S. B. (1977). Management of childhood non-Hodgkin's lymphoma. Cancer Treat. Rep., 61, 1161-1173.

Musshoff, K. (1977). Clinical staging classification of the non-Hodgkin's lymphomas. Strahlentherapie, 153, 218-221.

Nathwani, B. N., H. Kim and H. Rappaport (1976). Malignant lymphoma, lymphoblastic. Cancer, 38, 964-983.

Nathwani, B. N., H. Kim, H. Rappaport, J. Solomon and M. Fox (1978). Non-Hodgkin's lymphomas. A clinicopathologic study comparing two classifications. Cancer, 41, 303-325.

Nkrumah, F. K. and I. V. Perkins (1976). Burkitt lymphoma. A clinical study of 110 patients. Cancer, 37, 671-676.

Olumide, A. A., B. O. Osonkoya, V. A. Ngu (1971). Superior mediastinal compression: A report of five cases caused by malignant lymphoma. Cancer, 27, 193-202.

Patchefsky, A. S., H. S. Brodovsky, H. Menduke, M. Southard, J. Brooks, D. Nicklas, and W. C. Hoch (1974). Non-Hodgkin's lymphomas - a clinicopathologic study of 293 cases. Cancer, 34, 1173-1186.

Pinkel, D., W. Johnson and R. J. A. Aur (1975). Non-Hodgkin's lymphomas in children. Br. J. Cancer, 31 (Suppl. II), 298-324.

Rappaport, H., W. J. Winter, E. B. Hicks (1956). Follicular lymphoma. A re-evaluation of its position in the scheme of malignant lymphoma, based on a survey of 253 cases. Cancer, 9, 792-821.

Ree, H. J. and L. A. Leone (1978). Prognostic significance of parafollicular small lymphocytes in follicular lymphoma. Clinicopathologic studies of 82 cases of primary nodal origin. Cancer, 41, 1550-1510.

Rosenberg, S. A., H. D. Diamond, H. W. Dargeon and L. F. Craver (1958). Lymphosarcoma in childhood. N. Eng. J. Med., 259, 505-512.

Rosenberg, S. A. (1975). Bone marrow involvement in the non-Hodgkin's lymphomata. Br. J. Cancer, 31 (Suppl. II), 261-264.

Rosenberg, S. A. (1977). Validity of the Ann Arbor Classification for the non-Hodgkin lymphomas. Cancer Treat. Rep., 61, 1023-1027.

Schein, P. S., V. T. DeVita, Jr., S. Hubbard, B. A. Chabner, G. P. Canellos, C. Berard and R. C. Young (1976). Bleomycin, adriamycin, cyclophosphamide, vincristine and prednisone (BACOP) combination chemotherapy in the treatment of advanced diffuse histiocytic lymphoma. Ann. Intern. Med., 85, 417-422.

Schneider, B. K., G. R. Higgins, V. Swanson, H. Isaacs, B. H. Tindle and R. J. Lukes (1978). Malignant lymphomas of childhood (in preparation).

Stein, H., N. Petersen, G. Gaedicke, K. Lennert and G. Landbeck (1976). Lymphoblastic lymphoma of convoluted or acid phosphatase type - a tumor of T precursor cells. Int. J. Cancer, 17, 292-295

Sternberg, C. (1916). Leukosarcoma and myeloblastic leukemia. Beitr. Pathol., 61, 75-100.

Sullivan, M. P. (1973). Non-Hodgkin's lymphoma in childhood. In W. W. Sutow, T. J. Vietti and D. Fernbach, (Eds.), Clinical Pediatric Oncology. C. V. Mosby Co., St. Louis. pp. 313-336.

Sullivan, M. P. (1975). Treatment of lymphoma. Cancer, 35, 991-995.

Taylor, C. R. (1976). *Hodgkin's disease and the lymphomas, Vol. 1* Eden Press, Montreal. pp. 119-124.

Taylor, C. R. (1977). *Hodgkin's disease and the lymphomas. Vol. 2.* Eden Press, Montreal. pp. 195-204.

Ultmann, J. E. (1977). Discussion I. (S. A. Rosenberg, Chairman). Proceedings of the Conference on Non-Hodgkin's lymphomas, San Francisco, 1976. *Cancer Treat. Rep.*, 61, 1029-1036.

Warnke, R. H., H. Kim, Z. Fuks and R. F. Dorfman (1977). The coexistence of nodular and diffuse patterns in nodular non-Hodgkin's lymphomas. Significance and clinicopathologic correlation. *Cancer, 40*, 1229-1233.

Watanabe, A., M. P. Sullivan, W. W. Sutow and J. R. Wilbur (1973). Undifferentiated lymphoma, non-Burkitt type - meningeal and bone marrow involvement in children. *Am. J. Dis. Child., 125*, 57-61.

Webster, R. (1961). Lymphosarcoma of the thymus: its relation to acute leukemia. *Med. J. Australia, 16*, 583.

Williams, A. H., C. R. Taylor, G. R. Higgins, J. J. Quinn, B. K. Schneider, V. Swanson, J. W. Parker, P. K. Pattengale, S. B. Chandor, D. Powars, T. L. Lincoln, B. H. Tindle and R. J. Lukes (1978). Childhood lymphoma - leukemia. I. Correlation of morphology and immunologic studies. *Cancer, 42*, 171-181.

Wright, D. H. (1971). Burkitt's lymphoma - a review of the pathology, immunology and possible etiologic factors. *Path. Annu., 6*, 337-362.

Wollner, N., J. H. Burchenal, P. Exelby, P. H. Lieberman, G. D'Angio and M. L. Murphy (1975). Non Hodgkin's lymphoma in children: a review of 104 cases. In L. F. Sinks and J. O. Godden, (Eds.), *Conflicts in childhood cancer: an evaluation of current management. Progression Clinical and Biological Research*, Vol. 4, Alan Liss, Inc., New York. pp. 179-223.

Wollner, N., J. H. Burchenal, P. H. Lieberman, P. Exelby, G. D. D'Angio and M. L. Murphy (1976). Non-Hodgkin's lymphoma in children. A comparative study of two modalities of therapy. *Cancer, 37*, 123-134.

Ziegler, J. L. (1977). Treatment results of 54 American patients with Burkitt lymphoma are similar to the African experience. *N. Engl. J. Med., 297*, 75-80.

Zech, L., U. Haglund, K. Nilsson and G. Klein (1976). Characteristic chromosomal abnormalities in biopsies and lymphoid-cell lines from patients with Burkitt and non-Burkitt lymphomas. *Int. J. Cancer, 17*, 47.

Survival of Non-Hodgkin's Malignant Lymphomas according to Two Histopathologic Classifications

M. Barcos, U. Kim, J. Pickren, P. Reese, A. Freeman and
L. Stutzman

Roswell Park Memorial Institute, Buffalo, N.Y., U.S.A.

ABSTRACT

Biopsies of 268 previously untreated patients with non-Hodgkin's malignant lymphomas seen from 1971-5 were classified according to the nomenclatures of Rappaport and Lukes-Collins. The nodular (follicular) lymphomas were subdivided into grades (Butler-Stryker-Schullenberg): Grade I: exclusively follicular; Grade II: intermediate; Grade III: focally nodular. Among 95 with nodularity, 56% lived 80 months, while the median survival of 173 with the diffuse pattern was 25 months (p < 0.001). Although 22 Grade III lymphomas showed a less favorable trend than 28 Grade I and 43 Grade II cases, the differences were statistically insignificant. Diffuse lymphomas were significantly unfavorable relative to Grade III lesions.

In the Rappaport classification, high survival (59% at 78 months) occurred with poorly differentiated lymphocytic lymphomas (69 cases). Mixed cell lymphomas (45 cases) had a median survival of 36 months and histiocytic lymphomas (107 cases) 15 months. In the Lukes-Collins classification, high survival (51% at 78 months) was seen with cleaved (small and large) follicular center cell lymphomas (66 cases). The median survivals among mixed (cleaved and non-cleaved) cell (44 cases), small non-cleaved cell (36 cases), and large non-cleaved cell lymphomas (80 cases) were 44, 27 and 15 months, respectively. Thus, statistically significant prediction of survival was achieved by both the Rappaport and Lukes-Collins classifications.

*Keywords: Poorly differentiated lymphocytic lymphoma
Histiocytic lymphoma
Nodular (follicular) lymphoma*

The historical development of morphologic concepts regarding non-Hodgkin's malignant lymphomas has been reviewed by Lukes (1968), who emphasizes the inappropriateness and ambiguity implicit in the terms "lymphosarcoma" and "reticulum cell sarcoma". The terms have been generally abandoned in favor of the classification of Rappaport (1966). This classification defines criteria for distinguishing nodular lymphomas from reactive follicular hyperplasia and serves to resolve the long debated "borderline" lesion known as Brill-Symmers disease. The prognostic validity of the classification has been amply documented (Jones and colleagues, 1973; Schein and colleagues, 1974). However, with the introduction of immunologic assays the developmental origin or nodular lymphomas, including those of the

"histiocytic" type, has been tentatively assigned to follicular center cells. Because of the presence of receptors for complement (Jaffe and colleagues, 1974) and
apparent capacity to synthesize monoclonal immunoglobulin (Levy and colleagues,
1977), nodular lymphomas are considered to represent a neoplastic proliferation
of B lymphocytes. A series of new classifications of lymphomas has appeared
(Bennett, 1974; Dorfman, 1974; Lukes, 1974; Gerard-Marchant, 1974). Among these,
the one proposed by Lukes and Collins (1974) has been used concurrently with the
Rappaport system (1966) in the staging of lymphomas at Roswell Park Memorial Institute. The following data partially summarizes our experience with these
classifications over a recent five-year period.

Methods. An analysis is presented of the histopathologic and prognostic features
of 268 previously untreated patients with non-Hodgkin's malignant lymphomas who
were referred to Roswell Park Memorial Institute between 1971 and 1975. Lymph
node biopsies were classified without prior knowledge of the clinical history
according to the classifications of Rappaport (1966) and of Lukes and Collins
(1974). The nodular (follicular) lymphomas were subtyped into three grades using
the criteria of Butler, Stryker and Schullenberg (1974). Grade I follicular lymphomas are exclusively follicular, Grade II follicular lymphomas show early diffuse
lymphomatous dissemination in the interfollicular areas, and Grade III follicular
lymphomas show predominantly a diffuse pattern with either a focal or vague residual nodularity. The data was studied by life table analysis and Breslow test of
death rates (Breslow, 1970).

Results. There were 31 patients in the age range 3-20 (12%) and 237 adults (88%).
Five of six cases with convoluted lymphocytic lymphoma were previously reported
(Barcos and Lukes, 1975). Sixteen patients in the second decade of life fared
poorly (median survival of 30 months) as compared with 15 patients in the first
decade (66% survival at 72 months); eight patients in the third decade fared best
with a survival of 87% at 77 months (Fig. 1). The median survivals for patients
in decades 4, 5, 6, 7 and 8 were 75, 69, 44, 17 and 35 months respectively.

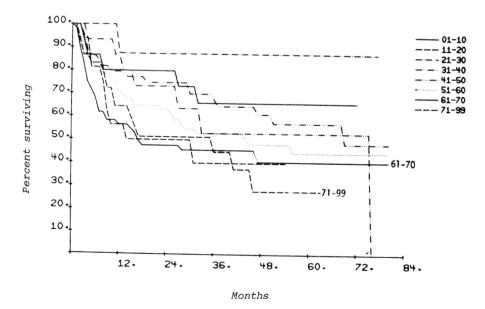

Fig. 1. Survival for patients with malignant lymphoma by decade (years).

*The numbers of male and female patients were 150 (56%) and 118 (44%), respective-
ly. Among males 45 had a follicular pattern with a survival of 51% at 80 months
and 105 had a diffuse pattern with a median survival of 27 months. Among females,
49 had a follicular pattern with a survival of 61% at 78 months and 69 had a diffuse pattern with a median survival of 23 months. The differences in survivals
between male and females in these two major pattern classes were statistically
insignificant.*

*Life tables of survival from the times of admission were constructed for the vari-
ous cell types. There was a statistically significant difference (p<0.001) in the
distribution of survivals among patients with nodular (follicular) versus diffuse
lymphomas, and also among the major cell classes of lymphomas, as defined by the
criteria of Rappaport and of Lukes and Collins, when analyzed with the Breslow
test. The survival of patients (95 cases) with follicular lymphomas at 80 months
was 56%. This was significantly higher than the median survival of 25 months seen
among patients with diffuse lymphomas (173 cases) (Fig. 2). Although a somewhat
less favorable trend was apparent with Grade III follicular lymphomas (22 cases)
compared to Grade I (28 cases) and Grade II (43 cases) lymphomas, the differences
within the three grades were not statistically significant. However, the prognostic importance of distinguishing Grade III lesions from the significantly less
favorable diffuse lymphomas is supported by the data (Fig. 2).*

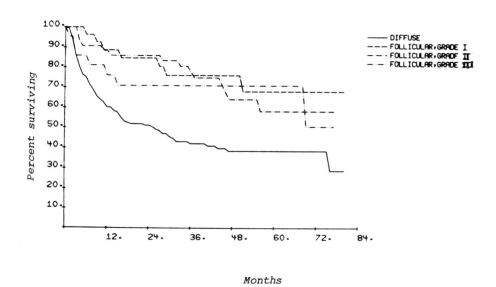

Fig. 2. Survival of patients according to pattern and grade of nodularity.

*Within the three major groups of the Rappaport classification the highest survival
(59% at 78 months) occurred with poorly differentiated lymphocytic lymphomas (69
cases)(Fig. 3). Mixed cell lymphomas (45 cases) had a median survival of 36 months
and histiocytic lymphomas (107 cases) a median survival of 15 months. Among the
four major groups of the Lukes-Collins classification, the highest survival (51%
at 78 months) was seen with cleaved (small and large) cell lymphomas (66 cases)
(Fig. 4). The median survivals among mixed (cleaved and non-cleaved) cell lymphomas (44 cases), small non-cleaved cell lymphomas (36 cases), and large non-cleaved
cell lymphomas (80 cases) were 44, 27 and 15 months, respectively.*

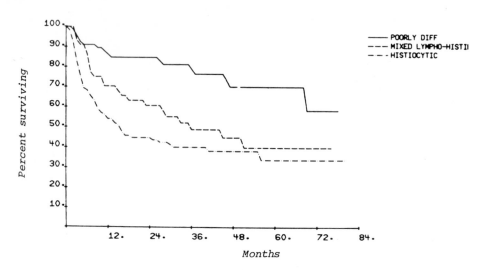

Fig. 3.   *Survival of patients according to Rappaport classification.*

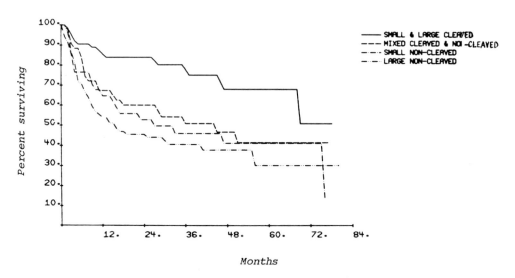

Fig. 4.   *Survival of patients according to Lukes-Collins classification.*

Discussion.   The value of predicting the probability of survival with major cyto-
logic classes of lymphomas as defined by Rappaport and Lukes-Collins was confirmed.
Moreover, when considering these cytologic classes as a group, even minor degrees
of nodularity were predictive of longer survivals than seen with diffuse patterns
of lymph node involvement (Fig. 2).   Our sample size of 95 nodular lymphomas did
not permit a statistical correlation of survival with grade of nodularity in each

cytologic category, but our findings appear to support those of Bagley and others
(1972), Butler and others (1974) and Warnke and others (1977) who reported that
diffuse areas of infiltration did not impart an unfavorable prognosis to poorly
differentiated lymphocytic or cleared cell lymphomas. Patchefsky and others (1974)
however, reported poorer survivals in poorly differentiated lymphocytic lymphomas
of diminished or minimal nodularity. In agreement with Butler and others (1974)
and Nathwani and others (1978) we find that the distinction made by Lukes and
Collins between large cleaved and large non-cleaved follicular center cell lymphomas facilitates the classification of histiocytic lymphomas into groups of favorable and unfavorable prognosis. The equivalence between certain cytologic classes
in the two classifications is not always clear, however, and is problematic.

Acknowledgement. This study was supported in part by grant CA 16065 from the
National Cancer Institute. We thank Joan Solomon and Debra Walsh for their expert
assistance in the collection and processing of the data. This study was also supported in part under contract NIH Nol-CM-67114.

References

Bagley, C. M., V. T. DeVita, Jr., C. W. Berard and G. P. Canellos (1972). Advanced lymphosarcoma - intensive cyclical combination chemotherapy with cyclophosphamide, vincristine, and prednisone. Ann. Intern. Med., 76, 227.

Barcos, M. P. and R. J. Lukes (1975). Malignant lymphoma of convoluted lymphocytes: a new entity of possible T cell type. In L. F. Sinks and J. O. Godden (Ed.), Conflicts in Childhood Cancer. Progress in Clinical and Biological Research, Vol. 4, Alan R. Liss, Inc., New York, p. 147.

Bennett, M. H., G. Farrer-Brown, K. Henry and A. M. Jelliffe (1974). Classification of non-Hodgkin's lymphomas. Lancet, II, 406.

Breslow, N. (1970). A generalized Kruskal-Wallis test for comparing K samples subject to unequal patterns of censorship. Biometrica, 57, 579.

Butler, J. J., J. A. Stryker and C. C. Schullenberg (1974). A clinicopathologic study of stages I and II non-Hodgkin's malignant lymphomata using the Lukes-Collins classification. Br. J. Cancer, 31: Suppl. II, 208.

Dorfman, R. F. (1974). Classification of non-Hodgkin's lymphomas. Lancet, I, 1295.

Gerard-Marchant, R., I. Hamlin, K. Kennett, F. Rilke, A. G. Stansfeld and J. A. M. Van Unnik (1974). Classification of non-Hodgkin's lymphomas. Lancet, II, 406.

Jaffe, E. S., E. M. Shevach, M. M. Frank, C. W. Berard and I. Green (1974). Nodular lymphoma-evidence for origin from follicular B lymphocytes. N. Engl. J. Med., 290, 813.

Jones, S. E., Z. Fuks, M. Bull, M. D. Kadin, R. F. Dorfman, H. D. Kaplan, H. Kim and S. A. Rosenberg (1973). Hodgkin's lymphomas, IV Clinico-pathologic correlation in 405 cases. Cancer, 31, 806.

Levy, R., R. Warnke, R. F. Dorfman, J. Haimovich (1977). The monoclonality of human B-cell lymphomas. J. Exp. Med., 145, 1014.

Lukes, R. J. (1968). The pathologic picture of the malignant lymphomas. In C. J. D. Zarafonetis (Ed.), Proceedings of the International Conference on Leukemia-Lymphoma. Lea and Febiger, Philadelphia. p. 333.

Lukes, R. J. and R. D. Collins (1974). Immunologic characterization of human malignant lymphomas. Cancer, 34, 1488.

Nathwani, B. N., H. Kim, H. Rappaport, J. Solomon and M. Fox (1978). Non-Hodgkin's lymphomas. A clinicopathologic study comparing two classifications. Cancer, 41, 303.

Patchefsky, A. S., H. S. Brodovsky, H. Menduke, M. Southard, J. Brooks, D. Nicklas and W. S. Hoch (1974). Non-Hodgkin's lymphomas - A clinicopathologic study of 293 cases. Cancer, 34, 1173.

Rappaport, H. (1966). Tumors of the hemopoietic system. In Atlas of Tumor Pathology, Sec. III, Fasc. 8, Armed Forces Institute of Pathology, Washington.

Schein, P. S., B. A. Chabner, G. P. Canellos, R. C. Young, C. W. Berard and V. T. DeVita (1974). Potential for prolonged disease-free survival following combination chemotherapy of non-Hodgkin's lymphomas. Blood, 43, 181.

Warnke, R. A., H. Kim, Z. Fuks and R. F. Dorfman (1977). The coexistence of nodular and diffuse patterns in nodular non-Hodgkin's lymphomas. Significance and clinicopathologic correlation. Cancer, 40, 1229.

Malignant Lymphomas: an Exercise in Immunopathology

C. R. Taylor, J. W. Parker, P. K. Pattengale and R. J. Lukes

Department of Pathology, Los Angeles County/University of Southern California Medical Center, Los Angeles, California, U.S.A.

ABSTRACT

The belief that neoplastic cells mimic the morphology and behavior of their normal progenitor cells is implicit in most classifications of neoplastic disease. The aim of this paper is to relate the various histological and clinical types of malignant lymphoma to current knowledge of the morphology and behavior of the lymphocyte. There is evidence that several aspects of normal lymphocyte function govern the histological appearances and behavioral patterns of lymphocytic neoplasms. These include:
 (1) The division of lymphocytes into two separate functioning subgroups (B cells and T cells);
 (2) The radical morphologic and functional changes occurring in the course of lymphocyte transformation, a physiologic response of the lymphocyte to antigen;
 (3) Lymphocyte circulation;
 (4) Lymphocyte 'homing' to specific areas of the lymphoid organs.
In addition, malignant lymphomas frequently develop against the background of an abnormal or sustained immune response, supporting the concept that lymphomas occur as aberrations of normal lymphocyte proliferation.

This paper seeks to re-examine some of the extablished morphologic concepts of lymphoma with reference to the results of studies attempting to correlate the morphologic and immunologic characteristics of the neoplastic cells. The relationship of the various neoplastic cell types to current knowledge of the variation in form and function of the lymphocyte, according to its state of physiological activation, is given particular emphasis.

key words: surface markers, lymphoma, leukemia, immunoperoxidase

INTRODUCTION

Changes in the nomenclature and classification of malignant neoplasms of the lymphoreticular system follow closely upon changing concepts of the nature of the lymphoreticular system and its component cells (Taylor, 1977). The purpose of this paper is to consider our current understanding of the nature and interrelations of the malignant lymphomas in the light of present day immunologic theories of the function of the lymphocyte.

125

BACKGROUND

Implicit in all the classifications of neoplasia, including lymphoma, is the assumption that the neoplastic cells mimic the morphologic forms and behavioral patterns of the normal cell population from which they are derived.

>   "There occur tumours corresponding to almost all kinds of normal tissues, and clearly our classification of tumours will run parallel with our classification of normal tissues." (Willis, 1948)

The concept of the reticulum cell as the central hemopoietic stem cell provided the basis for many classifications of lymphoreticular neoplasms (Ewing, 1928; Ross, 1932; Callender, 1934; Robb-Smith, 1938; Warren and Picena, 1942; Jackson and Parker, 1948; Marshall, 1956;—cited in Taylor, 1977, 1978d), some of which endured for many years (Robb-Smith, 1964). The publication of Rappaport's classification in 1956 (Rappaport, Winter and Hicks, 1956) signified the beginning of the end of the reticulum cell and introduced a new era of histologic diagnosis of lymphoma based upon the concept of two principal neoplastic cell types (lymphocyte and histiocyte). This classification gained wide acceptance over a period of 10 years for its ease of application and its clinical usefulness, but was in turn rendered obsolete by advances in basic immunology that resulted in a radical revision of previous concepts concerning the role and potentialities of the small lymphocyte. This presaged a profound change in our understanding of the functioning of the lymphoreticular system and its component cells. Inevitably, the rapid expansion of knowledge in basic immunology spilled over into clinical pathology, resulting in a rash of new lymphoma classifications (Bennett and colleagues, 1974; Diebold, 1975; Dorfman, 1974; Lennert, Stein and Kaiserling, 1975; Lukes and Collins, 1975; Mathe and Rappaport, 1976), as pathologists attempted to integrate the concepts of the immunologists with preexisting ideas of the nature and interrelations of lymphoreticular cells and their neoplastic derivatives.

Immunologically-Based Classifications

The translation of the methods of the experimental immunologist into clinical pathology has furthered the study of human lymphoproliferative diseases and has permitted critical examination of the biologic validity of recently proposed classifications (Taylor, 1977, 1978d). As a result of such studies, two of these schemes, namely those of Lennert and colleagues (1975) and Lukes and Collins (1975) have attained some degree of popular acceptance in different parts of the world. This paper presents a critical examination of the concepts underlying one of these schemes (that of Lukes and Collins) with a view to achieving a more logical understanding of the process of lymphoid neoplasia. Immunologic and morphologic studies performed on a leukemia/lymphoma cell population at Los Angeles County/University of Southern California Medical Center provide the basis of this analysis and discussion.

MATERIALS AND METHODS

The case population studied has been described in detail elsewhere. At the end of 1976, 299 cases had been studied (Lukes and colleagues, 1978a). In September, 1977, the number had risen to 425 (Lukes and colleagues, 1978b). Patients were drawn from the Los Angeles County/University of Southern California Medical Center, from Children's Hospital of Los Angeles, and from the 28 participating hospitals of the Southern California Lymphoma Group.

Tissue, blood, or bone marrow specimens were obtained in all cases and were examined by orthodox histological and cytological techniques for the purposes of diagnosis and classification. Immunologic cell surface marker techniques (Table 1) (Taylor, 1977, 1978a) were applied to suspensions of neoplastic cells, obtained from tissue homogenates, bone marrow, blood or other tissue fluids prior to therapy. A panel of cytochemical stains (Lukes and colleagues, 1978a, 1978b) was employed on cell imprints or smears of each case, and formalin fixed paraffin embedded tissues were

examined for the presence of monoclonal cytoplasmic immunoglobulin or lysozyme by
an immunoperoxidase method. Details of the practical procedures employed have been
published elsewhere (surface markers: Lukes and colleagues, 1978a, 1978b; Taylor,
1977, 1978a; immunoperoxidase methods: Taylor, 1974, 1978b, 1978c) and for this
reason will not be reiterated here.

TABLE 1   Techniques Most Commonly Used For Identification
of T Cells, B Cells, and Histiocytes

	T cells	B cells	Histiocytes Monocytes	Comments
Sponteneous sheep red cell (E) rosette	+	-	-	Most useful T cell marker
EAC (IgM) (complement receptor) rosette	(+)	+	+	Probably some T cells. Convoluted T cell lymphomas are observed with complement receptors
EA (IgG) (Fc receptor) rosette	-	+	+	Limited usefulness
Surface Ig*	-	+	(+)	By immunofluorescence. Monocytes may mark because of Fc receptors
Cytoplasmic Ig	-	+	-	Immunoperoxidase more useful than immunofluorescence in lymphomas because can be used on paraffin sections
Cytochemistry α-Naphthyl butyrase (NSE)	(+)	-	+	Focal staining reported in T cells. Specificity for T cells is not proved
Acid phosphatase	(+)	-	-	Reported in convoluted T cell and T cell ALL
Tartrate-resistant acid phosphatase	-	(+)	-	Hairy cell leukemia
Muramidase (lysozyme)	-	-	+	Immunoperoxidase method on paraffin sections or imprints

*T cells have a small amount of surface Ig not detected by immunofluorescence methods.

Ig = immunoglobulin; NSE = nonspecific esterase; parentheses indicate that
the finding lacks specificity, is controversial, or is only seen with certain
types of lymphoma-leukemia.

Methodology is described in detail elsewhere (Lukes and colleagues, 1978a,
1978b; Taylor, 1977, 1978a, 1978b, 1978c).

C. R. Taylor *et al.*

TABLE 2   Morphologic/Immunologic Classification of
Lymphocytic Neoplasia

Morphologic Division[1] (cell type)	Immunologic Division		
	B cell	T cell	'Non-marking'*
Small lymphocyte	lymphocytic lymphoma/ leukemia (includes B-CLL)	lymphocytic lymphoma/ leukemia (includes T-CLL)	*
Follicular center cell (FCC)	FCC lymphoma/leukemia[2] (cleaved or non-cleaved)	—[3]	*
Convoluted lymphocyte[4] (Lymphoblast)[4]	— —[5]	convoluted lymphocytic lymphoma/leukemia lymphoblastic lymphoma/ leukemia	* ALL
Immunoblast	immunoblastic sarcoma	immunoblastic sarcoma	*
Plasmacytoid lymphocyte	plasmacytoid lymphocytic lymphoma/leukemia	—	*
Plasma cell	plasmacytoma/myeloma	—	*
Hairy cell	hairy cell leukemia	—	*
Small lymphocyte with epithelioid cells	—	lymphoepithelioid cell lymphoma	*
Cerebriform lymphocyte	—	Sezary/mycosis fungoides	*
Unclassified	+	+	+

[1]Modified from Lukes and Collins (1975).

[2]Small cleaved and small non-cleaved FCC lymphomas frequently show early peripheral blood and marrow involvement (see footnote 5).

[3]Nodular T cell lymphomas occur rarely. These probably should be considered as distinct from follicular center cell tumors which, be definition, are of B cell type. In FCC lymphoma large numbers of reactive T cells may be found in the follicles along with neoplastic B cells (Jaffe and colleagues, 1977).

[4]This category is difficult to define due to the continuing controversy over whether or not convoluted cells are always recognizable in this form of lymphoma, in which leukemic manifestations are common (Barcos and Lukes, 1975; Nathwani, Kim and Rappaport, 1976). ALL (acute lymphoblastic leukemia) appears to be a related process. The use of the term 'lymphoblastic' implying a relationship with ALL thus seems a reasonable compromise, though it lacks strict morphologic definition (Taylor, 1978a, 1978d).

[5]The Burkitt-like lymphoma/leukemia (small non-cleaved cell), though typically morphologically distinct, should also be considered related to the lymphoblastic category of lymphoma/leukemia.

*Non-marking category includes 'undefined' cell type of Lukes and Collins (1975) and the broader 'null' cell group of other investigators. Cases falling in the non-marking category are relatively uncommon except for ALL.

RESULTS

A modified version (Table 2) of the original Lukes/Collins morphologic classification has been used in this report, to specifically include plasmacytoma/myeloma,
which appears to be closely related to other B cell neoplasms in terms of cellular
derivation (Taylor, 1974, 1978a, 1978c, 1978d), although its clinical behavior is
distinct. Similarly, lymphoepithelioid cell lymphoma has been included, for it appears to relate to other neoplastic conditions of the T cell series (Lukes and colleagues, 1978a, 1978b). The non-marking group includes the "null" cell category of
other investigators and the "undefined" group of Lukes and Collins. In its original
usage (Lukes and Collins, 1975) the undefined cell group referred to cases in which
neoplastic cells "lacked discriminating membrane markers or cytochemical indicators."
The majority of cases in the non-marking group fell into the clinical category of
acute lymphoblastic (lymphocytic) leukemia, the residuum consisting of a small number of cases of immunoblastic sarcoma, together with some histologically unclassifiable cases. In addition, the neoplastic cells of other morphologic types sometimes showed low marker scores for unresolved technical or biologic reasons. Interpretation of such cases as of B or T cell type was sometimes difficult, and was
only accomplished by the combined use of morphologic and immunologic parameters
(Lukes and colleagues, 1978a).

The results of combined morphologic and immunologic studies of malignant lymphoma
and leukemia offer substantial support to the concept that lymphocytic neoplasms
can be related to normal lymphocyte morphology and function. Of 425 lymphocytic
neoplasms studied by combined morphologic, cytochemical, immunohistologic and surface marker methods, 68% appeared to be of B cell type and 18% of T cell type. In
13% the cell type remained undefinable by the techniques employed. Only one case
showed surface marker and enzyme staining characteristics consistent with a histiocytic origin. These studies have been reported in full elsewhere (Lukes and colleagues, 1978b). The morphologic subtypes of the 425 cases of lymphoma/leukemia
(Lukes and colleagues, 1978b), classified according to the modified Lukes/Collins
classification, and their B and T cell derivations are summarized in Table 3. The
results of immunoperoxidase studies of 444 cases (Taylor, 1978c) are summarized in
Table 4. The immunoperoxidase study included some cases (e.g. cases of multiple
myeloma) in which fresh material was not available for study by surface marker
methods. The results of 113 cases upon which both surface marker and immunoperoxidase studies were performed are summarized in Table 5.

DISCUSSION

It has been postulated that neoplastic lymphocytes may mimic the morphology and
behavior of the normal lymphocyte population from which they are derived (reviews—
Taylor, 1977, 1978a, 1978d). The results of the studies reported here, and the
results of others drawn from the literature, will be discussed in conjunction with
four facets of normal lymphocyte behavior and function that may be expressed, to a
greater or lesser degree, by neoplastic lymphocytes:
  (1) The functional separation of lymphocytes into B cells and T cells;
  (2) The morphological and behavioral changes occurring in lymphocyte transfor-
      mation;
  (3) Lymphocyte circulation;
  (4) Lymphocyte homing.

(1) The Functional Division into T Cells and B Cells

The division of malignant lymphomas into B or T cell functional subtypes was proposed in the initial classification of Lukes and Collins (1975). Subsequent application of surface marker techniques to the study of lymphoproliferative disease in
man has confirmed the essence of this proposition, and has contributed to a clearer

C. R. Taylor *et al.*

TABLE 3 Percentage Distribution of Morphologic Subtypes of
425 Cases of Lymphoma Studied by Combined Morphologic
and Surface Marker Methods[1]

	B cell	T cell	Undefined cell[2]
Small lymphocyte	9.1	2.3	*
Follicular center cell	45.0	—	*
Convoluted lymphocyte (Lymphoblast)[3]	—[4]	9.6 —	*(12.9)
Immunoblast	3.5	3.5	*
Plasmacytoid lymphocyte	6.8	—	*
Plasma cell	none studied		
Hairy cell	3.3	—	*
Small lymphocyte with epithelioid cells	—	0.9	*
Cerebriform lymphocyte	—	2.1	*
	69%	18%	13%

One non-lymphocytic tumor of probable histiocytic origin was identified.

---

[1]Modified from Lukes and colleagues (1978b).

[2]The 'undefined' category includes only those 'non-marking' cases which could not be assigned to B or T cell class on the basis of morphology, e.g. a morphologically typical case of FCC lymphoma or plasmacytoid lymphocytic lymphoma would, by definition, be assigned to the B cell group, even if it failed to show clear immunologic marking. It is recognized that 'non-marking' or 'low marking' may occur for technical reasons, or it may reflect the biology of the tumor cell, as is thought to be the case in ALL.

[3]See footnote 4, Table 2.

[4]See footnote 5, Table 2. The percentage figure for FCC small non-cleaved lymphoma/leukemia was 6.8%.

TABLE 4   Results of Immunoperoxidase Studies in Non-Hodgkin
Lymphomas[1]

	Total	Tumor Cell Ig Negative[2]	Tumor Cell Ig Positive[2] (Monoclonal)	(Anomalous)[3]	Poor Quality[4]
Immunoblastic sarcoma (IBS)	122	53	38	14	17
Follicular center cell lymphoma	132	58	44	11	19
Plasmacytoid lympho-cytic lymphoma	28	2	17	4	5
Myeloma	29	0	18	8	3
'Reticulum cell sarcoma brain'[5]	24	5	11	2	6
Lymphoepithelioid lymphoma	6	6	0	0	0
Convoluted lymphoma	6	6	0	0	0
Secondary Carcinoma/ Anaplastic tumor	40	22	0	5	11
Reactive lymphade-nopathy		57 cases, variable numbers of plasma cells with polyclonal pattern, 3 possible monoclonal			
Total	444				

[1]Modified from Taylor (1978c).

[2]Ig positive reactive plasma cells were present in almost all cases, together with variable proportions of immunoglobulin positive immunoblasts in some cases. These stained with a polyclonal pattern, but their presence made the detection of an associated underlying monoclonal population difficult or impossible in some cases.

[3]Pattern of tumor cell staining not consistent with usual concepts of monoclonality.

[4]Includes cases in which there were inadequate numbers of cells for study, or in which fixation was apparently poor. In some cases this could be attributed to necrosis or extensive autolysis; in others the nature of the fixation process was unknown.

[5]The archaic term 'reticulum cell sarcoma' can be considered to include cases now classified as immunoblastic sarcoma. These cases are described in detail elsewhere (Taylor and colleagues, 1978).

C. R. Taylor *et al.*

TABLE 5   Summary of Combined Immunoperoxidase and Surface
Marker Studies Showing Marking of
Recognizable Tumor Cells

| Classification Category (Table 2) | No. | Ig in Cytoplasm | | | Surface Ig | | | E Rosette Positive[3] |
		Neg.	Mono-clonal[1]	Poly-clonal	Mono-clonal[1]	Poly-clonal or low[2]	Neg.	
Immunoblastic sarcoma-B	7	0	7	0	5	1	1	0
Immunoblastic sarcoma-T	13	11	1	1	0	10	3	13
Immunoblastic sarcoma-'non-marking'	2	1	0	1	0	2	0	0
Follicular center cell lymphoma	57	26	28	3	38	19	0	0[4]
Plasmacytoid lymphocytic lymphoma	12	0	11	1	10	2	0	0
Small lympho-cyte - B	8	7	1	0	7	1	0	0
Small lympho-cyte - T	5	5	0	0	0	3	2	5
Small lympho-cyte with epithelioid cells	3	3	0	0	0	3	0	3
Convoluted lymphoma	6	6	0	0	0	3	3	6
	113	59	48	6	60	44	9	27

[1]Monoclonal: cases in which the tumor cell population stained exclusively for one light chain and one heavy chain.

[2]Polyclonal or low: cases in which the SIg pattern was not obviously monoclonal, including those cases with very low percentages of SIg positive tumor cells.

[3]Lymphomas were designated E rosette positive when lymphoma cells formed spontaneous rosettes with sheep erythrocytes as viewed in stained cytocentrifuge preparations.

[4]Three nodular T cell tumors were observed; these are considered to be distinct from FCC lymphomas which, by definition, are of B cell type.

definition of B and T cell lymphocytic neoplasms (Jaffe and colleagues, 1977; Lennert, 1975; Lukes and colleagues, 1978a, 1978b; Stein, 1976).

Normal B and T lymphocytes cannot be distinguished reliably by morphological criteria, but only by surface marker methods. It might be expected that the corresponding neoplastic cells of B or T cell type might also be indistinguishable by morphology alone. However, in examining neoplastic cells by light microscopy, one assesses and compares cell populations rather than individual cells. On this basis there appear to be some real distinctions between certain B and T cell neoplasms.

The distinguishing morphological features of the B lymphocyte in the follicular center phase of its life cycle were the first to be clearly recognized (Kojima, Imai and Mori, 1973; Lennert, 1973; Lukes and Collins, 1973), and the recognition of follicular center cell lymphomas in fact preceded more comprehensive T and B cell subclassifications of lymphoma. Several other B and T cell lymphomas have since been distinguished by surface marker techniques, but are more difficult to identify by morphology alone. Distinctive morphological features (convoluted cell type) were ascribed to an aggressive lymphoma/leukemia particularly prevalent in young males and presenting as a mediastinal mass, as lymphadenopathy or as acute lymphocytic leukemia (Barcos and Lukes, 1975). The characteristic convoluted morphology has been observed in a varying proportion of cells, with varying degrees of facility by different observers, according to the precise criteria employed (Nathwani, Kim and Rappaport, 1976). Cases of this pathological entity are now accepted, on the basis of surface marker studies, as being of T lymphocytic origin (Jaffe and colleagues, 1977; Lukes and colleagues, 1978a, 1978b).

Finally, with regard to B cell/T cell distinction by morphology, there is growing evidence that immunoblastic sarcoma is also divisible into B and T cell subtypes. This condition, that previously passed under the terms reticulum cell sarcoma (Robb-Smith, 1964) or malignant lymphoma histiocytic (Rappaport, Winter and Hicks, 1956), appears to represent the neoplastic analogue of the transformed lymphocyte (vide infra). Surface marker and immunoperoxidase studies have revealed a B and T cell subdivision of tumors of this basic morphologic type, and have led to the recognition of several morphological criteria for distinguishing B immunoblastic sarcoma from T immunoblastic sarcoma in most cases (Lukes and colleagues, 1978b; Robb-Smith and Taylor, 1978; Taylor, 1978a, 1978c).

(2) The Morphological Changes Associated with Lymphocyte Transformation

Formerly the small lymphocyte was regarded as a quiescent end stage cell. Its potential for radical morphological and functional changes following antigenic stimulation was revealed in the process of lymphocyte transformation, and the small B lymphocyte was recognized as the precursor of the plasma cell series (Nossal and Ada, 1971). In fact, following specific antigenic stimulation, B lymphocytes bearing immunoglobulin receptors undergo metamorphosis to large transformed lymphocytes (or immunoblasts) (Dameschek, 1963) prior to maturation to the plasma cell (Fig. 1). These large transformed lymphocytes (immunoblasts) have no morphological resemblance to the lymphocytes from which they are derived. Prior to the advent of cellular immunology, such cells were considered to constitute a class entirely separate from lymphocytes and were regarded as varieties of reticulum cells or histiocytes. Thus the malignant counterparts of these cells formerly were designated as either reticulum cell sarcoma or malignant lymphoma histiocytic (Taylor, 1977, 1978a, 1978d). However, using immunological marker methods, these cells may now be recognized as transformed B or T lymphocytes (Jaffe and colleagues, 1977; Lennert, 1975; Lukes and colleagues, 1978a, 1978b; Stein, 1976; Taylor, 1974). The corresponding neoplasms are thus properly termed immunoblastic sarcomas, and further can be subdivided into B or T cell subtypes as described above.

C. R. Taylor *et al.*

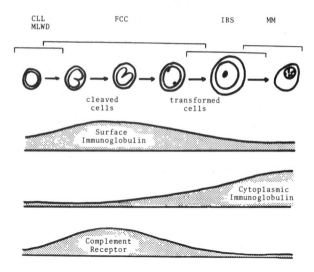

Fig. 1. Schematic representation of principal
B cell lymphomas to the process of B lymphocyte
transformation (including the follicular center
stage) and maturation to the plasma cell.
Variations in the expression of surface immunoglobulin, cytoplasmic immunoglobulin and complement receptor are indicated by the shaded areas.
The neoplastic cells mimic the morphology and
behavior of their normal counterparts (from
Taylor, 1977).

The different morphological types of lymphoma can be related to this transformation-
maturation process according to the concept that neoplastic lymphocytes mimic the
morphology and behavior of their corresponding normal counterparts (Fig. 1). Thus
small lymphocytic lymphoma, follicular center cell lymphoma, immunoblastic sarcoma,
and plasmacytoma/myeloma can now be seen to be various expressions of neoplasms of
a single cell type, the B lymphocyte, rather than four entirely distinct neoplasms
as implied by earlier classification schemes (Taylor, 1978a, 1978d). This is not
to imply that morphological distinctions between these neoplasms are valueless, for
there are real differences in clinical behavior which influence the prognosis and
the choice of therapy. However, it may ultimately be of more value to both pathologist and clinician to recognize the essential common origin of these four neoplasms, realizing that intermediate forms may occur, rather than to continue to
consider these diseases to be entirely separate processes. The radical differences
in histological appearance between the four B cell tumors listed above may then be
explained on the basis of a predominance of one or another of the different morphological variants of the B lymphocyte (Taylor, 1977, 1978a, 1978d). The concept is
summarized in Fig. 2.

A similar scheme to that proposed above may be prepared for the T cell lymphomas,
taking account of the transformation of the small T lymphocyte to the T immunoblast.
However, the product of T lymphocyte transformation, namely the sensitized effector
T cell, is not distinguishable on morphologic grounds from the small T cell prior
to transformation. In addition, a further complication in defining the various
stages of T cell transformation is the lack of a good immunological or immunohistological marker in the T cell series, corresponding to surface or cytoplasmic immunoglobulin in the B cell series.

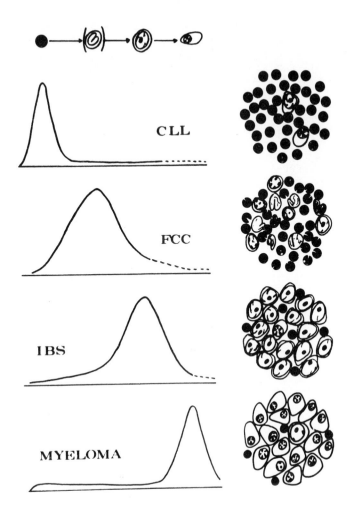

Fig. 2. Interrelations of B cell neoplasms.
Schematic depicts four different B cell neoplasms as
composed of the same three basic morphologic forms of
the B cell, namely the small lymphocyte, the immunoblast and the plasma cell, illustrated at the top of
the figure as morpholgic phases in B cell transfor-
mation/maturation (Fig. 1). The different histologic
pictures are produced simply by changes in the proportions of the different forms of the B cell within the
neoplastic clone. FCC lymphoma forms a partial exception in that a special variant of the B cell (the
cleaved cell), representing an intermediate stage of B
cell transformation in the follicle, is also present.
CLL=chronic lymphocytic leukemia/small lymphocytic
lymphoma; FCC=follicular center cell lymphoma; IBS=
immunoblastic sarcoma (B cell type).

(3) Lymphocyte Circulation

The work of Gowans and Knight (1964) demonstrated that small lymphocytes circulate extensively throughout the blood, lymph and peripheral lymphoid organs. The process of lymphocyte circulation appears to constitute an essential part of the function of the lymphocyte in the immune system (Nossal and Ada, 1971). In the resting non-antigenically stimulated host the majority of the circulating lymphocytes have the morphological appearance of small lymphocytes. However, following antigenic stimulation, increased numbers of partially transformed cells enter the efferent lymph and hence the peripheral blood (Hall and colleagues, 1967) and serve to disseminate the immune response to all the lymphoid tissues of the body.

Again, following the hypothesis that neoplastic lymphocytes mimic the behavior of their normal counterparts, it is possible to relate the clinicopathological course of various lymphocytic neoplasms to the behavior of the corresponding normal lymphocyte types. For example, lymphocytic neoplasms composed primarily of small lymphocytes frequently show a large or even predominating circulating cell component, and appear as chronic lymphocytic leukemia. In other cases, a non-circulating cell component predominates and the disease manifests as lymphocytic lymphoma well differentiated, though in many cases examination of peripheral blood by surface marker methods reveals that part of the neoplastic clone is in fact circulating. In this respect, CLL and lymphocytic lymphoma may be regarded as two ends of a spectrum of disease with many intermediate expressions (Braylan and colleagues, 1976) depending upon the proportion of the neoplastic cells in the circulating phase.

A similar situation appears to exist in relation to acute lymphoblastic leukemia (ALL) of childhood. Combined immunologic and morphologic studies reveal a continuous spectrum of disease from the overt leukemic to the frankly lymphomatous (Coccia and colleagues, 1976; Williams and colleagues, 1978). Immunological studies show that the leukemic forms are mostly non-marking (null cell), while the lymphomas most often show B (small non-cleaved, Burkitt-like) or T (convoluted or lymphoblastic) cell markers (see Tables 2 and 3).

In follicular center cell lymphoma the great majority of the neoplastic cells are confined to the tissues. Nevertheless, examination of peripheral blood, using surface marker methods, has revealed that circulating lymphoma cells are present in a proportion of cases (Gajl-Peczalska and colleagues, 1975; Garrett, Newton and Scarffe, 1977), and carry the same monoclonal immunoglobulin markers as shown by the tissue lymphoma cells. In some of these cases the circulating cell component is recognizable by morphological criteria (cleaved cells). In immunoblastic sarcoma and plasmacytoma/myeloma the predominant neoplastic cells, resembling the immunoblast or plasma cell respectively, are rarely detected in the circulation in a morphologically recognizable form. However, studies of idiotypic immunoglobulin markers in multiple myeloma (Mellstedt, Hammarstrom and Holm, 1974; Mellstedt, Petterson and Holm, 1976) have revealed that some cells of the neoplastic clone do in fact circulate, though these are not recognizable by morphologic criteria as they are cytologically indistinguishable from normal small lymphocytes.

Thus with reference to certain B cell lymphomas the overall disease presentation, as lymphoma or leukemia, appears to be governed by the degree to which the neoplastic lymphocytes reproduce the behavior of their normal counterparts (circulation, homing, etc.). However, as illustrated in Fig. 2, not all of the neoplastic cells necessarily display the same morphologic and behavioral characteristics, and in many cases (e.g. myeloma and follicular center cell lymphoma) subpopulations of the neoplastic clone may manifest morphologic and behavioral attributes at variance with the predominant cell type upon which classification is based (Taylor, 1978a, 1978d).

Again, less evidence is available with reference to T cell lymphomas, but in general small lymphocytes may manifest primarily as leukemia, large immunoblastic neoplasms manifest primarily as lymphoma, and neoplasms of cells of intermediate type may present anywhere along the spectrum of lymphoma to leukemia or may show mixed manifestations. These patterns of behavior correlate to those anticipated by analogy with the corresponding normal cell types.

(4) Lymphocyte Homing

Studies of lymphocyte depleted animals following thymectomy, bursectomy, and a variety of lymphocyte reconstitution experiments, reveal not only that lymphocytes circulate, but also that B and T lymphocytes preferentially "home" to certain anatomical regions or zones within the peripheral lymphoid tissue (Nossal and Ada, 1971). Thus within the lymph node, B lymphocytes particularly localize in follicular center cell areas (cortex), and T lymphocytes localize within the deep cortex (paracortex). Within the spleen the corresponding areas are the B cell follicle and the pariarteriolar lymphocyte sheath (T zone) (Nossal and Ada, 1971). In addition, T lymphocytes show a propensity to localize within the superficial dermis.

The pattern of tissue involvement by B or T cell lymphocytic neoplasms may in many cases be more easily understood with reference to these normal patterns of B and T lymphocyte circulation and homing. Thus lymphomas of follicular center cells not surprisingly, form follicles, and the loss of obvious follicle formation as occurs in diffuse follicular center cell lymphomas, might then be interpreted as giving evidence of some loss of functional differentiation. T cell lymphocytic neoplasms appear particularly to involve the paracortical areas of the lymph node (T zone lymphoma, Lennert) (Lennert, 1975; Stein, 1976), or when composed of small T lymphocytes with a prominent circulating component, often seem also to involve the skin (Sezary syndrome, T cell CLL) (Brouet and colleagues, 1975).

CONCLUSIONS

Lymphocytic neoplasms may best be understood by reference to the behavior of the corresponding normal lymphocyte (Taylor, 1978a, 1978d). This is not a novel idea, and in fact represents nothing more than the application to lymphocytic neoplasms of principles applied to neoplasia in general (Willis, 1948). Knowing the morphology of a lymphocytic neoplasm, it is possible to predict the probable pattern of nodal involvement, whether or not it is likely to circulate (leukemia), whether or not it is a rapidly proliferating tumor (the proportion of transformed lymphocytes), and whether it is of B or T cell subtype. The converse is also true, that knowing something of the immunologic, clinical, and behavioral patterns of a neoplastic lymphocyte population, it is possible to some degree to predict its morphology.

REFERENCES

Barcos, M. P. and R. J. Lukes (1975). Malignant lymphoma of convoluted lymphocytes:
   a new entity of possible T-cell type. In L. F. Sinks and J. O. Godden (Eds.),
   Conflicts in Childhood Cancer: An Evaluation of Current Management. Alan R.
   Liss, Inc., New York. p. 147.

Bennett, M. Y., G. Farrer-Brown, K. Henry and A. M. Jeliffe (1974). Classification
   of non-Hodgkin's lymphomas. *Lancet* 2, 405-406.

Braylan, R. C., E. S. Jaffe, J. W. Burbach, M. M. Frank, R. E. Johnson and C. W.
   Berard (1976). Similarities of surface characteristics of neoplastic well-
   differentiated lymphocytes from solid tissues and from peripheral blood. *Cancer
   Res* 36, 1619-1625.

Brouet, J. C., G. Flandrin, M. Sasportes, J. L. Preud'homme and M. Seligmann (1975).
   Chronic lymphocytic leukaemia of T-cell origin. Immunological and clinical evaluation in eleven patients. *Lancet* 2, 890-893.

Coccia, P. F., J. H. Kersey, J. Kazamiera, K. J. Gajl-Peczalska, W. Krivit and
   M. E. Nesbit (1976). Prognostic significance of surface marker analysis in
   childhood non-Hodgkin's lymphoproliferative malignancies. *Am J Hematol* 1, 405-
   417.

Dameshek, W. (1963). "Immunoblasts" and "Immunocytes"—An attempt at a functional
   nomenclature. *Blood* 21, 243-245.

Diebold, J. (1975). Classifications morphologiques des hématosarcomes lymphoides
   non hodgkiniens. *Nouv Presse Med* 4, 1046, 1048.

Dorfman, R. F. (1974). Classification of non-Hodgkin's lymphomas. *Lancet* 1, 1295-
   1296.

Gajl-Peczalska, K. J., C. D. Bloomfield, P. F. Coccia, H. Sosin, R. D. Brunning and
   J. G. Kersey (1975). B and T cell lymphomas. Analysis of blood and lymph node
   in 87 patients. *Am J Med* 59, 674-685.

Garrett, J. V., R. K. Newton and J. H. Scarffe (1977). Abnormal blood lymphocytes
   in non-Hodgkin's lymphoma. *Lancet* 1, 542.

Gowans, J. L. and E. J. Knight (1964). The route of re-circulation of lymphocytes
   in the rat. *Proc R Soc London Ser B* 159, 257-282.

Hall, J. G., B. Morris, G. Moreno and M. Bessis (1967). The ultrastructure and
   function of the cells in lymph following antigenic stimulation. *J Exp Med* 125,
   91-110.

Jaffe, E. S., R. C. Braylan, K. Nanba, M. M. Frank and C. W. Berard (1977).
   Functional markers: a new perspective on malignant lymphomas. *Cancer Treat Rep*
   61, 953-962.

Kojima, M., Y. Imai and N. Mori (1973). A concept of follicular lymphoma. A pro-
   posal for the existence of a neoplasm originating from the germinal center. In
   Malignant Diseases of the Hematopoietic System. *Gann Monograph on Cancer
   Research 15*. University of Tokyo Press, Tokyo. p. 195.

Lennert, K. (1973). Follicular lymphoma. A tumor of the germinal centers. In
   Malignant Diseases of the Hematopoietic System. *Gann Monograph on Cancer
   Research 15*. University of Tokyo Press, Tokyo. p. 217.

Lennert, K. (1975). Morphology and classification of malignant lymphomas and so-
    called reticuloses. *Acta Neuropathol Suppl* 6, 1-16.

Lennert, K., H. Stein and E. Kaiserling (1975). Cytological and functional criteria
    for the classification of malignant lymphomata. *Br J Cancer* 31, *Suppl* 2, 29-43.

Lukes, R. J. and R. D. Collins (1973). New observations on follicular lymphoma. In
    *Malignant Diseases of the Hematopoietic System. Gann Monograph on Cancer
    Research 15*. University of Tokyo Press, Tokyo. p. 209.

Lukes, R. J. and R. D. Collins. New approaches to the classification of the lympho-
    mata. *Br J Cancer* 31, *Suppl* 2, 1-28.

Lukes, R. J., C. R. Taylor, J. W. Parker, T. L. Lincoln, P. K. Pattengale and B. H.
    Tindle (1978a). Morphologic and immunologic surface marker study of 299 cases
    of non-Hodgkin's lymphomas and related leukemias. *Am J Pathol* 90, 461-485.

Lukes, R. J., J. W. Parker, C. R. Taylor, B. H. Tindle, A. D. Cramer and T. L.
    Lincoln (1978b). Immunologic approach to non-Hodgkin's lymphoma and related
    leukemias. An analysis of the results of multiparameter studies of 425 cases.
    In E. J. Freireich and E. M. Hersh (Eds.), *Seminars in Hematology, the Immuno-
    logical Aspects of Leukemia and Lymphoma*. Grune & Stratton, Inc., New York.
    (in press).

Mathe, G. and H. Rappaport (1976). Histological and cytological typing of neoplastic
    diseases of haematopoietic and lymphoid tissue. In *International Histological
    Classification of Tumours, No. 14*. World Health Organization, Geneva.

Mellstedt, H., S. Hammarstrom and G. Holm (1974). Monoclonal lymphocyte population
    in human plasma cell myeloma. *Clin Exp Immunol* 17, 371-384.

Mellstedt, H., D. Pettersson and G. Holm (1976). Monoclonal B-lymphocytes in
    peripheral blood of patients with plasma cell myeloma. Relation to activity
    of the disease. *Scand J Haematol* 16, 112-120.

Nathwani, B. N., H. Kim and H. Rappaport (1976). Malignant lymphoma, lymphoblastic.
    Cancer 38, 964-983.

Nossal, G. J. V. and G. L. Ada (1971). *Antigens, Lymphoid Cells and the Immune
    Response*. Academic Press, New York.

Rappaport, H., W. J. Winter and E. B. Hicks (1956). Follicular lymphoma. A reeval-
    uation of its position in the scheme of malignant lymphoma, based on a survey
    of 253 cases. *Cancer* 9, 792-821.

Robb-Smith, A. H. T. (1964). The classification and natural history of the lympha-
    denopathies. In G. T. Pack and I. M. Ariel (Eds.), *Treatment of Cancer and
    Allied Diseases*, Vol. 9, 2nd ed. Hoeberg, New York.

Robb-Smith, A. H. T. and C. R. Taylor (1978). *An Approach to Lymph Node Diagnosis*.
    Harvey Miller Publishers, Ltd., London. (in press).

Stein, H. (1976). Klassifikation der malignen Non-Hodgkin-Lymphome aufgrund
    gemeinsamer morphologischer und immunologischer Merkmale zwischen normalen und
    neoplastischen lymphatischen Zellen. *Immunität Infektion* 4, 52-69.

Taylor, C. R. (1974). The nature of Reed-Sternberg cells and other malignant
    "reticulum" cells. *Lancet* 2, 802-807.

140   C. R. Taylor *et al.*

Taylor, C. R. (1977). *Hodgkin's Disease and the Lymphomas*, Vol. 1. *Annual Research Review, 1976.* Eden Press, Montreal; Churchill, Longman, Livingstone, London/ Edinburgh.

Taylor, C. R. (1978a). *Hodgkin's Disease and the Lymphomas*, Vol. 2. *Annual Research Review, 1977.* Eden Press, Montreal; Churchill, Longman, Livingstone, London/ Edinburgh.

Taylor, C. R. (1978b). Immunoperoxidase techniques: theoretical and practical aspects. *Arch Pathol Lab Med* 102, 113-121.

Taylor, C. R. (1978c). Immunocytochemical methods in the study of lymphoma and related conditions. *J Histochem Cytochem* 26, 495-512.

Taylor, C. R. (1978d). Classification of lymphomas: "new thinking" on old thoughts. *Arch Pathol Lab Med* (in press).

Taylor, C. R., R. Russell, R. J. Lukes and R. L. Davis (1978). An immunohistological study of immunoglobulin content of primary CNS lymphomas. *Cancer* 41, 2197-2208.

Williams, A. N., C. R. Taylor, A. R. Higgins, J. J. Quinn, B. K. Schneider, V. Swanson, J. W. Parker, P. K. Pattengale, S. B. Chandor, D. Powars, T. L. Lincoln, B. H. Tindle and R. J. Lukes (1978). Childhood leukemia and lymphoma. I. Correlation of morphology and immunological studies. *Cancer* 42, 171-181.

Willis, R. A. (1948). *The Pathology of Tumours*. Butterworths, London.

Cytologic Classification of Non-Hodgkin's Lymphomas based on Morphology, Cytochemistry and Immunology

H. Stein, G. Tolksdorf, M. Burkert and K. Lennert

Institute of Pathology, University of Kiel, Hospitalstr. 42, D-2300 Kiel,
West Germany

ABSTRACT

By combining the simultaneous application of various immunologic techniques with subtle cytomorphologic and cytochemical analyses, substantial advances have been made in the classification of malignant non-Hodgkin's lymphomas. Using this approach it was possible to distinguish a lymphocytic tumor with immunoglobulin (Ig)-secreting cells (plasma cells or plasmacytoid cells), which was called malignant lymphoma, lymphoplasmacytoid, or LP immunocytoma, from chronic lymphocytic leukemia (CLL). A minority of the cases of LP immunocytoma revealed the same immunologic markers as CLL, whereas the majority showed a marker constellation similar to that of lymphomas of germinal center cell (GCC) origin. GCC lymphomas are the most common ones. They may consist of GCC with cleaved nuclei (centrocytes), of GCC with non-cleaved and GCC with cleaved nuclei (centroblasts and centrocytes), or of GCC with non-cleaved nuclei (centroblasts). GCC bear large amounts of surface Ig and express a large number of C3b and C3d receptors. Centroblastic/centrocytic lymphomas, which mostly show a follicular (nodular) growth pattern, contain numerous T lymphocytes as well as GCC. T-cell lymphomas are much less common that B-cell lymphomas. The most frequent type of T-cell lymphoma is T-lymphoblastic lymphoma, which in most cases appears as the "convoluted cell type." Four subtypes of T-lymphoblastic lymphoma can be distinguished by immunologic and cytochemical (acid phosphatase and acid esterase) markers. About half the cases previously called "reticulosarcoma" could be identified as "immunoblastic" lymphomas of the B type. The other half did not reveal B-cell markers or lysozyme.

KEYWORDS

Malignant non-Hodgkin's lymphoma - surface markers - enzyme cytochemical markers - B- and T-cell maturation.

INTRODUCTION

It is generally agreed that the best classification of non-Hodgkin's lymphomas would be a classification according to etiology. At present, however, it is still impossible to make such a classification. In tumor pathology, neoplasms are commonly classified according to the cells or tissue from which they arise. Until 1970, a cell origin-related classification of non-Hodgkin's lymphomas was also not possible, because it was not known that the morphologically uniform lymphoid cells show great

141

PAA	+	+	−	−	−	−	−	−	+		
cALLA	+	−	−	−	−	−	−	−	−		
Ia	+	+	−	−	−	−	−	−	+		
Tdt	+	+	+	+	+	−	−	−			
C3bR	−	(+)	+ +	+	−	−	−				
C3dR	−	(+)	+ +	+	−	−	−				
IgM-FcR	−	−	−	−	−	+	+	−	−		
IgG-FcR	(+)	(+)	−	−	−	−	−	+			
acP	−	−	+ + +	+ + +	+	+	+	+/−	+/−		
acE	−	−	−	−	−	+	+	−	−		
SHEEP-E 37°	−	−	−	−/+	+	−	−	−			
SHEEP-E 4°	−	−	−	+	+	+	+	+	+		
HTLA	−	−	+	+ +	+ + +	+ +	+ +	+ +	+ +		

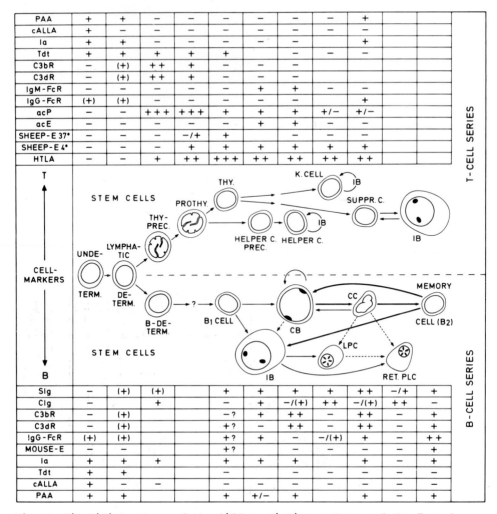

SIg	−	(+)	(+)		+	+	+	+	+ +	−/+	+
CIg	−	(+)	+		−	+	−/(+)	+ +	−/(+)	+ +	−
C3bR	−	(+)			−?	+	+ +	−	+ +	−	+
C3dR	−	(+)			+?	−	+ +	−	+ +	−	+
IgG-FcR	(+)	(+)			+?	+	−	−/(+)	+	−	+ +
MOUSE-E	−	−			+?		−	−	−	−	+
Ia	+	+	+		+	+	+		+	−	+
Tdt	+	+			−		−	−	−	−	−
cALLA	+	−	−		−	−	−	−	−	−	−
PAA	+	+			+	+/−	+		+	−	+

Fig. 1. Simplified scheme of the differentiation pathways of the T- and
B-cell systems and their immunologic and cytochemical markers.
Abbreviations in text.

diversity in origin and function. The detection of various immunologic markers in
the past eight years has led to the identification and description of a large number
of distinct subpopulations of the lymphoid cell system. The identification of these
markers has also made it possible to search for neoplastic equivalents of the
various subpopulations.

In contrast to other classifications, for example, the important one of Rappaport
(1966), which use terms that are not related to known lymphoid subpopulations,
the foremost aim of our approach to the classification of non-Hodgkin's lymphomas
was to separate entities whose cells correspond to normal lymphoid subpopulations.
To achieve this goal, we compared the morphologic features, enzyme cytochemical
properties, and immunologic markers of more than 250 non-Hodgkin's lymphomas with
those of normal lymphoid cells. A second aim of our work was to find morphologic
criteria for identifying the non-Hodgkin's lymphoma entities without the aid of
other techniques.

Since our classification is mainly based on the correlation between non-Hodgkin's lymphomas and normal B and T cells at different stages in their differentiation pathway, this presentation will begin with a brief description of the differentiation and maturation of the cells in the lymphoid cell system.

ORIGIN AND DIFFERENTIATION OF THE T- AND B-CELL SERIES IN RELATION TO THEIR IMMUNOLOGIC, MORPHOLOGIC, AND ENZYME CYTOCHEMICAL PROPERTIES

As outlined in the diagram in Fig. 1, it is generally presumed that a pluripotent undetermined stem cell of the bone marrow gives rise to lymphoid-determined stem cells (Van Bekkum and co-workers, 1971). These become T- or B-determined stem cells in response to as yet unknown stimuli. The pluripotent stem cell probably bears Ia-like antigen and common ALL antigen (cALL) and contains terminal deoxynucleotidyl transferase (Tdt). With the differentiation towards lymphoid stem cells, the cALL is quickly lost and the cells begin to express complement receptors (data reviewed by Stein, 1978).

The T-determined stem cells, which we call "thymocyte-precursor cells," enter the thymus anlage in the 9th to 10th gestational week. Thymocyte precursor cells are characterized by the expression of both complement receptor subtypes (C3b and C3d), focal acid phosphatase reactivity, small amounts of human T-lymphocyte antigen (HTLA), and the absence of sheep-erythrocyte (E) receptors and acid esterase. Thymocyte precursor cells develop into prothymocytes, which have the same markers plus sheep-E receptors. With increasing fetal age, the complement receptors disappear, the sheep-E receptors become stable at $37^{\circ}C$, and the amount of HTLA increases (data reviewed by Stein, 1978).

The differentiation of T cells into specialized cells, such as cytotoxic cells, suppressor cells, helper cells, etc., might begin in the thymus or just after emigration. Emigrated T cells differ from thymocytes in the absence of Tdt, the instability of the sheep-E receptors at $37^{\circ}C$, and the smaller amount of HTLA (data reviewed by Stein, 1978). It has been found that T-helper cells contain dot-like acid esterase (AE) activity (Grossi and co-workers, 1978) and express receptors for IgM (Moretta and co-workers, 1977). T-suppressor cells are AE-negative, but they contain azurophil granules and exhibit IgG receptors (Grossi and co-workers, 1978) and, notably, Ia-like antigen (Basten and co-workers, 1978). Ia-like antigen is not found in other T-cell subsets.

From studies on the AE (Tötterman and co-workers, 1977) and glycoprotein patterns (Andersson and Gahmberg, 1978) of blast cells induced by different means, we concluded that all T-cell subsets and probably B-cell subsets can regenerate themselves via a blast cell stage, generally called an immunoblast. In other words, each lymphoid cell subset appears to have its own immunoblast. Accordingly, we define an immunoblast as a lymphoid cell that is transformed for division and, in some instances, for differentiation. Immunoblasts exhibit a uniform "blastic" morphology, but differ in origin and fate.

There is little information about the differentiation pathway of the B-cell series, outlined at the bottom of the diagram in Fig. 1. It is speculated that the B-determined stem cell develops into an antigen-reactive B cell, which is called the B_1 cell. There are merely assumptions about the markers of B_1 cells, drawn from findings in chronic lymphocytic leukemia (CLL) of the B-cell type.

We have more information about the cells of the germinal center reaction (GCR) (reviewed by Müller-Hermelink and Lennert, 1978; Stein, 1978). The GCR plays an important role in the production of both B_1 and B_2 cells. B_2 cells are the cells

TABLE 1 Morphologic Classification of Non-Hodgkin's Lymphomas,
Established on Morphologic, Immunologic,
and Enzyme Cytochemical Criteria

Low-grade malignancy

ML lymphocytic
  Chronic lymphocytic leukemia, B type (B-CLL)
  Chronic lymphocytic leukemia, T type (T-CLL)
  Prolymphocytic leukemia
  Hairy cell leukemia
  Mycosis fungoides and Sézary's syndrome
  T-zone lymphoma

Secretory immunoglobulin-producing lymphomas
  ML lymphoplasmacytic/-cytoid (LP immunocytoma)
  ML plasmacytic (primary lymph node plasmacytoma)

Germinal center cell lymphomas
  ML centroblastic/centrocytic
  ML centrocytic

High-grade malignancy

ML centroblastic

ML lymphoblastic
  Burkitt type
  Convoluted cell type
  Unclassified

ML immunoblastic

ML = malignant lymphoma

that develop directly from the GCR. The starter cells of the GCR are both B_1 and B_2 cells, although B_2 cells predominate. In the GCR, B_1 and B_2 cells migrate to the lymph node cortex, where they transform into centroblasts. The centroblasts divide actively and develop into centrocytes. Their nuclei become round, and the centrocytes leave the germinal center. Some of them circulate in the blood as B_2 memory cells; others migrate to the submarginal areas of the same and other lymph nodes (such cells are called "marginal zone cells"), where they give rise to cells of the plasma cell reaction (PCR).

A majority of GCC bear surface immunoglobulin (SIg), and only a few (mostly centrocytes) contain cytoplasmic immunoglobulin (CIg). GCC have not only cytologic, but also other distinct immunologic features: they express a large number of receptors for both the C3b and the C3d fragment of the third complement component (C3). The GCC that migrate to the blood as memory B_2 lymphocytes retain both complement receptor subtypes, although the density of the receptors appears to diminish.

Usually, the PCR starts with marginal zone cells, which are predominantly derived from B_2 cells, but also from B_1 cells. Under appropriate antigenic stimuli, the marginal zone cells transform into immunoblasts, which show active mitosis. The immunoblasts migrate to the pulp cords and transform into plasmablasts and plasma cells. During the blast phase, there is a switch from the synthesis of SIg to that of secretory Ig. Thus, SIg and CIg are simultaneously demonstrable in B immunoblasts. After the immunoblast phase, the cells (plasmablasts and plasma cells) lose their SIg and complement receptors and contain increasing amounts of secretory Ig in their cytoplasm (data reviewed by Stein, 1978).

Cytologic	Immunologic	
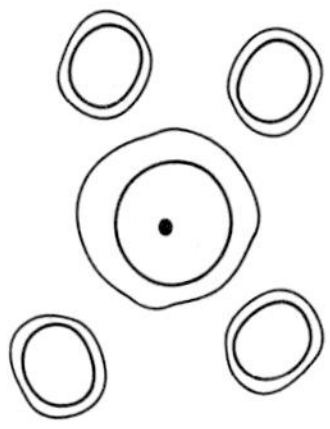	SIg classes	$\mu\delta > \mu > \gamma > \delta$ +
	SIg density	low
	Capping	highly reduced
	Cytoplasmic Ig	−
	C3b receptors	+/−
	C3d receptors	+++
	IgG-Fc receptors	+
	Mouse-E receptors	+++
	T-cell content: low ($\bar{X}=5\%$)	

Cytologic	Immunologic/enzyme cytochemical	
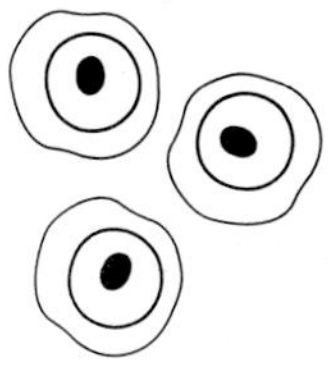	SIg density	very high
	C3b receptors	++
	C3d receptors	++
	IgG-Fc receptors	++
	Mouse-E receptors	−/(+)
	Sheep-E receptors	−
	Tartrate resistant acid phosphatase	+/−

Fig. 2. Properties of chronic lymphocytic leukemia of the B-cell
type (B-CLL).

Fig. 3. Properties of prolymphocytic
leukemia of the B-cell type.

CLASSIFICATION OF NON-HODGKIN'S LYMPHOMAS IN RELATION TO CELL ORIGIN

Our classification of non-Hodgkin's lymphomas is shown in Table 1. Only the most common entities and the most important cell markers will be discussed here. The data are reviewed in detail elsewhere (Lennert and Mohri, 1978; Stein, 1978).

Lymphocytic Lymphomas

The heading "ML lymphocytic" covers a group of lymphomas that consist of small lymphoid cells, only occasionally interspersed with large blast cells. These tumors are chronic lymphocytic leukemia (CLL), prolymphocytic leukemia, hairy cell leukemia, mycosis fungoides, Sézary's syndrome, and T-zone lymphoma.

Chronic lymphocytic leukemia, B-cell type (B-CLL). The most common entity in the group of lymphocytic lymphomas is B-CLL. As shown in Fig. 2, B-CLL cells are characterized by the presence of small amounts of SIg, the consistent absence of CIg, the constant presence of mouse-E receptors, and a predominance of C3d receptors over C3b receptors. Only a small number of T cells are found in the lymph node.

Cytologically, the predominant cells are small lymphocyte-like cells. They are generally interspersed with larger cells, called prolymphocytes and paraimmuno-blasts. Paraimmunoblasts have a central prominent nucleolus and abundant, weakly basophilic cytoplasm. In more than 80% of the cases of B-CLL, the prolymphocytes and paraimmunoblasts are gathered in clusters, which causes the so-called pseudo-follicular pattern. We have not seen such a pattern in sections from T-CLL.

Prolymphocytic leukemia. Prolymphocytic leukemia is a rare disorder. As more is known about the markers of prolymphocytic leukemia, however, its incidence appears to increase. Approximately 90% of the cases are of the B-cell type. Prolymphocytic leukemia cells (see Fig. 3) of the B type differ from B-CLL cells by a high density of SIg, the absence of mouse-E receptors, the presence of both complement receptor subtypes, and occasional tartrate-resistant acid phosphatase reactivity. Cytologically, prolymphocytic leukemia cells differ from B-CLL cells by their larger size, more abundant cytoplasm, and particularly their prominent nucleoli.

Chronic lymphocytic leukemia of the T-cell type (T-CLL), mycosis fungoides, and Sézary's syndrome.

Lymphocytic lymphomas of the T type can be reliably diagnosed only by immunologic markers. Certain cases of T-CLL and mycosis fungoides and Sézary's syndrome can be identified, however, by the content and reaction pattern of acid phosphatase and AE in the tumor cells. The cells of these disorders usually contain small granules of acid phosphatase and a few medium-sized or large granules of AE (Tolksdorf and Stein, submitted for publication). It has been shown that T cells containing one or two large granules of AE exhibit a helper-cell capacity (Grossi and co-workers, 1978). This finding strongly suggests that all T-cell neoplasms with large intracytoplasmic granules of AE are proliferations of cells in the T-helper cell series. Functional studies have revealed that the tumor cells in most cases of Sézary's syndrome are indeed T-helper cells.

Secretory Immunoglobulin-Producing Lymphomas

The next main group of lymphomas in our classification are the secretory Ig-producing lymphomas, namely, lymphoplasmacytic/lymphoplasmacytoid lymphoma (LP immunocytoma) and primary lymph node plasmacytoma. We shall discuss only LP immuno-cytoma, because primary lymph node plasmacytoma resembles multiple myeloma in cytology and immunologic properties, and multiple myeloma has been well character-ized.

LP immunocytoma.

In contrast to B-CLL, which is a purebred proliferation of non-secretory B cells arrested in a certain stage of differentiation, and to plasma-cytoma, which is a purebred proliferation of secretory cells, we have defined LP immunocytoma as a proliferation of a mixture of nonsecretory (lymphocyte-like) B cells and secretory B cells (plasma cells or their direct precursors). The secretory B cells, i.e., the plasma cells, are characterized by their content of easily detectable Ig in the cytoplasm (CIg). The CIg can be specifically demonstrated with the immunoperoxidase technique on paraffin sections in nearly all cases. The CIg is usually of the IgM class. Only 20-25% of the cases show secretion of the CIg. IgM-producing and -secreting LP immunocytoma is identical with macroglobulinemia of Waldenström.

It should be pointed out that, in most instances, the diagnostic secretory cell component, i.e., the plasma cells, can be identified only by cytologic criteria. An important aid in the rapid detection of secretory cells is the PAS reaction. Intranuclear and/or intracytoplasmic PAS-positive globules are found in more than 50% of the cases of LP immunocytoma.

Subtypes of LP immunocytoma.

LP immunocytoma is not a homogeneous entity. Three sub-types are discernible by morphology (see Fig. 4). The lymphoplasmacytoid subtype contains only a few blast cells. Its secretory cell component is made up of so-called lymphatic plasma cells, which resemble lymphocytes in nuclear structure, but plasma cells in their content of ergastoplasm. In the polymorphic subtype, there is a signif-icant number of blast cells, which may resemble immunoblasts or centroblasts. The lymphoplasmacytic subtype contains secretory cells that are similar to plasma cells of the bone marrow, the so-called Marschalkó plasma cells. In all three subtypes, Ig inclusion bodies are often detectable in the cisternae of the ergastoplasm.

The three subtypes of LP immunocytoma differ not only in morphology, but also in immunologic markers. The nonsecretory cells of the polymorphic and lymphoplasmacytic subtypes are C3b and C3d receptor-positive, like GCC, whereas the cells of the lympho-plasmacytoid subtype exhibit only C3d receptors, like B-CLL cells (Tolksdorf and Stein, 1978, unpublished data). Features common to all three subtypes are the constant presence of SIg on a large proportion of the cells and the presence of CIg in at least some of the neoplastic cells.

Cytologic	Immunologic			
		Subtype		
		„Cytoid"	„Poly-morphic"	„Cytic"
„Cytoid" subtype	SIg	+	+	+
	CIg	+	+	+
	C3b rec.	+/−	++	++
	C3d rec.	+++	++	++
	IgG–Fc rec.	+	+	+
	Mouse–E rec.	+++	+	−/+
„Polymorphic" subtype	T-cell content:	↓	↑	↑ a)
„Cytic" subtype				

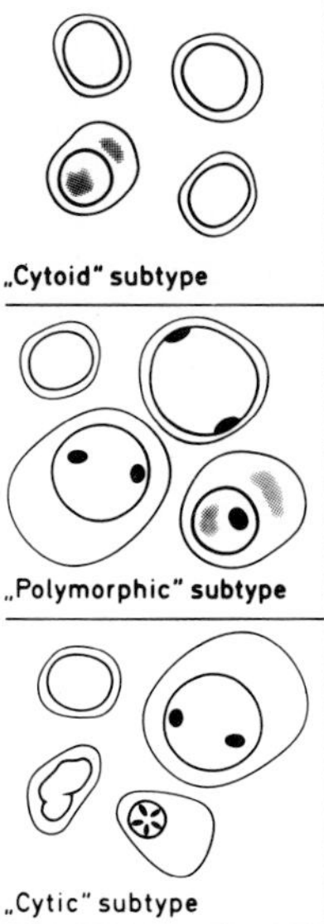

a) ↓ or ↑ = low or relatively high T-cell content

Fig. 4. Properties of the three subtypes of ML lymphoplasma-
cytic/-cytoid (LP immunocytoma).

Germinal Center Cell Lymphomas

The most common malignant lymphomas are derived from GCC. We group these tumors
together as GCC lymphomas. As symbolically demonstrated in Fig. 1, there are two
main types of GCC. The centroblast is characterized by a large pale nucleus with two
or three membrane-associated nucleoli and sparse basophilic cytoplasm. The centro-
cyte is characterized by a small or medium-sized, irregularly shaped or cleaved
nucleus and pale cytoplasm. The separation of two types of lymphoid GCC has proved
to be sufficient for describing all GCC lymphomas we have observed so far. We have
found three subtypes, viz.: centroblastic/centrocytic lymphoma, centrocytic lymphoma,
and centroblastic lymphoma.

Centroblastic/centrocytic lymphoma is a GCC lymphoma that imitates follicular hyperplasia. Centroblasts and centrocytes always proliferate side by side, but with a
predominance of centrocytes (see Fig. 5). The growth pattern is usually, but not
always follicular. Because of its cytologic composition, we call this type of
lymphoma "centroblastic/centrocytic."

Centroblastic/centrocytic lymphoma resembles follicular hyperplasia not only in
cytology, but also in immunologic markers. The neoplastic cells of centroblastic/
centrocytic lymphoma show a moderate to high density of SIg. In most cases there are
some CIg-positive cells, usually distributed around the neoplastic follicles, as
seen in follicular hyperplasia. The most important markers of GCC are the complement
receptor subtypes. The cells of the neoplastic follicles express receptors for both
C3b and C3d, like reactive GCC. Another characteristic of centroblastic/centrocytic
lymphoma is the relatively high percentage of mouse-E rosette-forming cells. There
are about 30% T cells; a similar proportion of T cells is found in follicular hyperplasia.

Cytologic	Immunologic	
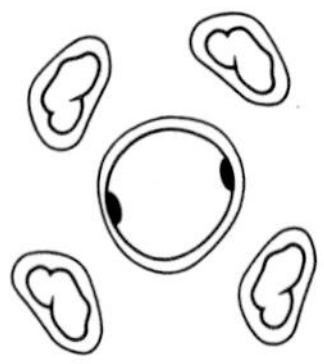	SIg classes	μ,γ, rarely δ +
	SIg density	medium
	Cytoplasmic Ig	(+)/−
	C3b receptors	++
	C3d receptors	++
	IgG-Fc receptors	+/−
	Mouse-E receptors	+
	T-cell content: relatively high ($\bar{X}$=30%)	

Cytologic	Immunologic	
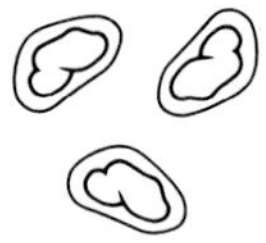	SIg classes	μ,γ ++, rarely δ+
	SIg density	high
	Capping	+++
	Cytoplasmic Ig	−/(+)
	C3b receptors	++
	C3d receptors	++
	IgG-Fc receptors	+/−
	Mouse-E receptors	−/(+)
	T-cell content: low ($\bar{X}$=7%)	

Fig. 5. Properties of ML centroblastic/centrocytic.

Fig. 6. Properties of ML centrocytic.

Centrocytic lymphoma. The second type of malignant lymphoma that we consider to be derived from GCC is called "centrocytic lymphoma," because it is composed only of cells that resemble reactive centrocytes, as symbolically demonstrated in Fig. 6. Centroblasts are consistently absent. The growth pattern is usually diffuse. The close relationship between the tumor cells of centrocytic lymphoma and small GCC is supported not only by their morphologic similarity, but also by the demonstration of both complement receptor subtypes on the centrocyte-like tumor cells.

Besides the difference in cytology, the separation of centrocytic lymphoma from centroblastic/centrocytic lymphoma is justified by the following immunologic findings: (1) centrocytic lymphoma contains no, or only a few cells that are capable of binding mouse E, and (2) there are only a few T cells in centrocytic lymphoma. Furthermore, the survival time of patients with centrocytic lymphoma is much shorter than that of patients with centroblastic/centrocytic lymphoma.

Centrocytic lymphoma cells differ in immunologic features from B-CLL cells by their high density of SIg, the presence of both complement receptor subtypes, and their inability to bind mouse E. Centrocytic lymphoma is more similar to prolymphocytic leukemia in immunologic markers.

Centroblastic lymphoma. The third malignant lymphoma that we regard as derived from GCC is characterized by a predominance of cells resembling centroblasts (see Fig. 7). The assumption of a close relationship between this tumor, which we call "centroblastic lymphoma," and GCC is based not only on the similarity in morphology, but also on (1) the observation that centroblastic lymphoma often develops out of a centroblastic/centrocytic lymphoma and (2) the demonstration of both complement receptor subtypes on the tumor cells. In centroblastic lymphoma, however, the expression of surface markers proved to be less constant than in the other two types of GCC lymphoma. Centroblastic lymphoma has the poorest prognosis among the GCC lymphomas; thus, we have grouped it with the malignant lymphomas of high-grade malignancy.

Lymphoblastic Lymphomas

Under the heading "lymphoblastic lymphoma," we have included all malignant lymphomas that consist of medium-sized "blast cells." One of the lymphoblastic entities, namely, lymphoblastic lymphoma of the Burkitt type, has been well characterized; thus, it will not be discussed here. The other cases of lymphoblastic lymphoma present great problems for morphologists, because only a minority of the cases can be classified

Cytologic	Immunologic	
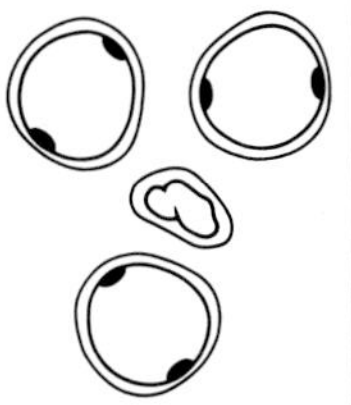	SIg	+/−
	Cytoplasmic Ig	−/+
	C3b receptors	+ CC ≫ CB
	C3d receptors	+ CC ≫ CB
	IgG-Fc receptors	−/+
	Mouse-E receptors	−/+
	T-cell content: low	

Cytologic	Immunologic/enzyme cytochemical	Subtype		
		B	T	O
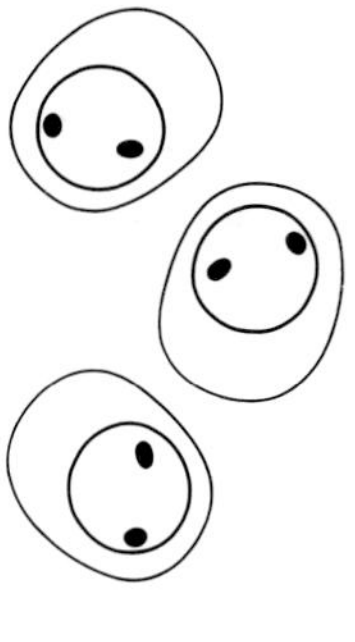	SIg	+	−	−
	Cytoplasmic Ig	+	−	−
	C3 receptors	−/+	−	−
	Mouse-E receptors	−/+	−	−
	Sheep-E receptors	−	+	−
	Lysozyme	−	−	−
	Immunophagocytosis a)	−	−	−
	Nonspecific esterase b)	−	−	−

a) rapid phagocytosis of IgG and/or C3b-coated particles
b) or only weak granular reaction

Fig. 7. Properties of ML centroblastic. Fig. 8. Properties of ML immunoblastic.

TABLE 2   Morphologic, Cytochemical, and Immunologic Features of the Three Main Subtypes of Lymphoblastic Lymphoma Other than the Burkitt Type

Marker	T type	B type	Null type
Convoluted nuclei	+ in some cases	−	−
Intensely basophilic cytoplasm	−/(+)	+	−/(+)
Granular PAS staining	+ in some cases	?	+ in most cases
Focal acid phosphatase activity	+ in most cases	−	−/(+)
Dot-like acid esterase activity	− in most cases[a]	−	−
Surface immunoglobulin	−	+	−
Sheep-erythrocyte receptor	+ in 80%	−	−
Complement receptor	+ in 50%[b]	+/−	−
Adherence of polyacryl acid beads	−	+	+
Ia-like antigen	−	+	+
Human T-lymphocyte antigen	+	−	−
Common-ALL antigen	−	−	+

[a] Positive in rare cases of T-lymphoblastic lymphoma probably derived from (peripheral) T cells determined for helper-cell functions.

[b] Present in lymphoblastic lymphomas derived from thymocyte precursors and prothymocytes, but absent in cases derived from postnatal thymocytes.

by morphologic criteria – these are lymphoblastic lymphomas of the convoluted cell type. We include all lymphoblastic lymphomas that are not morphologically classifiable under the heading "lymphoblastic lymphoma, unclassified type."

By applying enzyme cytochemical and, in particular, immunologic techniques, it is possible to separate lymphoblastic lymphomas into three main subtypes, namely, the T, the B, and the null type. The morphologic, enzyme cytochemical, and immunologic

features of these subtypes are summarized in Table 2. Convoluted nuclei are found in
the T type. It should be stressed, however, that convoluted nuclei are not a reliable marker of this type of lymphoma, since they are often inconspicuous or even
absent. The most intense basophilic staining of the cytoplasm is usually found in
the B type, and granular PAS staining is more common in the null type than in the
other types. Strong, focal acid phosphatase reactivity is a very characteristic,
although not specific feature of the T type; a strong reaction is not found in all
cases of the T type. The acid phosphatase and AE reaction patterns make it possible
to separate the lymphoblastic lymphomas of the T type into those derived from thymocytes and those derived from peripheral T cells (see below).

The third group of features in Table 2 are the immunologic markers that are sufficient for subtyping lymphoblastic lymphomas and can be applied by anyone, since the
reagents are commercially available. SIg is restricted to the B type. The presence
of sheep-E receptors proves the T-cell origin. Complement receptors may occur on
cells of both the B and the T type. The simultaneous presence of receptors for
complement and sheep E is indicative of a prothymocytic origin. Adherence of poly-
acryl acid beads and the expression of Ia-like antigen is found on cells of the B
and null types, but not on those of the T type (Jäger and co-workers, 1977). A
specific marker of the T type is HTLA, and a specific marker of most cases of the
null type is cALL antigen.

If all the available markers are considered together, the lymphoblastic lymphomas of
the T type have to be further subdivided into four subtypes (Stein, 1978), whose
cells correspond to different differentiation stages of the thymocyte and T-cell
lineages (see Fig. 1):

Lymphoblastic lymphoma of the thymocyte precursor subtype is characterized by strong,
focal acid phosphatase activity, complement receptors, moderate amounts of HTLA,
and Tdt. The cells are devoid of sheep-E receptors and AE.

Lymphoblastic lymphoma of the prothymocyte subtype has the same markers as the thymocyte precursor type, but, in addition, shows sheep-E receptors that are stable at
37°C in a majority of cases.

The cells of lymphoblastic lymphoma of the mature thymocyte subtype bear sheep-E
receptors that are stable at 37°C and large amounts of HTLA, but no complement
receptors. They contain Tdt and usually reveal focal acid phosphatase activity, but
lack AE.

The cells of lymphoblastic lymphoma of the peripheral T-cell subtype are different
from thymocytes and similar to peripheral T cells in their low density of HTLA, their
capacity to form sheep-E rosettes only at 4°C, and their focal AE activity.

The division of the group of lymphoblastic lymphomas into the B type, the null type,
and the T type and its subtypes is important, because these subtypes also differ in
clinical behavior, survival time, and response to therapy.

Immunoblastic Lymphoma

The last entity of our classification is immunoblastic lymphoma. An important feature
of the tumor cells is their large size. For this reason, such tumors are called
large-cell lymphomas by some authors. These tumors used to be interpreted as neoplastic proliferations of reticulum cells or histiocytes. We must point out here
that we classify only the large cell lymphomas whose cells resemble reactive immunoblasts with Giemsa staining as immunoblastic lymphoma. The group of immunoblastic
lymphomas defined by our classification does not include large cell lymphomas that
can be morphologically recognized as derived from histiocytes and that are known
as malignant histiocytosis (Byrne and Rappaport, 1973) or histiocytic medullary
reticulosis (Scott and Robb-Smith, 1939).

TABLE 3   Intracytoplasmic Immunoglobulin, Lysozyme, and
Albumin in 50 Cases of Large Cell Lymphoma Whose
Cells Resemble Reactive Immunoblasts in Morphology
with Giemsa Staining

	Incidence	(%)
Immunoglobulin	26/50	52
Monotypic (restriction to one light chain)	19/50	38
ϰ	13/50	26
λ	6/50	12
Bitypic (presence of both light chains)	7/50	14
Lysozyme	0/50	0
Albumin	0/50	0

Our earlier analysis of tissue extracts from immunoblast-like large cell lymphomas
showed an increase in the Ig content in 60% of the cases. This finding suggested
Ig production and thus a B-cell nature of the lymphomas. To substantiate our assumption, we investigated sections from 50 cases of immunoblast-like large cell lymphoma
for the presence of light chains and lysozyme in the cytoplasm by means of the
immunoperoxidase (PAP) technique (Burkert and colleagues, 1978). The results are
shown in Table 3. In 52% of the cases, we detected light chains in the cytoplasm of
tumor cells. Specification of the light chain type showed staining for only one
type in 38% of the cases, which strongly suggests synthesis of the Ig chains by the
tumor cells and thus their B-cell origin. It is remarkable that in 14% of the cases
both light chain types were detectable in tumor cells. It is difficult to explain
this finding. Phagocytosis seems to be an unlikely explanation, however, since we
always found lysozyme in neutrophils, monocytes, and histiocytes, but never in
tumor cells.

Figure 8 summarizes the available information about immunoblastic lymphoma. By
applying immunologic markers, the morphologically uniform group of immunoblastic
lymphomas can be subdivided into at least three types. The B type is most common.
It is characterized by the simultaneous presence of SIg and CIg; the cells thus
resemble reactive B immunoblasts. We shall not discuss any other markers here,
because they do not show a constant expression. According to data of Seligmann and
co-workers (1977) and Braylan and co-workers (1977) and to our own findings, immunoblastic lymphomas with T-cell properties appear to account for less than 10% of the
cases. In 30-40% of the cases, the immunoblastic lymphoma cells do not exhibit any
of the known markers. We would like to mention here that none of the immunoblastic
lymphomas of the null type that we have investigated so far showed features of
macrophages, such as immunophagocytosis or lysozyme. New markers are needed to
clarify the true nature of the null-type immunoblastic lymphomas.

FINAL REMARKS

The abundance of data presented here is not supposed to obscure the fact that there
are still some lymphomas that do not fit into our classification as it presently
stands. Examples of such lymphomas are alkaline phosphatase-positive lymphoma and
certain types of T-cell lymphoma. About 10% of the non-Hodgkin's lymphomas cannot
be classified at all, even when we apply immunologic methods. Much more work will
have to be done before we can answer all the remaining questions.

REFERENCES

Andersson, L. C., and C. G. Gahmberg (1978). Surface glycoprotein patterns of normal and malignant human lymphocytes. VI. International Conference on Lymphatic Tissues and Germinal Centers in Immune Reactions, June 1978, Damp/Kiel. Plenum Press, New York, in press.

Basten, A., J. F. A. P. Miller, R. Loblay, P. Johnson, J. Gamble, E. Chia, H. Pritchard-Briscoe, R. Callard, and I. F. C. McKenzie (1978). T cell dependent suppression of antibody production. I. Characteristics of suppressor T cells following tolerance induction. Eur. J. Immunol., 8, 360-370.

van Bekkum, D. W., M. J. van Noord, B. Maat, and K. A. Dicke (1971). Attempts at identification of hemopoietic stem cell in mouse. Blood, 38, 547-558.

Braylan, R. C., E. S. Jaffe, R. B. Mann, M. M. Frank, and C. W. Berard (1977). Surface receptors of human neoplastic lymphoreticular cells. In S. Thierfelder, H. Rodt, and E. Thiel (Eds.), Immunological Diagnosis of Leukemias and Lymphomas. Haematology and Blood Transfusion, Vol. 20. Springer, Berlin-Heidelberg-New York. pp. 47-52.

Burkert, M., H. Stein, H. Boumann, and K. Lennert (1978). Demonstration of intracytoplasmic immunoglobulin, lysozyme and albumin and isoelectric focusing pattern of tissue immunoglobulin in so-called reticulum-cell sarcoma (immunoblastic or large-cell lymphoma). VI. International Conference on Lymphatic Tissues and Germinal Centers in Immune Reactions, June 1978, Damp/Kiel. Plenum Press, New York, in press.

Byrne, E., Jr., and H. Rappaport (1973). Malignant histiocytosis. In K. Akazaki, H. Rappaport, C. W. Berard, J. M. Bennett, and E. Ishikawa (Eds.), GANN Monograph on Cancer Research, Vol. 15. University of Tokyo Press, Tokyo. pp. 145-162.

Grossi, C. E., S. R. Webb, A. Zicca, P. M. Lydyard, L. Moretta, M. C. Mingari, and M. D. Cooper (1978). Morphological and histochemical analyses of two human T-cell subpopulations bearing receptors for IgM or IgG. J. exp. Med., 147, 1405-1417.

Jäger, G., C. Pachmann, H. Rodt, and D. Huhn (1977). Polyacrylsäure-Kügelchen als Nachweis von B-Lymphocyten. Blut, 35, 335.

Lennert, K., and N. Mohri (1978). Histopathology and diagnosis of non-Hodgkin's lymphomas. In K. Lennert, Malignant Lymphomas Other than Hodgkin's Disease. Springer, New York. pp. 111-469.

Moretta, L., S. R. Webb, C. E. Grossi, P. M. Lydyard, and M. D. Cooper (1977). Functional analysis of two human T-cell subpopulations: help and suppression of B-cell responses by T cells bearing receptors for IgM or IgG. J. exp. Med., 146, 184-200.

Müller-Hermelink, H. K., and K. Lennert (1978). The cytologic, histologic, and functional bases for a modern classification of lymphomas. In K. Lennert, Malignant Lymphomas Other than Hodgkin's Disease. Springer, New York. pp. 1-71.

Scott, R. B., and A. H. T. Robb-Smith (1939). Histiocytic medullary reticulosis. Lancet, ii, 194-198.

Seligmann, M., J.-C. Brouet, and J.-L. Preud'Homme (1977). The immunological diagnosis of human leukemias and lymphomas: an overview. In S. Thierfelder, H. Rodt, and E. Thiel (Eds.), Immunological Diagnosis of Leukemias and Lymphomas. Haematology and Blood Transfusion, Vol. 20. Springer, Berlin-Heidelberg-New York. pp. 1-15.

Stein, H. (1978). The immunologic and immunochemical basis for the Kiel classification. In K. Lennert, Malignant Lymphomas Other than Hodgkin's Disease. Springer, New York. pp. 529-657.

Tötterman, T. H., A. Ranki, and P. Häyry (1977). Expression of the acid α-naphthyl acetate esterase marker by activated and secondary T lymphocytes in man. Scand. J. Immunol., 6, 305-310.

Tolksdorf, G., and H. Stein (1978). Acid α-naphthyl acetate esterase in hairy cell leukemia. Submitted for publication.

On the Problems and the Tasks of the Clinical Non-Hodgkin Lymphoma Research Today*

K. Musshoff**

*Supported by "Kampf dem Krebs" of the German Cancer Society
**Radiological Centre, Department of Radiotherapy of the
Albert-Ludwig's-University, Freiburg im Breisgau, Hugstetter St. 55,
D-7800 Freiburg, West Germany (F.G.R.)

ABSTRACT

Three diagnostic principles are available for the histopathological diagnosis of the Non-Hodgkin Lymphomas (NHL): (1) the
older, clinically insufficiently relevant classification with
concepts such as lymphosarcoma, reticulum-cellsarcoma etc., (2)
more recent morphological classifications including, in particular,
that of Rappaport and co-workers; the latter is clinically
significant and reproducible but scientifically inaccurate, and
(3) the functional-morphological classifications based on the
immunology of Lennert (Kiel Classification) and of Lukes and
Collins. These have proved, after the first, especially retrospective,
examinations with the Kiel Classification, to be clinically
significant and reproducible. Scientifically, they correspond to
the modern conception of the NHL as neoplasmes of the immune system.
Comparative examinations of the Rappaport and the Kiel Classifications
have proved that these classifications only partly correspond, not
only in the comparison of the individual pathohistological types
but also in the comparison of the principal subgroups of "good and
poor prognosis" of the Rappaport Classification in the definition
of Rosenberg and Kaplan (1975) and the "low and high grade
malignancy" of the Kiel Classification.
  The Ann Arbor Classification, which was conceived for the
Hodgkin Lymphomas, is generally applied today to the clinical
diagnosis of the NHL. It is not optimal for the diagnosis of NHL,
but as long as no better classification is available and
internationally in use, it is suitable as a clinically satisfying
principle of classification. The formulation of a new and unique
clinical NHL classification presupposes that agreement in the field
of the pathohistological classification is at our disposal.

KEYWORDS: Comparison of:

          older pathohistological classifications,
          morphological Rappaport Classification,
          functional-immunological Kiel Classification.

       Ann Arbor Classification.

We are going to talk to day about lymphomas other than
Hodgkin's disease. The hope of obtaining the very successful,
one could almost say, dramatic results of the Hodgkin Lymphomas
research by applying their proved diagnostic criteria and
therapeutic procedures to the Non-Hodgkin Lymphomas (NHL) has only
been partly realized, for example, with children's lymphoblastic
leukemia (Pinkel and co-workers, 1972). There has been no therapeuti
break-through, on a wide scale, comparable with that of the Hodgkin
Lymphomas (HL) (Ultmann, 1978). The reasons for this disappointment
are to be seen in the diverging and still partly obscure nosology
of the NHL and in the greater diversity of this group, the lack of
a generally recognized histopathological and also clinical classification principle.

ON THE NATURAL HISTORY OF NHL

The HL and NHL differ from one another in the following
fundamental points:
- The NHL develop in a quarter to a third of all cases extranodally,
  a place of origin which can not be demonstrated, with absolute
  certainty, in a single case of HL (Brown and co-workers, 1975;
  Johnson and co-workers, 1975; Musshoff and co-workers, 1971,
  1975; Peters and co-workers, 1968).
- Whereas the HL show a tendency towards a more centrifugally
  limited distribution - which is, indeed, the precondition for
  the successful therapeutic concept of the central lymphatic
  irradiation in the form of the mantle and inverted Y-field
  technique (Kaplan, 1972) - the NHL show a stronger tendency
  towards the centripetal distribution and dissemination (Jones
  and co-workers, 1973; Goffinet and co-workers, 1977), as well as,
  and this is probably the most important difference, the frequent
  transition to leukemia and invasion in the central nervous
  system (Jaffe and co-workers, 1977; Lennert, 1978; Murphy,1977;
  Pinkel and co-workers, 1972; Rosenberg, 1975).

ON THE CLINICAL STAGING CLASSIFICATION

Since the non-leukemic NHL like the HL seem to follow the
classic laws of malignancy, i.e. the laws of the normally uni-
centrical origin and of the invasive, lymphogenic and/or
hematogenic extension, all the clinical stages can be classified
according to the Ann Arbor Classification system (Carbone, Kaplan,
Musshoff and co-workers, 1971). Leukemias with primary sarcoma can
by classified as a special form of the Dissemination Stage IV. By
this, I mean to say that until a better staging classification
becomes available it will be possible to continue working quite
successfully with the Ann Arbor Staging Classification, in spite
of the fact that, as Rosenberg (1977) said in San Francisco in
1976, this classification which was conceived for the Hodgkin
Lymphomas is of only limited value for the Non-Hodgkin Lymphomas.

ON THE PATHOHISTOLOGICAL CLASSIFICATION AND NOMENCLATURE

The greatest difficulties at the moment facing a clinical
mastering of the NHL problems lie in the field of pathohistological
diagnostics and classification. Today we are working with three
principles of classification:

- Up to about a decade ago the so-called "older nomenclature" which
  is, even today, still widely applied, was generally valid, with

terms such as lymphosarcoma, reticulumcell-sarcoma and others. Comparative examinations with the Rappaport and Kiel Classifications reveal that these older pathohistological disease terms do not describe entities but diseases of different malignancy and prognosis (Jones and co-workers,1973; Musshoff,1978). Thus, these terms, as Lukes said in 1968, have no specific meaning.

- In 1956 Rappaport and co-workers (Rappaport, Winter and Hicks, 1956; Rappaport,1966) brought a great deal of order into the histological and, thus, into the clinical diagnosis of the lymphomas by means of a classification of the lymphomas into "lymphocytic" and "histiocytic" cells, into "well" and "poorly differentiated" according to the degree of their differentiation, and into "nodular" and "diffuse" according to their distribution pattern. Our knowledge today of the clinical diagnostics of the NHL and their treatment and prognosis rest primarily on the findings based on the Rappaport Classification.

   The Rappaport Classification, according to the opinion of the conference in San Francisco in 1976 (Jones and Godden,1977) summarized by DeVita (1977), is clinically significant and reproducible but scientifically inaccurate.

- Recent morphological, cytochemical and immunological examinations have established that the malignant lymphomas are neoplasmes of the immune system (Hansen and Good,1974; Seligmann, Brouet and Preud'homme, 1977) and that the histiocytes of Rappaport are, on the whole, not histiocytes but transformed lymphocytes. Our modern understanding of NHL, as the result of a morphological and functional approach, has been formulated in two classifications: In that of Lukes and Collins (1974) and in the Kiel Classification (Gerard-Marchant and co-workers, 1974), which is based on the concept of Lennert and co-workers (1967, 1975).

PRELIMINARY RESULTS OF A COMPARISON OF THE KIEL AND RAPPAPORT CLASSIFICATIONS

   If we compare the diagnoses of a patients' collective as both Rappaport and Lennert have done retrospectively with a small Freiburg collective according to their respective principles, we can see that the Rappaport and Kiel types are only partially identical diseases. Neither do the prognostic judgements in about 25% of all the cases coincide, when a synopsis is made of the cases into both prognostic principal groups (1) the "good" and "poor prognosis" of the Rappaport Classification (Rosenberg and Kaplan, 1975) and (2) the "low" and "high grade malignancy" of the Kiel Classification (Tab. 1).

   The differences are particularly great in the Rappaport type, "poorly differentiated lymphocytic diffuse " (PDL D). This group belongs, according to the Kiel Classification, about half and half to the "low" and "high grade malignancy" subgroups whose prognoses are significantly different. This finding argues that this group defined by Rappaport contains at least two prognostically diverging entities (Fig. 1a).

   Contrary to the diffuse form, Rappaport's nodular form of the "poorly differentiated lymphocytic" lymphomas (PDL N) shows, on corresponding subdivision into both the subgroups "low and high grade malignancy", no prognostic differences in the survival rates, whereby of course, the small number of only three patients in the subgroup of high malignancy is to be taken into consideration as a limiting factor (Fig. 1b).

TABLE 1　Comparative corrdination of the histopathological diagnoses according to the Rappaport Classification (on the abscissa) and according to the Lennert (Kiel) Classification (on the ordinate) subdivided respectively into both the subgroups of "good" and "poor prognoses" according to the definition of Rosenberg and Kaplan (1975) and of "low" and "high grade malignancy". (80 cases from the Pathological Institute of Freiburg University reclassified by H.Rappaport, K.Lennert and W.Sandritter[1]) (Joint investigations with H. Schmidt-Vollmer, W.v.Stotzingen and H.Umbach)

		RAPPAPORT CLASSIFICATION											
		WDL N	WPL D	PDL N	PDL N&D	M N	PDL D	H N	M D	H D	Lb CV	U	No of patients
KIEL CLASSIFICATION	LC	0	2	0	0	0	0	0	0	0	0	1	2
	LP	0	1	1	0	1	8	0	1	0	0	1	13
	CC	0	1	0	0	0	3	0	0	0	0	1	5
	CB-CC	0	0	7	1	0	0	0	1'	0	0	1	10
	CB	0	0	1	0	1	0	0	0	1	0	0	3
	LB	0	0	0	2	0	5	0	0	5	5	2	19
	IB	0	0	0	0	0	2	0	1	22	1	0	26
	U	0	0	0	0	0	0	0	0	1"	0	0	1
	No of patients	0	4	9	3	2	18	0	3	29	6	6	80

low grade malignancy (n = 31)
high grade malignancy (n = 49)

Good Prognosis (n = 18)　　　　　Poor Prognosis (n = 56)

'= Lennert diagnosis: CB-CC, follicular and diffus with sclerosis　　"= Lennert diagnosis: U, high grade malignancy

Abbreviations:

WDL N = well diff.lymphoc.nod.　　　H N = histiocytic nod.
WDL D = well diff.lymphoc.diff.　　　H D = histiocytic diff.
PDL N = poorly diff.lymphoc.nod.　　Lb-cv = lymphoblastic convoluted
PDL D = poorly diff.lymphoc.diff.　　U　 = unclassified
PDL N = poorly diff.lymphoc.nod.　　P Q = poor quality
　et D　　　　　　　　and diff.

LC　　 = lymphocytic　　　　　　　　　CB　 = centroblastic
LP　　 = lymphoplasmocytoid　　　　　LB　 = lymphoblastic
CC　　 = centrocytic　　　　　　　　　IB　 = immunoblastic
CB-CC = centroblastic-centrocytic　　U　　 = unclassifiable

[1] I wish to thank Prof. Dr. W. Sandritter for placing the slides and blocks of the Pathological Institute of Freiburg University at my disposal for this investigation. I should also like to thank him and Prof. Dr. H. Rappaport and Prof. Dr. K. Lennert for reclassifying the old slides and blocks.

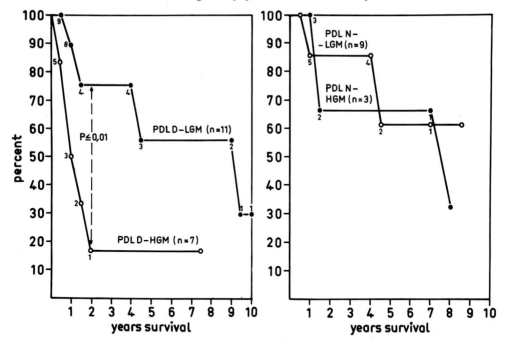

Fig. 1   The life expectancy (survival rates) of the disease groups
          (a) "poorly differentiated lymphocytic diffuse" lymphomas
          (PDL D) and (b) "poorly differentiated lymphocytic nodular"
          (PDL N) lymphomas of the Rappaport Classification subdivided
          respectively according to their attachment to the "low
          grade malignancy" (LGM) or "high grade malignancy" (HGM)
          lymphomas of the Kiel Classification.
               In brackets the number of patients at risk.(Joint
          examinations with H. Schmidt-Vollmer, W.v.Stotzingen and
          H. Umbach).

          On the   other hand, within the low grade malignant lymphomas
of the Kiel Classification the 10 patients with follicular lymphomas
(one of them: "follicular and diffuse with sclerosis") which
correspond up to 80% to the nodular form of Rappaport (of Rappaport
8 were diagnosed as nodular, 1 as histiocytic diffuse (H D) and 1
as unclassified (U)) have absolutely the same prognosis as the rest
of the 21 patients of the low grade malignant group, which according
to the Lennert definition have diffuse character (16 were likewise
diagnosed by Rappaport as diffuse, 2 as nodular and 1 as unclassified
(see also Table 1)) (Fig. 2).

DISCUSSION
          In the long run, for the histo-morphological and histofunctional
diagnosis of the NHL, a histopathological classification system must
be aimed at, which is not only clinically significant and reproducible
but also scientifically exact. The new morphological functional
classifications of Lukes and Collins (1974) and the Kiel Classification
(Gerard-Marchant and co-workers, 1974) which is based on the works
of Lennert, Mohri, Stein and co-workers (1967, 1975) do more justice
to the character of the NHL as neoplasmes of the lymphatic immune

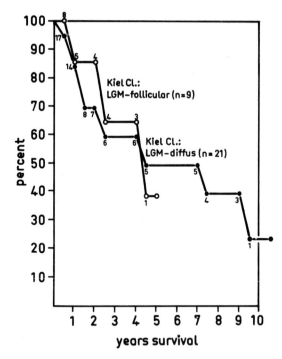

Fig. 2   The life expectancy (survival rates) of the low grade
           malignant lymphomas divided into the subgroup of the
           follicular type (centroblastic-centrocytic) and into the
           subgroup of the diffuse types (lymphocytic, lympho-
           plasmocytoid, centrocytic).
                In brackets the number of patients at risk. (Joint
           examinations with H. Schmidt-Vollmer, W.v. Stotzingen
           and H. Umbach).

system than the old morphological classifications were capable of.
The few retrospective examinations available up to now using the
Kiel Classification, one of the two morphological-functional
classifications, have proved their clinical and prognostic
significance (Musshoff and co-workers, 1975/76; Brittinger and co-
workers, 1976; Stacher and co-workers, 1976; Dühmke and co-workers,
1977). The first prospective examinations have confirmed these
findings (Brittinger and co-workers, 1978). My own examinations
carried out together with Schmidt-Vollmer, von Stotzingen and Umbach
revealed that the prognostic evidence of the Rappaport and Kiel
Classifications is, on the whole, of equal value (Musshoff,1978b;
v. Stotzingen, 1978). On the other hand Meugé and co-workers (1978)
asserted the superiority of the Kiel Classification. Nevertheless,
it is still an open question, which of both of these classifying
types best correspond to the real disease entities. One is inclined
to assume that the new classifications of Lukes and Collins as well
as of Lennert and co-workers (Kiel Classification) with their
additional immunological examination methods must do more justice
to reality, than was possible for Rappaport and co-workers twenty
years ago with purely morphological diagnostics. In fact, the above-
mentioned observation that the morphological type "poorly differentiated lymphocytic diffuse" Lymphoma (PDL D) can be divided into

two groups of low and high grade malignancy with different
prognoses argues in favor of the view of Lukes and co-workers (1977)
that the traditional cytological types of Rappaport are heterogenous.

Although the generally recognized favourable prognosis of the
nodular pattern of lymph node involvement of the Rappaport
Classification is caused primarily through its preponderant
attachment to the low grade malignant cell species, it still cannot
be precluded today that there is also a favourable variant of this
nodular pattern in the cell group of the high grade malignancy.

The diagnosis of the nodular patterns of lymph nodes (a) as
regards their prognosis in connection with cells of different
malignancy and (b) as regards their partial agreement with the
follicular pattern of the Kiel Classification is still an unsolved
problem and requires further comparative investigations.

The insufficient agreement, on the whole, of the Rappaport
and Kiel Classifications, both in the comparison of the individual
types with one another and in the comparison of both of the
respective principle subgroups of "good and bad prognoses" and
"low and high grade malignancy" makes a simple transference to
the Kiel Classification of the great clinical and therapeutic
stock of experience that was gained with the Rappaport Classification
only possible with a certain amount of qualification. Consequently,
we can hardly agree with the view that is often taken that the
morphological classification of Rappaport and the morphological-
functional classifications which are represented here by the Kiel
Classification designate the same diseases. (The same is probably
true of the Lukes and Collins Classification.)

In the course of our efforts to establish a new clinical
classification for the NHL instead of the present Ann Arbor
Classification we should recollect the four important reasons for
a valid clinical staging classification (Rosenberg, 1977): "(1)
the provide important prognostic information for different sites
and extent of the disease, (2) to assist the physician in
selecting the most appropriate therapeutic program, (3) to provide
a standardized system which permits comparison of therapeutic
results and (4) to provide an accepted descriptive system which
communicates the extent of the disease".

As long as our knowledge of the natural history of the NHL
remains limited, we should aim at a differentiated and not at a
simplifying classification. This differentiated classification
would put us in the position to be able to classify many findings
and would best fulfil the demand to document the topographical
calculation as carefully as possible. Together with Schmidt-
Vollmer we made such an attempt in 1975. With careful topographical documentation, we will do justice at the same time to
the demand for prognostic information, in as far as the prognosis
is predominantly determined by the distribution stage. While that
is the case to a large extent with malignant tumours and also
with HL in general, we see in some NHL early dissemination stages
with high survival rates, and in other lymphomas with loco-
regionally limited distribution, significantly shorter survival
rates.

Without a generally acceptable histopathological classification
comparable to the Hodgkin Lymphomas classification, it is difficult
even to imagine the highly desirable revision of the clinical Ann
Arbor Classification. The peculiar fact that the clinical distribution and the histopathological degree of malignancy can behave
controversely in single lymphomas (for example: early dissemination

in the favorable lymphocytic types (Jones and co-workers, 1973))
makes a close combination of pathohistological and clinical
diagnoses and classifications necessary.

In the face of the fundamental importance of pathology for our
modern understanding of lymphomas, it must be said, with all due
recognition of the valuable progress which functional pathology has
made in recent years, that the greatest hindrance, at the moment,
in the clinical lymphomas research is the lack of consensus as
regards a unifying histopathological classifying principle.

After the Airlie House workshop for the planning of retrospective and prospective studies to delineate optimal classifications
of the Non-Hodgkin Lymphomas, 1975, the National Cancer Institute
(NCI) decided to sponsor a study to examine leading histopathological
classifications as to their accuracy and reproducibility and their
connection with all the available clinical findings. It is very
much to be hoped that this investigation will bring us a unified
and optimal histopathological classification (DeVita, 1977).

Only afterwards will we be able to turn successfully to a
new clinical staging classification. But, in this connection, the
question seems to me to be fully open as to whether it will be
possible to formulate a single generally valid staging classification
for all NHL, or whether it will be necessary, and perhaps more
useful, to formulate separate classifications for individual NHL
groups to which adjustments could be made in a suitable form, as
has already been done with success in childrens' oncology (Murphy,
Auer and Hustu, 1978).

REFERENCES

Airlie House Warrenton, Virginia (1975): Invitational workshop for
the planning of retrospective and prospective studies to
delineate optimal classifications of the Non-Hodgkin's lymphomas,
September 4-5.
Brittinger,G., H.Bartels, A.Burger, E.Dühmke, H.H.Fülle, U.Gunzer,
R.Heinz, D.Huhn, G.W.Löhr, K.Musshoff, L.Nowicki, M.Pfloch,
H.Pralle, U.Schmalhorst (Kieler Lymphomgruppe) (1978). Grund-
lagen und bisherige Ergebnisse der prospectiven Studie der
Kieler Lymphomgruppe über Non-Hodgkin-Lymphome. In A.Stacher
und P.Höcker (Ed.), Lymphknotentumoren. Urban und Schwarzen-
berg, München-Wien-Baltimore, pp 193-200.
Brittinger,G., H.Bartels, K.Brehmer, E.Dühmke, U.Gunzer, E.König,
H.Stein (Kieler Lymphomgruppe) (1976). Klinik der malignen
Non-Hodgkin-Lymphome entsprechend der Kiel Klassifikation:
Centrocytisches Lymphom, centroblastisch-centrocytisches
Lymphom, lymphoblastisches Lymphom, immunoblastisches Lymphom.
In H.Löffler (Ed.), Maligne Lymphome und monoklonale Gammo-
pathien 18, 211-223.
Brown,T.C., M.V.Peters, D.E.Bergsagel and J.Reid (1975). A retro-
spective analysis of the clinical results in relation to the
Rappaport histological classification. Symposium on Non-
Hodgkin's Lymphomata, London, 8-12 October 1973. Br.J.Cancer,
31. Suppl.II, 174-186.
Carbone,P.P., H.S.Kaplan, K.Musshoff, D.W.Smithers, M.Tubiana
(1971). Report of the Hodgkin's disease staging classification
commitee. Conference on staging in Hodgkin's disease. Ann
Arbor, April 26-28, 1971. Cancer Res. 31, 1860-1861.

DeVita,V.T. (1977). Summary of Symposium. In: St.E.Jones and J.
    Godden (Ed.), Proceedings of the conference on Non-Hodgkin's
    lymphomas. Cancer Treat.Rep. 61, 1223-1227.
Dühmke,E., und J.Queck (1977). Retrospektive Analyse von malignen
    Non-Hodgkin-Lymphomerkrankungen der Radiologischen Klinik der
    Universität Kiel von 1969-1975. Strahlentherapie 153, 229-231.
Gerard-Marchant,R., J.Hamlin, K.Lennert, F.Rilke, A.G.Stansfeld
    and J.A.M. van Unnik (1974). Classification of non-Hodgkin's
    lymphomas. Lancet II, 405-408.
Goffinet,D.R., R.Warnke, N.R.Dunnick, R.Castellino, E.Glatstein,
    Th.S.Nelson, R.F.Dorfman,S.A. Rosenberg and H.S.Kaplan (1977).
    Clinical and Surgical (Laparotomy) evaluation of patients with
    non-Hodgkin's lymphomas. Cancer Treat.Rep. 61, 981-992.
Hansen,J.A., and R.A.Good (1974). Malignant disease of the lymphoid
    system in immunologic perspective. Hum.Pathol.5, 567-599.
Jaffe,N., D.Buell, J.R.Cassady, D.Traggis and H.Weinstein (1977).
    Role of staging in childhood non Hodgkin's lymphomas. Cancer
    Treat. Rep.61, 1001-1007.
Johnson,R.E., V.T.DeVita, L.E.Kun, B.R.Chabner, P.B.Chretien,
    C.W.Berard and S.K.Johnson (1975). Patterns of involvement
    with malignant lymphoma and implications for treatment decision
    making. Br.J.Cancer 31, Suppl.II, 237-241.
Jones,S.E., Z.Fuchs, M.Bull, M.E.Kadin, R.F.Dorfman, H.S.Kaplan,
    S.A.Rosenberg and H.Kim (1973). Non-Hodgkin's lymphomas
    IV. Clinicopathologic correlation in 405 cases. Cancer 31,
    806-823.
Jones,St.E., and J.Godden (Eds.) (1977). Proceedings of the
    conference on non-Hodgkin's lymphomas, Sept.30 to Oct.2, 1976,
    San Francisco. Cancer Treat. Rep. 61, 935-1230.
Kaplan,H.S. (1972). Hodgkin's Disease. Cambridge, Massachusetts
    Harvard University Press.
Lennert,K. (1967). Classification of malignant lymphomas (European
    concept). In Rüttimann,A. (Ed.), Progress in Lymphology, pp.
    103-109. G.Thieme Stuttgart.
Lennert,K. (1978). Some ideas for a modern lymphoma classification.
    In K.Lennert in collaboration with N.Mohri, H.Stein, E.Kaiser-
    ling, H.K.Müller-Hermelink, Malignant Lymphomas other than
    Hodgkin's disease. Springer, Berlin-Heidelberg-New York, pp.
    93-98.
Lennert,K., N.Mohri, H.Stein and E.Kayserling (1975). The histo-
    pathology of malignant lymphoma. Brit. J. Haemat. 31 (Suppl.),
    193-203.
Lukes,R.J. (1968). The pathologic picture of the malignant
    lymphomas. In Ch.J.D.Zarafonetis (Ed.), Proceedings of the
    International conference on leukemia-lymphoma. Lea Y.Feliger,
    Philadelphia, pp. 333-356.
Lukes,R.J., and R.D.Collins (1974). A Functional Approach to the
    Classification of Malignant Lymphoma. In K.Musshoff (Ed.),
    Diagnosis and Therapy of Malignant Lymphoma. Recent Results
    in Cancer Res. 46, Springer, Berlin-Heidelberg-New York,
    pp. 18-30.
Meugé, C., B.Hoerni, A.de Mascarel, M.Durand, P.Richaud, G.Hoerni-
    Simon, J.Chauvergne and C.Lagarde (1978). Non-Hodgkin
    Lymphomas. Clinico-pathologic correlations with the Kiel
    Classification. Europ.J.Cancer 14, 587-592.
Murphy,S.B. (1977). Management of childhood non-Hodgkin's lymphomas.
    Cancer Treat. Rep. 61, 1161-1173.

Murphy,S.B., R.J.A.Aur and H.O.Hustu (1978). Patterns of presentation
    and relapse in childhood non-Hodgkin's lymphoma. XII Inter-
    national Cancer Congress, Buenos Aires, Oct. 5-11, 1978. Panel
    No. 2, Non-Hodgkin Lymphoma. Pergamon Press Non-Hodgkin Lymphoma
    in this book.
Musshoff,K. (1978a). Voraussetzungen und Probleme der adjuvanten
    Chemotherapie in Verbindung mit der primären Strahlentherapie
    der Nicht-Hodgkin-Lymphome unter besonderer Berücksichtigung
    der Histologie. In H.Huber (Ed.), Adjuvante zytostatische
    Chemotherapie. Blut, Sonderband in press.
Musshoff,K. (1978b). Vergleiche der Kiel- und Rappaport-Klassifikation.
    1. Forumdiskussion in A.Stacher und P.Höcker (Ed.), Lymphknoten-
    tumoren. Urban und Schwarzenberg, München-Wien-Baltimore, pp
    288-290.
Musshoff,K., and H.Schmidt-Vollmer (1975). Prognosis of Non-Hodgkin's
    Lymphomas with special emphasis on the staging classification.
    Z.Krebsforsch.83, 323-341.
Musshoff,K., H.Schmidt-Vollmer, K.Lennert and W.Sandritter (1975/1976).
    Preliminary clinical findings on the Kiel Classification of
    malignant Lymphomas. Workshop for the classification of Non-
    Hodgkin Lymphomas, Airlie House, Warrenton,Virginia,Sept.4-5,
    1975- Z.Krebsforsch. 87, 229-238.
Musshoff,K., H.Schmidt-Vollmer and D.Merten (1971). Reticulum Cell
    Sarcoma, an oncological model for a system of classifying the
    malignant lymphoma. Europ.J.Cancer 7, 451-457.
Peters,M.V., R.Hasselback and T.C.Brown (1968). In Zarafonetis,C.J.D.
    (Ed.), Proceedings of the International Conference on Leukemia-
    Lymphoma. Philadelphia: Lea and Febiger, 357-370.
Pinkel,D., J.Simone, H.O.Hustu, R.J.A.Aur (1972). Nine years
    experience with "total therapy" of childhood acute lymphocytic
    leukemia. Pediatrics 50, 246-251.
Rappaport,H. (1966). Tumors of the hematopoitic system. Sect.3,fasc.8.
    Washington D.S. Armed Forces Institute of Pathology, 91-156.
Rappaport,H., W.J.Winter and E.B.Hicks (1956). Follicular lymphoma:
    A re evaluation of its position in the scheme of malignant
    lymphomas, based on a survey of 253 cases. Cancer 9, 729-821.
Rosenberg,S.A. (1975). Bone marrow involvement in the non-Hodgkin's
    lymphomata. Br.J.Cancer 31 (Suppl.II), 261-264.
Rosenberg,S.A. (1977). Validity of the Ann Arbor staging classification
    for the non-Hodgkin's lymphomas. Cancer Treat.Rep.61,1023-1027.
Rosenberg,S.A. and H.S.Kaplan (1975). Clinical trials in the non-
    Hodgkin's lymphomata at Stanford University experimental design
    and preliminary results. Brit.J.Cancer 31, Suppl.II, 456-464.
Seligmann,M., J.-C.Brouet and H.-L.Preud'homme (1977).Immunologic
    classification of non-Hodgkin's lymphomas: current status.
    Cancer Treat. Rep. 61, 1179-1183.
Stacher,A., R.Waldner und H.Theml (1976). Klinik der malignen Non-
    Hodgkin Lymphome entsprechend der Kieler Klassifikation: Lympho-
    plasmozytoides Lymphom (LPL) und chronische lymphatische Leukämie
    (CLL). In H.Löffler (Ed.) Haematologie und Bluttransfusion 18:
    Maligne Lymphome und monoklonale Gammopathien, 199-209.
Stotzingen,W.von (1979). Non-Hodgkin-Lymphome. Ein klinischer Ver-
    gleich der Klassifikationen von Rappaport und Lennert (Kiel
    Klassifikation). Inangural Dissertation der Mediz.Fakultät der
    Albert-Ludwigs-Universität Freiburg im Breisgau.
Ultmann,J.E. (1978). Zur Diagnose,Stadieneinteilung und Behandlung
    der Non-Hodgkin-Lymphome. In A.Stacher und P.Höcker (Ed.),
    Lymphknotentumoren. Urban und Schwarzenberg, München-Wien-Baltimore,
    pp. 1-6.

Clinical Implications of Pathological and Immunological Patterns in Non Hodgkin Lymphomas

V. Diehl, M. Schaadt and A. Georgii

Division of Hematology-Oncology and Department of Pathology,
Medizinische Hochschule Hannover, G.F.R.

A B S T R A C T

A reproducible, scientifically accurate and clinically relevant classification
for the non-Hodgkin's lymphomas (NHL) must be based not only on morphological
criteria as used in the Rappaport classification (33) but also on the newer
immunological concepts utilising surface marker and cytochemical techniques.
Although the Rappaport classification has best support for its clinical utility (22, 1)
this histopathological classification has received mounting criticism based on an
improved understanding of cytogenesis, differentiation pathways and cellular
interactions of the various lymphoid subpopulations present in NHL.

The Kiel classification (Table 1) has not yet been used as much as the
Rappaport classification for clinical studies but it does take into consideration
immunological cell marker analysis (using frozen sections, single cell suspensions
and cell extracts) in addition to cytological, histochemical and ultrastructural criteria
in order to delineate the different cell populations and differentiation represented
in NHL biopsy material (for review see K. Lennert: "Malignant lymphomas",
Springer Verlag, 1978).

This paper tries to summarise the increasing evidence for the scientific accuracy
of the Kiel classification and its clinical relevance relating   Lennert's classification
with retrospective clinical studies (6, 7, 11, 15, 16, 20, 30, 316, 42).   The report
refers to our own experience using the Kiel classification in a group of 143 NHL
patients treated in Hannover.

Patients:

For this study 89 patients with the histological diagnosis of NHL treated during the last 10 years in our institution were evaluated for clinical presentation, response to therapy and prognosis. Two patients did not receive therapy at all. These 89 patients were chosen out of a total number of 143 with NHL on the basis of representative sections of primary or re-biopsy material, classified according to the Kiel system. 54 patients could not be considered for this report, since they were either classified according to other than Kiel classification systems or because of incomplete followup data. The sections were judged by our local pathologists at time of diagnosis. Patients included in this study, that were diagnosed primarily before 1974 (initiation of the Kiel-system) were judged by re-biopsy material or re-evaluation of the primary slides according to the Kiel-system.

Clinical staging was done according to the protocol of the Kiel Lymphoma Study group, as reported by Brittinger and coworkers (6). The clinical staging classification was derived from the ANN ARBOR System (10).

The treatment was given according to the grade of malignancy of the biopsy material and the clinical stage: for patients with low grade malignant lymphomas (LGML) of stage I and II primary treatment was radiation (4.500 rad, extended fields). Patients with generalized disease (Stage III-IV) received primary chemotherapy (Vincristin, Cyclophosphamide and Prednisone, 6 cycles) followed by involved field radiation (2.500 rad). Patients with high grade malignant lymphomas (HGML) received initially aggressive chemothearapy (6 x COP-Mtx or 6 x CHOP) followed by involved field radiation. This combination therapy was given regardless of the clinical stage in HGML patients.

Survival was evaluated according to the life table analysis of Cutler and Ederer (13). Statistical significance was calculated using the chi-square test.

The sex ratio in our patient group showed a predominance of males: 52 males, 37 females; the males dominating in the low grade group (33 versus 20), whereas in the high grade group an even distribution was seen (19 versus 17).

The age distribution is demonstrated together with the data derived from the literature (6,7,30,31), reviewing a total of about 1.570 patients.

Comparison of the Kiel- and Rappaport-Classifications:

Table 1 tries to compare the different entities of the Kiel classification with the histological subgroups of the Rappaport-Classification. It is evident from this comparison that there is some agreement as far as the cytological subtypes are concerned: the LGML lymphocytic, lymphoplasmocytoid and centrocytic (small cell lymphomas) correspond to "lymphocytic well differentiated", (excluding CLL) (Rappaport), centrocytic paritally being indentical with NPDL. The HGML, categorized as "large cell lymphomas" = blastic, correspond to the celltypes: "histiocytic", "lymphocytic poorly differentiated" or "undifferentiated" (Rappaport). The architectural description nodular or diffuse (Rappaport) overlaps the border of low and high grade malignancy. The nodular (follicular)lymphomas (Rappaport) seem to be identical in a high proportion with the centroblastic-centrocytic entity (follicular center cells) (24).

Clinical presentation:

Table 2 demonstrates our own results in combination with the available information from the above cited studies (6,7,16,20,30,31,42), concerning age, primary stage, constitutional symptoms, dynamic of lymphnode enlargement, extranodal involvement and hematological parameters. A total of 1.570 patients was reviewed in these studies. The data of the "Kiel Lymphoma Group" (including about 250 cases in a prospective and 405 cases in a retrospective analysis), comprising several clinical groups at different centers in West Germany and Austria, served as the base line information. These data are used with kind permission by Prof.G Brittinger, Essen, the chairman of the Kiel-Lymphoma Group.

It becomes obvious from this survey that there are remarkable differences between the low and the high grade malignancy groups, whereas within these two main categories the incidence of the various clinical parameters was rather similar. More than 50% of the LGML patients presented with generalized disease (clinical stages III and IV), whereas in the HGML more than 50% of the patients were diagnosed with lokalised disease (stages I and II). The presence of constitutional symptoms was evenly distributed between both groups. The aggressive growth tendency of the HGML was reflected by the rapidity of lymphnode enlargement occuring in 2/3 of this patient group, versus 18 % in the low grade category. This phenomenon was also obvious from the duration of symptoms before diagnosis, which was significantly shorter in the high malignant group. Extranodal involvement (bone marrow and liver) and peripheral lymphocytosis were more frequent in patients with LGML. Primary lymphonodal involvement was seen in 84 % , equally distributed between the two groups (31), the infiltration of the Waldeyer lymphatic ring was observed more often in high grade lymphomas, according to Musshoff and coworkers (31). Meugé and coworkers (30) saw involvement of visceral locations and Waldeyers ring more frequently in LGML (lymphoplasmacytoid); mediastinal masses occured more often in high grade cases (lymphoblastic-convoluted type). The frequency of lymphnode involvement, visualized by lymphoangiography was higher in the LGML category (30). Leukemic presentation during evolution of the disease was observed most frequently in lymphocytic and lymphoblastic entities (3). The highest incidence of monoclonal dysproteinaemia was documented in lymphoplasmocytoid immunocytoma patients (26 %) followed by 8 % in immunoblastic lymphomas (7). Primary CNS involvement was rare. With progression of the disease it occured most frequently in childhood lymphoblastic lymphomas, in the low grade category in the centrocytic (2/5 in our series) and in the immunocytic polymorphous type. In summary: The cyto-histological discrimination between low and high grade malignancy lymphomas of the Kiel classification is paralleled by a dichotomy in some clinical patterns, like initial stage, duration of symptoms, and rapidity of tumorprogression. LGML occured in the older age (5 to 6 decade) and were rarely seen below the age of 30.

Correlation between prognosis and histological classification:

Despite the rather small number of patients in our own study there was a good agreeement, concerning therapy response and prognosis when compared with the above listed literature reports in which the Kiel system was also used as histopathological classification (6,7,16,20,30,31,42).
The survival for patients with LGML was significantly (p = 0,001) better than for those with HGML, showing a 50 % probability of survival at 22 months (fig.1). The LGML had at 5 years still 85 % probability of survival. If one breaks down the two main groups in histological subentities (excluding centrocytic and lymphoplasmocytoid lymphomas because of two small numbers) (fig. 2), lymphocytic lymphomas had the best prognosis, reaching a plateau at 94 % for up to 7.5 years. Centroblastic-centrocytic lymphomas (nodular, according to Rappaport) leveled off after 4 years at 65 % survival probability. The worst prognosis had lymphoblastic lymphomas (DUL, DPDL) with 30 % probability after 3 years, followed by centroblastic lymphomas with a plateau after 1.5 up to 7.5 years at 45 % survival probability. Immunoblastic lymphomas (DHL), in contrast to other reports (7,16,30,31), had an intermediate prognosis with a plateau of 55 % probability of survival up to 10.5 years. The number of cases is too small to speculate about the relevance of these findings. This entity might cover two prognostically different subtypes, as it is discussed for the histiocytic lymphomas in the Rappaport classification, or includes cases of lympho-epitheliomas (Schmincke - Regaud), as demonstrated by Musshoff (31b).

Response to therapy and duration of complete remission:

Patients with low grade malignant lymphomas responded with a complete disappearance of all tumor signs following first therapy in 75 %, versus 37.1 % in the HGML group (table 3). Criteria for complete remission in CLL were peripheral leukocyte count below 30.000/mm^3 and absence of disease induced symptoms. Partial remission (more than 50% reduction of all tumor parameters) was reached in about 20% in both categories. Failure of therapy was higher in the HGML group (42,9 %) compared with 1.9 % in the good prognosis group. The rates of response for all

patients together were: complete remission 59.8 %, partial remission 21.8 % and no
response 18.4 %. Duration of complete remission did not differ significantly between both groups with a median duration of 2 years for the HGML and 3 years for
the LGML (fig. 3). 6.5 years after start of therapy all patients with HGML had
terminated complete remission whereas 13 % of patients with LGML stayed in
complete remission up to 9 + years.

Correlation between prognosis and response to therapy: (Fig.4)
In HGML complete responders had a significantly better survival than those
achieving only a partial reduction of their disease, with a 50 % survival probability of 2.5 years (PR) versus 8 years (CR) (p = 0,009). Non-responders in
HGML survived significantly shorter (50 % probability of 9 months) than partial-
or complete-responders. The survival of patients with LGML achieving complete
remission did not differ significantly from that of HGML patients. Furthermore,
there was no statistically significant difference in survival between complete
and partial responders in the LGML group (p = 0.554).
Fig. 5 demonstrates as a trend analysis the duration of complete remissions for
the different histological entities. Statistical analysis was obsolete because
of the small number of patients in each group. It becomes obvious, however, that
lymphoblastic lymphoma not only comprises the lowest number of complete responders, but also has the shortest duration of complete remission. LP immunocytic lymphoma relapses earlier than the other low grade lymphomas, thus taking
an intermediate position between low and high grade malignancy, as it is also
shown by others (30). Lymphocytic and centroblastic-centrocytic lymphomas
terminate complete remission rather early inspite of their good overall prognosis
(fig. 2), supporting again the finding, that achievement and duration of CR in
LGML does not influence survival as much as in HGML.

Table 4 correlates immunological cell markers, demonstrated on in vitro cell
suspensions or frozen sections from NHL-biopsy-material to cytological subtypes and malignancy grading. As B-cell markers the presence of surface immunoglobulin and EAC-rosette positivity was taken. As T-markers rosetting with sheep
red blood cells was used (SRBC = E-rosettes) (tab. 5). These data are derived
from the studies of H. Stein (41), which created the immunological
basis of the Kiel classification. As it is shown in table 4, histological diagnoses expressing B-cell characteristics dominate as well in LGML as in HGML.
According to the results of Stein (41) and others (37) B-cell as well as T-cell
markers do not allow a sensitive and clinically relevant differentiation between
high and low malignant lymphomas as it is reflected by pure cyto-histological
criteria or cytokinetic characteristics as demonstrated by Silvestrini et al. (39).
T-cell proliferation of lymphoid tissue (tab. 4), comprising a minor proportion
of NHL, cyto-histologically, again, is represented in both, low and high malignant categories.
NHL, lacking B- or T-cell markers, the so-called Null- or unqualified-lymphomas,
exclusively are high malignant and occur most frequently in the age group below
30 years, comprising most of the cases with ALL (common ALL).

Table 5 correlates cyto-histological, immunological and clinical patterns with
prognosis in a synopsis according to own and literature findings.
From this survey it becomes evident that:
    1. Cyto-histo-morphological analysis of biopsy material according to the Kiel
       system offers the possibility to discriminate between a group of lympho-
       proliferative diseases with a malignant, rapidly progressive course
       (HGML) and a more benign variant with slowly progressing lymphopro-
       liferation and a good prognosis despite disseminated disease at time
       of diagnosis (75 %) (LGML).

2. B- and T-cell markers do not discriminate sensitively enough between disease entities of rapidly proliferating, highly malignant tumors and the benigne variants. The expression of immunological markers nevertheless, reflects to a certain degree the stage of differentiation of the lymphoproliferation: morphological entities which lack B- or T-cell markers (Null- or unqualified) exclusively belong to immature, rapidly growing, high malignant lymphoproliferations as demonstrated also by Bloomfield et. al (4) using cell marker analysis in combination with the Rappaport classification. Surface markers, in combination with cytological criteria however, do correlate with clinical patterns, i.e. T-cell-lymphomas involving predominantly mediastinal nodes, thymus and skin, whereas B-cellymphomas involve more often organs, possibly representing bursa equivalent areas as in liver, spleen, bone marrow and in Peyers plaques.
3. Response to therapy determines survival to a much greater extent in HGML than in LGML, the latter in which the achievement of complete remission does not improve survival significantly.
4. There seems to be a good correlation between the nodular lymphomas of the Rappaport classification and the centroblastic-centrocytic entity of the Kiel classification. Most diffuse lymphomas overlap the low-high grade malignancy border. There is some identity of well differentiated lymphomas whith the "cytic"-lymphomas (Kiel), and the poorly differentiated histocytic or undifferentiated lymphomas with the high grade -"blastic" cell types (Kiel).
5. It is concluded from this study, that the Kiel classification not only satisfies the endeavour for a scientifically accurate, cytologically and immunologically based nomenclature, but also offers the clinician the opportunity to foresee prognosis and decide in the future for a biologically relevant therapy at the time of primary diagnosis.

REFERENCES:

1. Anderson, T., R.A. Bender, R.J. Fisher, V.T. de Vita et al. (1977)
   Cancer Treatm. Rep. 61, 1057 - 1066
2. Aisenberg, A.C., K.J. Bloch (1972)
   N. Eng. J. Med. , 287, 272 - 7276
3. Bennet, M.H.
   Sclerosis in Non Hodgkin lymph. (1975)
   5th Congr. Europ. Soc. Path., Vienna
4. Bloomfield, C.D., J.H. Kersey et al. (1977)
   Cancer Treatm. Rep. 61, 963 - 970
5. Brittinger, G.H., Bartels et al. (Kieler Lymphomgrauppe) (1976)
   In: Mal. Lymph. u. monokl. Gammapath. (Löffler ed)
   In: Hämatologie und Bluttransf. 18, 211 - 233, München, Lehmanns
6. Brittinger, G., H. Bartels, K. Bremer et al. (1977)
   Strahlentherapie 153, 222 - 228
7. Brittinger, G. (1978)
   "Controversies in Cancer Treatment"
   Brussels, April 1978 (EORTC-Symposium)
8. Brouet, J.C., G. Flandrin et al. (1975)
   Lancet, II, 890 - 893
9. Buskard, N.A., D. Catovsky et al. (1976)
   In: Mal. Lymph. and. monoklon. Gammapath.
   Hämat. u. Bluttransf., Bd. 18, 237 - 253
10. Carbone, P.P., H.S. Kaplan et al. (1971)
    Ann Arbor, Cancer Res. 31, 1860 - 1861
11. Castellani, R.G., Bonadonna et al. (1977)
    Cancer, 40, 2322 - 2328

168 V. Diehl, M. Schaadt and A. Georgii

12a Catovsky, D., J.E. Pettit, D.A.G. Galton et al. (1974)
Leukaemic reticuloendotheliosis ("Hairy cell leuk.")
Brit. J. Haem., 26, 9 - 27
12 Coccia, F.P., H.J. Kersey et al. (1976)
Am. J. Hem. 1, 41505 - 417
13. Cutler, S.J., and F. Ederer
J. of chronic diseases, Dec. 1958, pp 699 - 712
14. Clifford, P. (1968)
Treatment of Burk. Lymph., Lancet, I, 599
15. Delbrück, H., H.C. Weichert, G. Schmitt et al. (1978)
Klin. Wochenschr. 56, 539 - 543
16. Dühmke, E. (1976)
Strahlentherapie, 152, 129 - 139 (2)
17. Fleischmayer, R., S. Eisenberg (1964)
Arch. Derm. 89, 69 - 79
18. Fuks, Z.Y., M.A. Bagshaw, E.M. Farber (1973)
Cancer, 32, 1385 - 1395
19. Galton, D.A., G. Goldman et al. (1974)
Brit. J. Haemat., 27, 7 - 23
20. Garwicz, S., T. Landberg et al. (1978)
Scand. J. Hematol., 20, 171 - 180
21. Gerard-Marchant, R., J. Hamlin, K. Lennert et al. (1974)
Clasific. of Non Hodgkin Lymph., Lancet, 2, 406 - 408
22. Jones, S.E., Z. Fuks, M. Bull et al. (1973)
Cancer, 31, 806 - 823
23. Lennert, K. (1975)
Acta Neuropath. Suppl., 6, 1 - 16
24. Lennert, K. (1978) (ed.)
Malignant Lymphomas, other than Hodgkin's disease.
Springer, Berlin
25. Levine, P.H., R.B. Cho et al. (1975)
Ann. Int. Med., 83, 31 - 36
26. Lukes, R.J., and Collins, R.D. (1974)
Cancer 34, 1488 - 1503
27. Lukes. R.J., K. Lennert (1974),
10.Int. Cong. Int. Acad. Path., Hamburg
28. Lumb, G (1954),
Tumors of lymph. tiss. Edinburgh-London, Livingstone
29. MacKenzie, M.R. Fudenberg, H.H. (1972).
Blood, 39, 874 - 889
30. Meugé, C., B. Hoerni, A. DeMascarel et al. (1978).
Europ. J. Cancer, 14, 587 - 592
31. Musshoff, K. H. Schmidt,Vollmer, K. Lennert, and W. Sandritter (1976),
Z. Krebsforschg. 87, 229 - 238
31b. Musshoff, K. (1978):
Vergleich der Kiel- und Rappaport Klassifikation. 1. Forumsdiskussion.
In: A. Stacher, P. Höcker (Ed.) "Lymphknotentumore"
32. Rappaport, H. W.J. Winter, E.B. Hicks (1956),
Cancer, 9, 792 - 821
33. Rappaport, H. (1966).
in: Atlas of Tum. Path., sect. 3, fasc. 8, Wash., D.C. US Armed Forc. Inst.
of Path.
34. Rieber, E.P., v. Heyden, H.W. et al. (1976).
Klin. Wschr., 54, 1011- 1019
35. Riehm, H. H. Gadner, K. Welte (1977).
Klin.Päd, 189, 89 - 102
36. Schrek, R. W.J. Donelly (1966).
Blood, 27, 199 - 211

37. Seligmann, M., J.C. Brouet, and J.L. Preud'homme (1977)
     Cancer Treatm. Rep. 61, 1179 - 1183
38. Seligmann, M. J.C. Brouet, J.L. Preud-Homme (1977).
     In: Imm. Diagn. of Leuk.and Lymph. Haemat. and Blood-Transf.
     Vol 20, 1 - 15, (Thierfelder ed.),
     Springer, Heidelberg
39. Silvestrini, R. R. Piazza, A. Riccardi, F. Rilke (1977).
     J. Nat. Canc. Inst., 58, 499 - 504
40. Stacher, A., and P. Höcker (ed.) (1978). Lymphknotentumore,
     München, Urban und Schwarzenberg, in press.
41. Stein, H. (1978),
     The immunolog. and immunochemical basis for the Kiel
     classification. In: Lennert, K. Malign. Lymph., other than Hodgkin Disease,
     Springer, Berlin
42. Takacsi-Nagy, L., G. Tarkovass et al. (1978).
     Folia Hematolog. Leipzig, 105, 79 - 92

V. Diehl, M. Schaadt and A. Georgii

Table 1

COMPARISON OF THE KIEL- AND THE RAPPAPORT HISTOLOGICAL CLASSIFICATION [*]

KIEL CLASSIFICATION 1974		RAPPAPORT'S CLASSIFICATION 1966	
Low-grade malignant lymphomas			
Lymphocytic	LC	M.L. lymphocytic, well dif- ferentiated, diffuse	DWDL
CLL and others	CLL		
Lymphoplasmacytoid (immunocytic)	LP	M.L. lymphocytic with dysproteinemia	DWDL with dysproteinemia
Centrocytic	CC	M.L. lymphocytic, well and poorly differentiated, nodular or diffuse	DWDL, NWDL DPDL, NPDL
Centroblastic/Centrocytic follicular follicular and diffuse diffuse	CB-CC	M.L. lymphocytic, well differentiated M.L. lymphocytic, poorly differentiated nodular or diffuse	NWDL, DWDL NPDL, DPDL NML, DPL NHL, DHL
with or without sclerosis		M.L. lymphocytic- histiocytic M.L. histiocytic	
High-grade malignant lymphomas			
Centroblastic	CB	M.L. histiocytic nodular or M.L. undifferentiated diffuse	NHL, NUL DHL, DUL
Lymphoblastic	LB	M.L. undifferentiated, diffuse M.L. lymphocytic, poorly differentiated, diffuse	DUL, DPDL
Burkitt-type	LB-BL		
convoluted-cell-type	LB-CONV		
others			
Immunoblastic	IB	M.L. histiocytic, diffuse	DHL

[*]according to Lennert, K. 1978

(24)

Table 2

NON-HODGKIN-LYMPHOMAS: CLINICAL IMPLICATIONS ACCORDING TO THE KIEL-CLASSIFICATION

	Histological entity	Median age	Primary stage (path. or clinical)	Consti- tutional symptoms	Rapid lymphnode enlarge- ment (<3 month)	Initial Bone marrow involve- ment	Initial Liver involve- ment	Lympho- cytosis >4000/mm³	Lympho- penia <1000/mm³	Thrombo- cytes <100.000 /mm³	Hb <10 g%
LOW GRADE MALIGNANCY	CLL	62	Rai-I 46 % II 36 % III 9 % IV 9 %	36 %	4 %	100 %	N.D.	100 %	0 %	10 %	6 %
	LP	63	75 % Stage III-IV		10 %	87 %	36 %	65 %	0 %	20 %	10 %
	CB-CC	52	50 % Stage III-IV	45 %	16 %	45 %	23 %	2 %	25 %	3 %	7 %
	CC	61	75 % Stage III-IV	44 %	45 %	76 %	45 %	24 %	36 %	16 %	4 %
	TOTAL			48 %	18 %	77 %	38 %	54 %	14 %	11 %	15 %
HIGH GRADE MALIGNANCY	CB	66	50 % Stage III-IV	50 %	69 %	24 %	8 %	0 %	17 %	6 %	6 %
	LB-Burkitt type	15 and	58 % Stage III-IV	17 %	67 %	0 %	N.D.	0 %	14 %	17 %	
	LB-Convoluted type	62	57 % Stage III-IV	54 %	91 %	64 %	N.D.	40 %	0 %	33 %	8 %
	LB-unclassi- fied	35		33 %	78 %	61 %	N.D.	11 %	22 %	17 %	
	Immuno- blastic	63	45 % Stage III-IV	56 %	75 %	31 %	17 %	6 %	22 %	28 %	22 %
	TOTAL			50 %	62 %	38 %	14 %	8 %	21 %	20 %	15 %

N.D.: Not documented

Table 3

NON HODGKIN LYMPHOMAS: RESPONSE TO THERAPY
==

LOW GRADE MALIGNANCY

Histological classification	Number of cases	Complete Remission	Partial Remission	No Response
lymphocytic, CLL + others	17	76,5 %	23,5 %	0,0 %
lymphoplasmacytoid, immunocytic	6	83,3 %	16,7 %	0,0 %
centrocytic	5	60,0 %	40,0 %	0,0 %
centroblastic-centrocytic	22	77,3 %	18,2 %	4,5 %
unclassified low malignant	2	50,0 %	50,0 %	0,0 %
TOTAL LOW GRADE MALIGNANCY	52	75,0 %	23,0 %	1,9 %

HIGH GRADE MALIGNANCY

centroblastic	12	33,3 %	33,3 %	33,3 %
lymphoblastic	10	30,0 %	0,0 %	70,0 %
immunoblastic	13	46,2 %	23,1 %	30,7 %
TOTAL HIGH GRADE MALIGNANCY	35	37,1 %	20,0 %	42,9 %

SUMMARY LOW AND HIGH GRADE MALIGNANCY

Low grade malignancy	52	75,0 %	23,1 %	1,9 %
High grade malignancy	35	37,1 %	20,0 %	42,9 %
TOTAL	87	59,8 %	21,8 %	18,4 %

Table 4

IMMUNOLOGICAL MARKERS IN CORRELATION TO HISTOLOGICAL ENTITIES

	B-CELL-TYPE	T-CELL-TYPE	NULL-CELL-TYPE (Non-B-Non-T)
LOW GRADE MALIGNANCY	B-CLL (lymphocytic) Prolymphocytic Hairy-cell leuk. LP immunocytoma Plasmocytoma Centroblastic-centrocytic Centrocytic	T-CLL (lymphocytic) T-type prolymphocytic Mycosis fungoides Sezary syndrome T-zone lymphoma	
HIGH GRADE MALIGNANCY	Centroblastic B-Immunoblastic B-lymphoblastic Burkitt-type B-Non-Burkitt-type B-ALL	T-Immunoblastic T-lymphoblastic convoluted type T-ALL	Null-Immunoblastic lymphoblastic (unqualified) Common-(Null)-ALL

Table 5a

LOW GRADE MALIGNANCY NON-HODGKIN-LYMPHOMAS: HISTOLOGY, IMMUNOLOG, CELL MARKERS, CLIN. IMPLICATION, PROGNOSIS

HISTOLOGICAL DESIGNATION		CELL TYPE	CELL CHARACTERISTICS				CLINICAL IMPLICATIONS AND PROGNOSIS				
KIEL-CLASSIFICATION	RAPPAPORT-CLASSIFICATION	% OF CASES	SMIG	EAC_d ROSETTES	SRBC (E) ROSETTES	REFERENCE FOR IMMUNOLOGICAL DETERMINATION	PRIMARY SITES, MEDIAN AGE	RESPONSE TO THERAPY	5 YEAR SURVIVAL	50 % SURVIVAL	REFERENCE FOR CLINICAL DATA AND SURVIVAL
B-CLL	DWDL	B-Cell-Type 97-100 %	+	+	-	37, 2, 41	Bone marrow involvement 100 %, lymphnode involvement 78 %, autoimmune phenomena 62 ys	good	44 %		5, 40, 42
B-PROLYMPHOCYTIC LEUKEMIA	DWDL	B-Cell-Type 95-99 %	+	+	-	9	Splenomegaly, no lymphadenopathy, Lymphocytosis (mean 355.000/mm³) 50-60 ys	poor	10		19
HAIRYCELL LEUKEMIA (phagocytosing lymphocytes)	DWDL	B-Cell-Type 95-99 %	++	+/-	-	34, 36	Splenomegaly, Panhemocytopenia, dry tap! 40-60 ys	Splenectomy, therapy of choice	50 %		12 a
LP IMMUNOCYTOMA	DWDL with dysproteinemia	B-Cell-Type 100 %	+	+	-	38	3 types: lymphnode-splenomegalic-oculocutaneous- dysproteinemia, monoclonal Ig, haemolyt. anemia 63 ys	good response / bad response	mean survival 49, 2 months / 24, 1 months		5, 24, 29 / 24, 29
CENTROBLASTIC - CENTROCYTIC	NWDL, DWDL, NPDL, DPDL, NML, DML, NHL, DHL	B-Cell-Type 100 %	++	++	-	41	Slowly progressing lymphnode enlargement, bone marrow involvement 45 %, B-symptoms + never below 20 ys 52 ys	good	40-60 %		5, 7, 28, 32
CENTROCYTIC	DWDL, NWDL, DPDL, NPDL	B-Cell-Type 100 %	++	++	-	41	Lymphnode involvement 70-80 %, bone marrow involvement 68 %, Splenomegaly 50 %, B-symptoms 50 %, leukemic variant 61 ys	moderate to good	leukemic variant 11 % (20)	48 months	5
T-CLL	DWDL	T-Cell-Type 1-3 %	-	-	+	37, 2, 41	Bone marrow involv. 80-100 %, Splenomegaly ++, Skinlesions +, lymphnode involvement rare, Neutropenia range 25-78 ys	moderate to good	like B-CLL		24
T-TYPE PROLYMPH. LEUKEMIA	DWDL	T-Cell-Type 2-5 %	-	-	+	9	like prolymphocytic leukemia	poor	10 %		24
MYCOSIS FUNGOIDES	DWDL	T-Cell-Type 80-100 %	-	-	+ (T-helper cells)	41	Involvement of skin, lymphnodes, organs stages of skin involvement: eczematous-erythematous- tumorous lymphopenia: bad progn. sign range 40-60 ys	good to moderate	8year survival: ekzem. stage 85 %, eryth. stage 39 %, tumor. stage 5 %		18
SEZARY SYNDROME	DWDL	T-Cell-Type 80-100 %	-	-	+ (T-helper cells)	41	Leukemic variant of myc. fung. with exfoliative erythrodermia, atyp. circulating lymphocytes, general lymphadenopathy, skin-tumors 60-70 ys	good; tumorous stage: poor response	like myc. fung.		17

V. Diehl, M. Schaadt and A. Georgii

Table 5b

HIGH GRADE MALIGNANCY NON-HODGKIN-LYMPHOMAS: HISTOLOGY, IMMUNOLOG. CELL MARKERS, CLIN. IMPLICATION, PROGNOSIS

HISTOLOGICAL DESIGNATION		CELL TYPE	CELL CHARACTERISTICS				CLINICAL IMPLICATIONS AND PROGNOSIS				
KIEL-CLASSIFICATION	RAPPAPORT-CLASSIFICATION	% OF CASES	SMIG	EAC ROSETTES	SRBC (E) ROSETTES	REFERENCE FOR IMMUNOLOGICAL DETERMINATION	PRIMARY SITES, MEDIAN AGE	RESPONSE TO THERAPY	5 YEAR SURVIVAL	50 % SURVIVAL	REFERENCE FOR CLINICAL DATA AND SURVIVAL
CENTROBLASTIC	NHL, NUL, DHL, DUL	too few cases	++	N.T.	N.T.	41	Bone marrow involv. 24 %, lymphocytosis rare, liver involvement 8 %, rapid progress of disease 66 ys	aggressive treatment necessary, cures possible in 20-25 %	20-25 %	9 months	7, 40
IMMUNOBLASTIC (with plasmoblastic or plasmocytic differentiation)	NHL, NUL, DHL, DUL	B-Cell-Type 50-60 %	++	N.T.	N.T.	38	<50 % stage IV at diagnosis, rapid lymphnode enlargement (cervical, mediastinal, abdominal) increase in monoclonal Ig. Paraproteinemia 5-10 %, 5 % leukemic Men > Women 63 ys	poor, even to aggressive treatment	stage I: 37% all stages: 7%	4-8 months	3, 5, 7
LYMPHOBLASTIC - BURKITT-TYPE (African + Non African)	DHL	B-Cell-Type 80-100 %	++	10	-	41	Extranodal tumors (jaw 55%, ovary 38 %), abdominal tumors 25 %, initial bone marrow involvement 0 % 5-20 ys	good; (African) chemotherapy most effect. poor (Non-African) 10-25 %	45-50 % ... 5	8 months	5, 7, 14, 25 ... 5
B-ALL	ALL	B-Cell-Type 2 %	N.T.	N.T.	-	24	Bone marrow involv. 100 %, lymphnode ++, lymphocytosis +, prognosis worse than C- and O-ALL 10-15 ys	poor		4 months	12, 24
LYMPHOBLASTIC - CONVOLUTED OR NON CONVOLUTED	DUL, DPDL	T-Cell-Type 80-100	-	(-)	+	41	Mediastinal mass (82 %), 50 % leukemic (ALL of acid phosph. type) extranodal involvement (testes, ovaries, CNS), lymphnode enlargement rapid 90 %, initial bone marrow involvement 64 %	poor, even to aggressive combination therapy	10-15 %	8-10 months	5, 24
T-ALL	ALL	T-Cell-Type 25 %	-	(-)	+	24, 12	thymic tumor, bone marrow involvement secondary, extreme lymphocytosis, hepatosplenomegaly 10-25 ys	poor	10-20 %		12, 24
IMMUNOBLASTIC (without plasmoblastic differentiation)	DHL	T-Cell-Type Minority	-	N.T.	+	27	SEE IMMUNOBLASTIC LYMPHOMA, B-CELL-TYPE				3
NULL-LYMPHOBLASTIC (COMMON ALL)	ALL	Null-Cell-Type 70-75 %	N.T. (C-All Ag -, Ia Ag +, Tdt +)	N.T.	N.T.	12	No thymic tumor, bone marrow involvement 100 %, no mass lesions two peaks: 2-25 and 60 ys	good	WBC <100 x 10^3/mm³: 65-85% WBC >100 x 10^3/mm³: 20-40%		35, 12
NULL-IMMUNOBLASTIC	DHL	Null-Cell-Type 30-40 %	-	-	-	27, 24	SEE IMMUNOBLASTIC LYMPHOMA, B-CELL-TYPE				3, 5

CUMULATIVE SURVIVAL OF PATIENTS WITH NON–HODGKIN–LYMPHOMAS

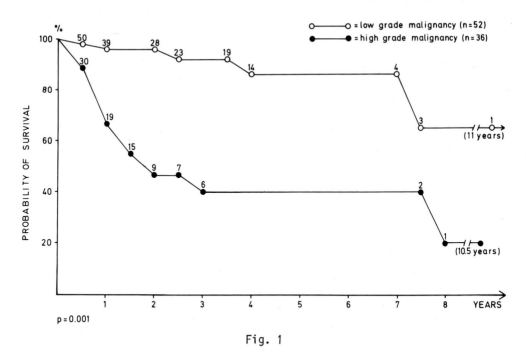

Fig. 1

CUMULATIVE SURVIVAL OF PATIENTS WITH NON–HODGKIN–LYMPHOMAS ACCORDING TO HISTOLOGICAL ENTITIES OF THE KIEL CLASSIFICATION[*)]

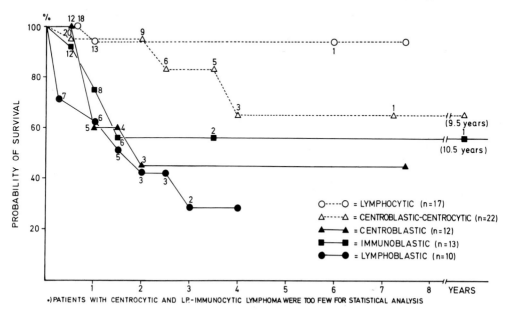

Fig. 2

DURATION OF COMPLETE REMISSION OF PATIENTS WITH NON–HODGKIN–
LYMPHOMAS FOLLOWING FIRST TREATMENT

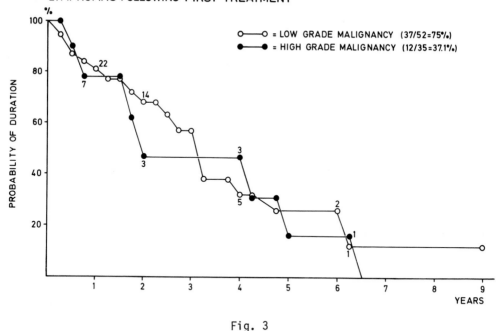

Fig. 3

CUMULATIVE SURVIVAL OF PATIENTS WITH NON–HODGKIN–LYMPHOMAS
BY RESPONSE TO THERAPY

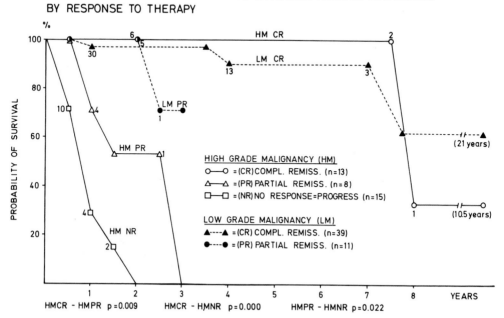

Fig. 4

DURATION OF COMPLETE REMISSION OF PATIENTS WITH NON–HODGKIN–LYMPHOMAS
BY HISTOLOGICAL CLASSIFICATION

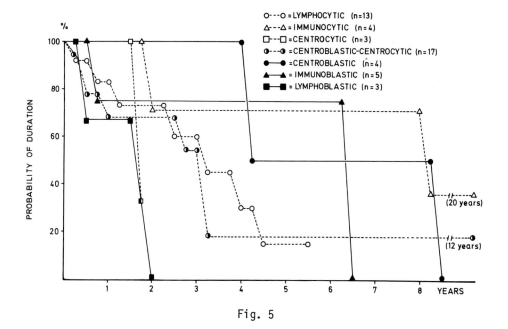

Fig. 5

Classification of Non-Hodgkin Lymphomas from Biopsies of the Bone Marrow with Special Emphasis to Their Spread

A. Georgii

*Institute of Pathology, Medizinische Hochschule Hannover,
Karl-Wiechert-Allee 9, 3000 Hannover 61, G.F.R.*

ABSTRACT

Histopathological examination of the bone marrow in patients with non-Hodgkin's lymphoma requires a careful technique of obtaining core biopsies. A further requirement is a histological technique which may be used in association with cytological studies in order to allow the distinction between normal haematopoiesis and malignant cells. In semi-thin sections from core biopsies, focal, extended or confluent infiltrations may be found. The primarily focal growth is correlated with lymphomas of low grade malignancy using the Kiel classification and with the well differentiated lymphocytic lymphomas (Rappaport classification). The centrocytic lymphomas (Kiel classification) which are classified as diffuse poorly differentiated lymphocytic lymphomas (Rappaport classification) are composed of small follicular center cells and have the lowest rate of focal involvement (50%) compared with more than 67% in the other low grade malignancies. The incidence of bone marrow involvement was higher in the low grade malignancies than in the high grade large cell lymphomas (70% versus 18-53% respectively). An exception to this was the group of follicular lymphomas of centroblastic-centrocystic type with a 55% of involvement. There were also differences in the 'prediagnostic time' between patients with focal and diffuse involvement of the bone marrow, however, this was not true for the immunoblastic types. The results of bone marrow biopsy changed the clinical stage to Stage IV in 19-60% of 210 patients. These results are compared and contrasted with those reported by Chabner and his colleagues.

The incidence of bone marrow involvement in patients with Non-Hodgkin-Lymphomas –
NHL's – differs considerably when comparing the findings of various authors. The incidence
of our own material in those cases which were biopsied at first admission to the hospital is
38 %, which is in good agreement with results from DICK et al. (1974) and STEIN et al.
(1976). Differences of incidence (JONES et al., 1972; PATCHEFSKY et al., 1974;
ROSENBERG et al., 1975; LIAO, 1977) could be caused by the different ways of obtaining
the biopsies or performing the histological processings. According to the results of
BRUNNING et al. (1975), that two fold, bilateral biopsies with the JAMSHIDI   technique
(1971) have yielded an over 50 % higher positive incidence than unilateral biopsies, it is
concluded that the positive findings largely depend on the size of the specimen.

Our own biopsies were done with a fraising instrument of BURKHARDT (1966) that produces cores of 4 to 30 mm size or by trephines with JAMSHIDI's needle technique which also
yields very good cores. The square of the bone marrow field available for diagnosis with these
two methods are 44 and 30 mm^2 respectively.

The preparative techniques of core embedding, cutting and staining must be adequately
to differentiate the neoplastic cells as well as by imprints, cytologically or by histological
sections from lymph nodes.

The cytological differentiation of lymphomas in the bone marrow by a highly elaborated
technique is essential to distinguish between lymphocytes and other blood cells for instance
normoblasts. Moreover among the small, lymphocytic lymphomas differentiation should be
possible between pure lymphocytic and centrocytic (GERARD-MARCHANT et al., 1974),
that means cleaved or small follicular center cells according to LUKES a. COLLINS (1975)
in order to extend RAPPAPORT's classification (KRÜGER, 1978). This has become of more
interest since the results of EVANS et al. (1978) have demonstrated the high rate of bone
marrow involvement in these patients.

Our own material of 727 bone marrow biopsies were resin-embedded and cut to 2 micron
sections includes so called primary lymphomas of the bone marrow. These 384 cases of primaries are the CLL's, the HCL's, the Waldenstrom's and plasmacytomas. The other 343
cases of lymphomas which are of nodal origin probably have an incidence of 53 % bone
marrow involvement. –

The subcategories of the Kiel-classification (GERARD-MARCHANT et al., 1974) are
given in the infiltrated versus all cases and their percentage. The results demonstrate a rather
high involvement of the low malignant subcategories which lies between 70 and 80 %,

except the follicular lymphomas from CB-CC-type. The high malignant, large cell lympho-ma subgroups lie between 20 and 50 % incidence only, not regarding the leukemias.

TABLE 1

KIEL-CLASSIFICATION	POSITIVE / TOTAL	PERCENT
lymphocytic	30 / 42	71
lymphocytic CLL	118 / 118	100
lymphocytic HCL	38 / 38	100
lympho-plasmacytic	21 / 29	72
lympho-plasmacytic with M. Waldenstrom	41 / 41	100
plasmacytoma	149 / 172	87
centrocytic	26 / 32	81
centrocytic-centroblastic	53 / 97	55
centroblastic	6 / 15	40
lymphoblastic	18 / 34	53
lymphoblastic ALL	27 / 27	100
immunoblastic	14 / 79	18
TOTAL	541 / 724	75

Table 1: Total incidence of bone marrow involvement in NHL

The infiltration of the bone marrow space is mostly localized and focally, which stays in that pattern for quite a long period, sometimes for years. This is the case even in autochtho-nous bone marrow lymphomas such as CLL, Waldenstroem's disease and in early plasmacyto-mas, but not in hairy cell leukemia. -

Depending on their localization in the bone marrow space it can be differentiated bet-ween central and paratrabecular sites, and intermediate types in which the infiltrates are localized in both sites simultaneously. The 3 types of localization are shown in Fig. 1,

A. Georgii

FIGURE   1

CENTRALLY

INTERMEDIATE

PARATRABECULAR

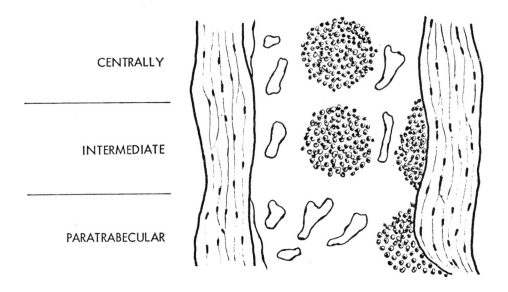

Fig. 1: Localization of NHL infiltrates within the bone marrow

with a central site in CLL seen best in a low magnification by Giemsa staining. Secondly
a paratrabecular involvement with a very distinct localization to the terminal sinuses along
the bone trabeculi can be observed in all types of follicular lymphomas and lympho-plasmacytoid lymphomas. Thirdly, the intermediate type is shown with focally infiltration in sites
along the trabeculi and in the center, whereby focal and extended patterns of infiltrates
are demonstrated in Fig. 2.

FIGURE 2

FOCALLY

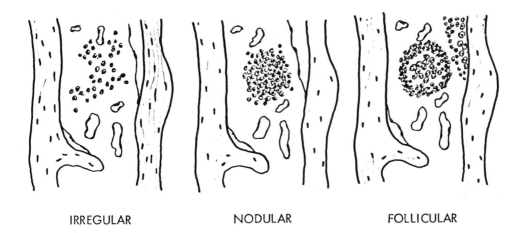

IRREGULAR   NODULAR   FOLLICULAR

EXTENDED

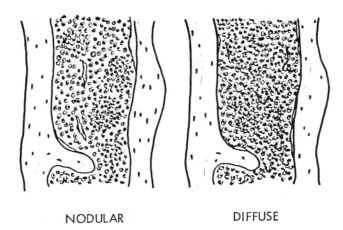

NODULAR   DIFFUSE

Fig. 2: Scheme of growth pattern

A. Georgii

These localizations of lymphoma infiltrates are related to the histological subcategories to some extent. CLL for instance is always centrally localized, and it is nodular in outline, as has been shown before.

T A B L E   2

KIEL-CLASSIFICATION	LOCALIZED PATTERN / INVOLVED BONE M		PERCENT
lymphocytic	21 / 30		70
lymphocytic CLL	38 / 118	P	32
lymphocytic HCL	0 / 38	P	0
lympho-plasmacytic	14 / 21		67
lympho-plasmacytic with M. Waldenstroem	29 / 41	P	71
plasmacytoma	27 / 149	P	18
centrocytic	13 / 26		50
centrocytic-centroblastic	50 / 53		94
centroblastic	4 / 6		67
lymphoblastic	4 / 18		22
lymphoblastic ALL	0 / 27	P	0
immunoblastic	6/ 14		43
TOTAL	206 / 541		38

Table 2: Incidence of focal involvement of the bone marrow

Follicular lymphomas that means - PDL - D - without plasmacytoid features and M - L a. H - N - according to RAPPAPORT's new classification (s. KRÜGER, 1978) can be found paratrabecular or in intermediate sites. The high grade malignant or poor prognosis lymphomas were never detected to be centrally localized, as it has been seen in those with good prognosis quite distinctively. The increasing proliferation will progress from the focal localized pattern of infiltrates to an extended complete involvement of the marrow space, which can be diffuse and very uniform, but also may retain some nodular outline (Fig. 2).

There is a correlation to histological subcategories at least to some degree as shown
in Table 2. A certain trend of irregular forms with intermediate localization of high malignant
lymphomas to change into extended diffuse patterns can be stated. However, also well
differentiated CLL can be diffuse as the slow proliferating hairy cell leukemia always is. On
the other hand nodular patterns of CLL or focally central localized patterns of lympho-plasmacytoid lymphomas stays in their focal and nodular patterns over long periods. The focal
arrangement of lymphoma infiltrates, which still remains constant during the further progression of disease there fore represents a characteristic feature for each case (see also Fig. 2).

CLINICAL CORRELATIONS

The question is wether there are correlations of this histomorphological patterns to clinical findings or to the course of the disease. The prediagnostic time between onset of first
clinical symptoms and bone marrow biopsy performed on first admission of the patient with
the exception of immunoblastic lymphomas that means according to RAPPAPORT histiocytic
diffuse or undifferentiated, a finding which needs further evaluation.

The values of peripheral blood counts reveal obvious divergenicies in cell counts and hemoglobin between nodular and diffuse growth pattern of bone marrow infiltration. The white
blood cells from patients with diffuse growth pattern are increased in alle 5 subcategories
illustrated here, but this differences are not significant statistically. The thrombocytes,
erythrocytes, and hemoglobin are reduced by the diffuse growth which is statistically   significant in some groups. For diffuse growing lymphomas of the bone marrow these findings
from peripheral blood therefore imply the tendency to anemic and leukemic clinical courses,
which is considerable different in the nodular type lymphomas. This result corresponds well
to the shorter prediagnostic time of diffuse growing lymphomas.

Bone marrow biopsies are an essential for clinical staging of lymphoma patients (JONES
et al., 1972; VINCIGUERRA a. SILVER, 1973; ROSENBERG et al., 1975; LIAO, 1977).
Several reports were given on diverse subcategories of lymphomas. In Burkitt lymphomas
of North-American children and young adults a surprising high incidence of bone marrow
involvement was demonstrated, although leukemic blood values are very rare (BRUNNING
et al., 1975). In well differentiated small cell lymphomas an extremely high bone marrow
involvement was reported by EVANS et al. (1978), which was of some influence to
survival times when anemia predominated.

The first gross comparison gives the number of patients from each of the 4 clinical stages before and after the bone marrow histology. By these findings from 210 patients a shifting from stage III into stage IV is obvious, while the stages I and II are lesser involved. The percentage of stage IV rises up from 19 to 60 % of these 210 cases. This phenomenon implies that the probability of bone marrow involvement is conspicuous higher in stage III than in the other two clinical stages with lesser nodal spread.

There is no difference of this phenomenon to the histological subcategories but it can be seen in low and highgrade malignant lymphomas likewise, that the most important shifting is from stage III to IV.

TABLE 3

CLINICAL STAGES		I %	II %	III %	IV %
Chabner et al., 1976	pre	13	21	42	24
n = 170	post	7	13	33	48
own cases, 1978	pre	10	13	58	19
n = 210	post	10	10	21	60

Table 3: Changes in staging of Non-Hodgkin-Lymphomas by bone marrow biopsies

And finally, comparing these results with those of De Vita's laboratory (CHABNER et al., 1976) as shown in Table 3 points to higher changes occuring in our own material. Whether this can be explained by staging procedures done earlier during the course of the diseases in CHABNER's patients or by a more successful bioptical procedure remains open sofar. The remarkable statement is in both studies the high compartment of shifting from lower stages into the final stage IV. The question arises therefore whether all patients should be included in the clinical stage IV if the bone marrow is infiltrated and if this should be done regardless and independant from grade and extend of bone marrow involvement.

ADDENDUM
Our research is supported by grant Ge 121/16 from the Deutsche Forschungsgemeinschaft. The corporation with Dr. K.F. Vykoupil, Dr. J. Thiele, Dr. H. Ostertag and H. Bartel in this project is acknowledged.

REFERENCES

BRUNNING, R.D., BLOOMFIELD, C.D., McKENNA, R.W., and PETERSON, L.A.:
Bilateral trephine bone marrow biopsies in lymphoma and other neoplastic diseases.
Annals of Internat. Medicine 82, 365 - 366 (1975)

BURKHARDT, R.:
Technische Verbesserungen und Anwendungsbereich der Histo-Biopsie von Knochenmark
und Knochen.
Klin.Wschr. 44, 326 - 334 (1966)

CHABNER, B.A., JOHNSON, R.E., YOUNG, R.C., CANELLOS, G.P., HUBBARD,
S.P., JOHNSON, S.K., and DeVITA, V.T.:
Sequential nonsurgical staging of non-Hodgkin's lymphoma.
Ann.Intern.Med. 85, 149 - 154 (1976)

DICK, F., BLOOMFIELD, C.D., and BRUNNING, R.D.:
Incidence, cytology, and histopathology of non-Hodgkin's lymphomas in the bone marrow.
Cancer 33, 1383 - 1398 (1974)

EVANS, H.L., BUTLER, J.J., and YOUNESS, E.L.:
Malignant lymphoma, small lymphocytic type. A clinicopathologic study of 84 cases with
suggested criteria for intermediate lymphocytic lymphoma.
Cancer 41, 1440 - 1454 (1978)

GERARD-MARCHANT, R., HAMLIN, I., LENNERT, K., RILKE, F., STANSFELD, A.G.,
and VAN UNNIK, J.A.M.:
Classification of non-Hodgkin's lymphomas.
Lancet II, 406 (1974)

JAMSHIDI, K., and SWAIM, W.R.:
Bone marrow biopsy with unaltered architectur - a new biopsy device.
J.Lab.Clin.Med. 77, 335 - 342 (1971)

JONES, S.E., ROSENBERG, S.A., and KAPLAN, H.S.:
Non-Hodgkin's lymphomas. I. Bone marrow involvement.
Cancer 29, 954 - 960 (1972)

KRÜGER, G.:
Internationale Untersuchung zur Wertigkeit verschiedener Klassifikationsschemata für Non-
Hodgkin-Lymphome.
Blut 36, 117 - 121 (1978)

LIAO, K.T.:
The superiority of histologic sections of aspirated bone marrow in malignant lymphomas.
A review of 1, 124 examinations.
Cancer 27, 18 - 628 (1977)

LUKES, R.J., and COLLINS, R.D.:
New approaches to the classification of the lymphomata.
Br.J.Cancer 31, 1 - 28, Suppl. II (1975)

PATCHEFSKY, A.S., BRODOVSKY, H.S., MENDUKE, H., SOUTHARD, M.,
BROOKS, J., NICKLAS, D., and HOCH, W.S.:
Non-Hodgkin's lymphomas: A clinicopathologic study of 293 cases.
Cancer 34, 1173 - 1186 (1974)

RAPPAPORT, H.:
Tumors of the hematopoietic system.
Atlas of Tumor Path. Section 3, Fascicle 8 (1966)

ROSENBERG, S.A., DORFMAN, R.F., and KAPLAN, H.S.:
A summary of the results of a review of 405 patients with non-Hodgkin's lymphoma at
Stanfort University.
Br.J.Cancer 31, 168 - 173, Suppl. II (1975)

STEIN, R.S., ULTMANN, J.E., BYRNS, G.E., MORAN, M.E., GOLOMB, H.M.,
and OETZEL, N.:
Bone marrow involvement in non-Hodgkin's lymphoma.
Cancer 37, 629 - 636 (1976)

VINCIGUERRA, V., and SILVER, R.T.:
The importance of bone marrow biopsy in the staging of patients with lymphosarcoma.
Blood 41, 913 - 920 (1973)

Present State of Clinical and Surgical Staging Procedures in Adult Non-Hodgkin's Lymphomas

H. Kasdorf

Dep. Oncología, Fac. de Medicina, C. Correo 930, Montevideo, Uruguay

ABSTRACT

Laparoscopy is a staging procedure which provides as much valuable information for treatment of non-Hodgkin's lymphoma as does routine laparotomy plus splenectomy. Its morbidity is definitively less. The only clear indication for staging laparotomy is in stage I and localized
stage II where curative radiotherapy is the treatment of choice.A complete clinical remission and the non necessity of a maintenance therapy can only be assessed by careful restaging.

KEYWORDS

Lymphomas, Non-Hodgkin's Lymphomas, Staging, Clinical Staging, Pathological Staging, Evaluation Staging Procedures, Restaging.

INTRODUCTION

Through accurate staging much valuable information is obtained in relation to a) the natural history of the different clinico-pathological
entities which constitute the non-Hodgkin's lymphomas (4,17,18,24,36);
b) the background required for an adequate therapeutic approach and -
post-treatment follow-up (4,11,17,18,24,36).

Quite enough experience has been gained about the biological behaviour
of most of the different non-Hodgkin's varieties and therefore, the importance of staging is now mainly focused on providing the necessary
information for a correct treatment and follow-up.

At the time of presentation, over a half of the patients have a generalized disease (4,11,17,18,24,36). Its anatomical extension can be determined by using, after a careful physical examination and radiological, scintigraphic and laboratory studies, some minor surgical procedures such as: iliac crest bone marrow and liver biopsies (1,2,5,7,10,
12, 17, 18).

The purpose of this paper is to stress the importance of the combination of all the different staging procedures, short of exploratory laparotomy and the limited value of the latter in these lymphomas.

SEQUENCE OF STAGING PROCEDURES

Table 1 summarizes the series of diagnostic procedures involved in
clinical staging and which are usually interrupted as soon as there
is evidence of an involvement of an extranodal site (lung, bone, liver, stomach, etc.).

TABLE 1 Staging Procedures

Physical Examination
        - lymph nodes, spleen, liver
        - nose and throat

Laboratory Studies
        - routine
        - liver and renal function tests

Radiological Studies

        - chest, tomogram
        - bipedal lymphography
        - intra-venous pyelogram (optional)
        - inferior venacavagram (optional)
        - bone, stomach (optional)
        - paranasal sinus and nasopharynx (optional)

Scintigraphic Studies
        - 99m Tc (liver, spleen, bone) (optional)
        - 67 Ga (lymph nodes) (optional)

If following the staging criteria of the Ann Arbor classification (9)
the patient is not staged as IV, one proceeds with the next investigations which then consist of a) bone marrow core biopsy (posterior
iliac crest, bilateral), b) liver biopsy (percutaneous or laparosco-
pic), c) if possible, laparoscopy-aided spleen and lymph node biop -
sies.

Patients in stages I-III and under 60 years of age may then be subjected to an exploratory laparotomy with splenectomy and with an extensive tissue sampling (needle and wedge biopsies of the liver, paraaor-
tic and mesenteric lymph node biopsies, open bone marrow iliac crest
biopsy) (4,5,17,18,36).

VALUE OF STAGING LAPAROTOMY

The value of the surgical abdominal exploration is much disputed. It
is fully accepted in most research centers when performing clinical -
investigationsinvestigations, as the final procedure of the sequence
of above mentioned studies and where findings change the treatment -
plans. However, its use as a routine staging practice is clearly not
indicated. There are many situations in which its value is seriously
questioned because the findings of the surgical exploration are either
not needed for an adequate and correct staging or are not reliable(2,
5,10,11,12,13,24,34).

The now quite large experience with systematic staging laparotomy has
shown:

- In nodular lymphomas[1] (those belonging to low grade malignancy and corresponding in general to centre-cytic or centre-blastic or cleaved follicular centre cell[3]) a high yield of about 80% positive abdominal findings (mesenteric and portal lymph nodes, liver, spleen) when lymphography is abnormal (12,18). Even with a negative lymphography, the incidence is still relevant and varies from 20-50% (12,18).

- In diffuse lymphocytic lymphomas[1] there is a pronounced trend to generalize early. These lymphomas should therefore always be considered as biologically stage IV (24), except perhaps when the disease is truly localized (stage I and II localized[4]).

- In extensive stage II[4] diffuse histiocytic lymphoma[1] (high grade malignancy[2], immunoblastic lymphoma[2]; non cleaved follicular centre cell lymphoma[3]) where a careful surgical exploration often fails to reveal occult disease and patients later relapse outside the radiation field (13,14).

The increasing use of chemotherapy in an attempt to improve survival and cure rates of radical radiotherapy in apparently localized lymphomas makes the staging laparotomy unnecessary (5,8).

The probably best and most agreed upon indication for laparotomy is stage I and localized stage II when radiotherapy is the only treatment given, particularly in patients with histiocytic lymphoma (5,13,32).

Laparotomy with splenectomy has an immediate morbidity which varies between 10 to 40% (5,14) and is clearly superior to the 3-4% complication rate of peritoneoscopy (1,5). Furthermore, delayed side effects due to splenectomy have been reported, such as depression of humoral immunity by intensive combined treatments (21), increased incidence of varicella-zoster infection (27), cases of fatal septicemia. Therefore, the risks of surgical staging are definitely higher (1,5).

RE-STAGING

After a radical treatment by radiotherapy and/or combination chemotherapy, patients entering a complete remission may harbor residual disease below the clinically detectable level. Restaging of non-Hodgkin's lymphoma patients has shown occult foci in 24% of the cases treated by intensive chemotherapy and in apparent clinical remission (23).

Clinical experience and investigations carried out show that all tests and studies which were abnormal at the initial staging, have to be repeated, particularly bone marrow biopsy and lymphography (apparently the most important and useful procedures for restaging) (22,23).

---

[1]Rappaport classification (30)

[2]Kiel classification (16)

[3]Lukes and Collins classification (26)

[4]Localized stage II is defined by the involvement of the primary site (nodal and extranodal) and the contiguous regional nodes. Non-contiguous involvement is classified as extensive stage II and these patients have a high risk of disseminated disease (3,8,28,29).

There is now an increasing general agreement that all clinical trials should include systematic restaging procedures after the patient has achieved clinical remission. Only in these conditions can one be fairly certain that the patient has no residual disease and needs no maintenance therapy (5,14,22,23,33,35). For the same reason, patients individually managed should probably also be submitted to a thorough restaging (23).

DISCUSSION

Though careful exploration of the abdominal cavity and splenectomy - allows the detection of occult lesions not found by laparoscopy, these findings modify the necessary staging for an adequate treatment only in a small percentage (5,18). Therefore, the combined use of peritoneoscopy and bone marrow core biopsy are procedures which permit the determination of the anatomical extension of the non-Hodgkin's lymphomas with an acceptable degree of accuracy. Furthermore, with laparoscopy, the complication rate is almost negligeable while laparotomy and splenectomy have a definite immediate morbidity (5,13) plus eventual delayed complications (5). Moreover, patients 60 years of age or older are most often medically not fit to be operated on. The advantages of laparoscopy and laparotomy have been summarized by Bonadonna and others (5) in a recent paper and are reproduced in table 2.

TABLE 2 Advantages of laparoscopy and laparotomy

Laparoscopy
- Detects liver involvement in most patients with hepatic infiltration.
- Detects spleen involvement in approximately one-third of patients with splenic infiltration, especially when tumor nodules are present on the surface.
- Can be easily repeated to assess the status of remission when liver is involved before chemotherapy.
- Can be performed under local anesthesia; operating room is not required.
- Produces minimal morbidity and recovery is rapid.
- Reduces costs and stay in hospital.

Laparotomy
- Allows accurate evaluation of abdominal involvement with particular reference to spleen, porta hepatis and mesenteric and para-aortic nodes.
- Can avoid excessive irradiation exposure to left kidney and left lung by removal of a large spleen.
- Can preserve ovarian function during pelvic irradiation.

As it has been emphasized by several authors, the focal distribution of the lymphomas require the performance of posterior crest biopsies bilaterally to assure a high degree of accuracy (5,7,35).

With the present state of knowledge, laparotomy in non-Hodgkin's lymphomas appears to be indicated only where curative local radiotherapy is the only treatment to be used. This corresponds to stage I and localized stage II and refers particularly to histiocytic lymphomas (5, 13,32). In all other stages, where usually systemic treatment modali-

ties are preferred (whole body irradiation, chemotherapy; either alone
or in combination with localized radiotherapy), an extensive and precise staging is not any more essential nor necessary for reaching a -
treatment decision. However, the documentation of the involvement of
different nodal and extranodal sites in non-Hodgkin's lymphomas does
maintain its importance, since an accurate restaging seems to be the -
only valid and objective criteria to assure a complete remission and to
withhold from maintenance therapy (5,22,23,34).

Additional procedures, such as computerized axial tomography (25,32) -
and ultrasonography (6) may be extremely useful for staging and restaging. The development of methods and techniques to detect minimal residual disease (tumour markers (15), cell sorting (15,19) and in vitro
assays of tumour stem cells (20)) will certainly increase in the future the precision in diagnosing the presence of disease. But, as pointed out by Herman and Jones (23), these ultrasensitive techniques will
only be of value if patients have been previously investigated by ri-
gorous conventional restaging procedures.

In conclusion: The combined use of all the different staging procedures short of laparotomy plus splenectomy are usually sufficient in providing the necessary information for an adequate treatment and a correct follow-up. Truly localized histiocytic lymphoma, stages I and II
localized, where radical radiotherapy constitutes the only treatment,
is probably the only clear indication for the surgical exploration of
the abdominal cavity.

REFERENCES

1 - Anderson, T., S.H. Rosenoff, R.A. Bender and others (1976). Peritoneoscopy: A useful tool in restaging lymphoma patients. Proc. Ann.
Assoc. Cancer Res, 17, 268 (abstr. C-125).
2 - Anderson, T., R.A. Bender, S.H. Rosenoff and others (1977). Peritoneoscopy: A technique to evaluate therapeutic efficacy in non -
Hodgkin's lymphoma patients. Cancer Treat. Rep., 61, 1017-1022.
3 - Banfi, A., G. Bonadonna, G. Buraggi and others (1965). Clinical -
staging and treatment of lymphosarcoma and reticulum cell sarcoma.
Tumori, 51, 153,178.
4 - Bonadonna, G., F. Pizetti, R. Musumeci and others (1975). Staging
laparotomy in non-Hodgkin's lymphomata. Br. J. Cancer (Suppl. II),
31, 252-260.
5 - Bonadonna, G., R. Beretta, R. Castellani and others (1978). Current
views on surgical staging in planning the treatment of malignant
lymphomas. In H.J. Tagnan and M.J. Staquet (Ed.) Recent Advances
in Cancer Treatment, Raven Press, New York. pp. 55-67.
6 - Brascho, D.J. and others (1978). Ultrasonography in Hodgkin's disease and non-Hodgkin's lymphomas. Radiology, 125, 485-487.
7 - Brunning, R.D., C.D. Bloomfield, R.W. McKenna and others (1975).
Bilateral trephine bone marrow biopsies in lymphoma and other neoplastic diseases. Ann. Intern. Med., 82, 365-366.
8 - Bush, R.S., M. Gospodarowicz, D.E. Bergsagel and others (1978). Radiation therapy for localized non-Hodgkin's lymphoma. Proceedings
XIIth International Cancer Congress, Buenos Aires, Argentina, Pergamon Press.
9 - Carbone, P.K., H.S. Kaplan, K. Musshoff and others (1971). Report
of the committee on Hodgkin's disease staging classification. Can
cer Res., 31, 1860-1861.
10- Chabner, B.A., R.E. Johnson, P.B. Chretien and others (1975). Per-

cutaneous liver biopsy, peritoneoscopy and laparotomy: An assessment of relative merits in the lymphomata. Br. J. Cancer (Suppl.II)
31, 242-247.
11- Chabner, B.A., R.E. Johnson, G.P. Young and others (1976). Importance of prelaparotomy staging in non-Hodgkin's lymphoma(NHL).Proc.
Ann. Assoc. Cancer Res., 17, (abstr. (-72).
12- Chabner, B.A., R.E. Johnson, V.T. De Vita and others (1977). Sequential staging in non-Hodgkin's lymphoma. Cancer Treat. Rep.,61,
993-997.
13- De Vita, V.T. (1977). Discussion. In S.E. Jones and J. Godden (Ed)
Proceedings of the conference on non-Hodgkin's lymphomas. Cancer
Treat. Rep., 61, 1032.
14- De Vita, V.T. (1977). Summary of Symposium. In S.E. Jones and J.
Godden (Ed), Proceedings of the conference on non-Hodgkin's lymphomas. Cancer Treat. Rep., 61, 1224.
15- Frei, E. III , S. Schlossman and M. Israel (1977). New approaches to
the treatment of non-Hodgkin's lymphoma. Cancer Treat. Rep., 61,
1209-1217.
16- Gerard-Marchant, R., I. Hanslin, K. Lennert and others (1974).Clas-
sification of non-Hodgkin's lymphomas. Lancet, 2, 406-408.
17- Goffinet, D.R., R.A. Castellino, H. Kim and others (1973). Staging
laparotomies in previously untreated patients with non-Hodgkin's
lymphomas. Cancer, 32, 672-681.
18- Goffinet, D.R., R. Warnke, N.R. Dunnick and others (1977). Clinical and surgical (laparotomy) evaluation of patients with non-Hodgkin's lymphomas. Cancer Treat. Rep., 61, 981-992.
19- Greaves, M.I. (1975). Clinical application of cell surface markers.
Prog. Hematol., 9, 255-303.
20- Hamburger, A.W. and S.E. Salmon (1977). Primary bioassay of human
tumor stem cells. Science, 197, 461-463.
21- Hancock, B.W., L. Bruce, A.M. Ward and others (1976). Changes in
the immune status in patients undergoing splenectomy for the staging of Hodgkin's disease. Br. Med. J., 1, 313-315.
22- Herman, T.S., and S.E. Jones (1977). Systematic restaging in the
management of non-Hodgkin's lymphomas. Cancer Treat. Rep., 61,1009
1015.
23- Herman, S.,and S.E. Jones (1978). Systematic restaging in patients
with Hodgkin's disease. Cancer, 42, 1976-1982.
24- Johnson, R.E., V.T. De Vita, L.E. Kun and others (1975). Patterns
of involvement with malignant lymphoma and implications for treatment decision making. Brit. J. Cancer (Suppl. II), 31, 237-241.
25- Jones, S.E., D.A. Tobias and R.S. Waldman (1978). Computed tomo -
graphic scanning in patients with lymphoma. Cancer, 41, 480-486.
26- Lukes, R.J. and R.D. Collins (1974). Immunologic characterization
of human malignant lymphomas. Cancer, 34, 1488-1503.
27- Monfardini, S., E. Barjetta, C.A. Arnold and others (1975). Herpes
Zoster - varicella infection in malignant lymphomas. Influence of
splenectomy and intensive treatment. Eur. J. Cancer, 11, 51-57.
28- Musshoff, K. and H. Schmidt-Vollmer (1975). Prognosis of non-Hodgkin's lymphomas with special emphasis on the staging classification. Z. Krebsforsch., 83, 323-341.
29- Peters, M.V., R.S. Bush, T.C. Brown and others (1975). The place
of radiotherapy in the control of non-Hodgkin's lymphomata. Br.J.
Cancer (Suppl. II), 31, 386-401.
30- Rappaport, H. (1966). Tumors of the hematopoietic system. In Atlas
of Tumor Pathology, section 3, fascicle 8, US Armed Forces Institute of Pathology, Washington D.C.
31- Redman, H.C., E. Glatstein, R.A. Castellino and others (1977).Com—

puted tomography as an adjunct in the staging of Hodgkin's disease
and non-Hodgkin's lymphomas. Radiology, 124, 381-385.
32- Rosenberg, S.A. (1977). Discussion. In S.E. Jones and J. Godden
(Ed), Proceedings of the conference on non-Hodgkin's lymphomas. Can
cer Treat. Rep., 61, 1032.
33- Scheni, P.S., V.T. De Vita, S. Hubbard and others (1976). Bleomycin, adriamycin, cyclophosphamide, vincristine and prednisone(BACOP)
combination chemotherapy in the treatment of advanced diffuse histiocytic lymphoma. Ann. Intern. Med., 85, 417-422.
34- Ultman, J.E. (1977). Discussion. In S.E. Jones and J. Godden (Ed)
Proceedings of the conference on non-Hodgkin's lymphomas. Cancer
Treat. Rep., 61, 1032.
35- Ultman, J.E. (1977). In S.E. Jones and J. Godden (Ed). Proceedings
of the conference on non-Hodgkin's lymphomas. Cancer Treat. Rep.,
61, 1034.
36- Veronesi, U., R. Musumeci, F. Pizzetti and others (1974). The value of staging laparotomy in non-Hodgkin's lymphomas(with emphasis on the histiocytic type). Cancer, 33, 448-459.

Major Ongoing Clinical Trials in Non-Hodgkin's Lymphoma

James G. Schwade, Eli Glatstein and Franco M. Muggia

*Radiation Oncology Branch and Cancer Therapy Evaluation Program,
National Cancer Institute, Bethesda, Maryland 20014, U.S.A.*

Keywords: Lymphoma, Non-Hodgkin's Lymphoma, Clinical Trials, Radiation, Radiation
Therapy, Chemotherapy

ABSTRACT

Currently, the Division of Cancer Treatment of the National Cancer Institute is
monitoring over 100 clinical trials of therapy for non-Hodgkin's lymphoma. The
relation of some of the more significant of these protocols to the important issues
in the treatment of non-Hodgkin's lymphoma is discussed.

INTRODUCTION

As progress continues to be made in the treatment of non-Hodgkin's lymphomas,
questions regarding the most rational therapeutic approach to this group of diseases
in its many manifestations require carefully designed clinical trials to obtain
useful answers. Among the leading controversies in the treatment of non-Hodgkin's
lymphoma are:

1. The influence of histology on prognosis and treatment results.
2. The role of radiation therapy in early (Stage I and II) disease.
3. The role of total body irradiation (TBI) and hemi-body irradiation (HBI),
    particularly in Stage III and IV disease.
4. The place of conservative therapy (single agents or deferred treatment)
    particularly in the nodular lymphomas.
5. The role of maintenance chemotherapy.
6. The role of cell cycle specific chemotherapy.
7. The role of sequential, non-crossresistant drug combinations.
8. The contribution of low-dose consolidation radiation therapy.
9. The role of nonspecific immunostimulation or immune modulation.
10. The utility of total parenteral nutrition (TPN).

Currently, the Division of Cancer Treatment of the National Cancer Institute is
monitoring well over 100 clinical trials of therapy for non-Hodgkin's lymphoma.
These range from Phase II studies, executed through Division of Cancer Treatment
(DCT) contractors, to identify new active chemotherapeutic agents, to multi-modality
randomized clinical trials, both by NCI supported sources as well as other major
groups or institutions in the United States and abroad.

The purpose of this paper is to examine the relationship to the above
issues of some of the more important trials currently open to patient
accrual.

197

The Influence of Histology on Prognosis and Treatment Results

Currently, the National Cancer Institute is supporting a contract study at Stanford University, the University of Minnesota, Tufts University, and Instituto Nacionale Tumori (Milan, Italy) which studies the clinicopathologic correlation between presentation, results of treatment, and survival of patients with NHL, according to each of six different histopathologic classification systems. The study involves 12 pathologists, 6 using his own system and 6 using all six systems of classification. Specimen reproducibility will be compared among pathologists. In addition, 20 percent of the specimens will be randomly repeated for each pathologist to assess individual consistency. Although other classifications, including those utilizing surface receptors may eventually prove to be superior, the Rappaport histopathologic classification appears to offer real correlation with prognosis, and is generally used as a standard for comparison.

The Role of Radiation Therapy in Early (Stage I and II) Disease

Currently, a number of protocols are exploring the place of radiation therapy, either alone or in combination with chemotherapy, in early stage disease. Some of the more significant of these protocols are shown in Table 1.

The Role of TBI and HBI

There has been a recent rekindling of interest in TBI and HBI, based largely on recent work by Johnson (1970) and Hellman (1977), despite the fact that the mechanism of action remains obscure. Randomized trials of these therapies are shown in Table 2.

Conservative or Deferred Therapy

Portlock and Rosenberg (1976), based on trials conducted at Stanford, have argued that patients with NLPD and other advanced stages of favorable subtypes of asymptomatic non-Hodgkin's lymphoma survive as well on continuous single-agent therapy as on more complex drug regimens. However, others have felt that a "watch and wait" policy with minimal palliative radiation therapy as needed may be more prudent than aggressive combination drug treatment at diagnosis (Lewis, 1978). This decision has been based on observations that a significant proportion (1/3) of the NLPD subtype eventually convert into DHL, a histologic subtype evolving from follicular center cells into a state more vulnerable to aggressive chemotherapy. Moreover, this policy may be superior to the use of long-term, single-agent treatment, which may interfere with the effectiveness of drug combinations for future use when NLPD patients ultimately relapse, and which may carry a finite risk of leukemogenesis. The schemata for the current Stanford and NCI protocols are in Table 3.

The Role of Maintenance Chemotherapy

While data from a number of trials suggest that patients with NLPD, DLPD, or patients with favorable subtypes who have previously relapsed or who attained less than complete remissions received benefit from maintenance chemotherapy (McKelvey, 1976; Portlock, 1976), the NCI experience would indicate that maintenance therapy does not prolong overall survival in patients with DHL or NML in complete remission after induction therapy for patients with advanced stage disease (Anderson, 1977; DeVita, 1975; Schein, 1974; Young, 1977). Trials addressed to the role of maintenance chemotherapy or comparing different forms of maintenance are shown in Table 4.

The Role of Cell Cycle Specific Chemotherapy

Recently, the Southeastern Oncology Study Group completed a randomized Phase III

study of BCNU, cyclophosphamide, vincristine, and prednisone versus cyclophosphamide, vincristine, and prednisone in non-Hodgkin's lymphoma, randomizing responders
to the same therapy or to cyclic methotrexate, cytosine arabinoside, and 6-Thioguan-
ine (SEG 349). This protocol was closed to accrual in early 1978. Current protocols
utilizing cell cycle specific agents are shown in Table 5.

The Role of Sequential, Non-crossresistant Drug Combinations

At the 1978 meeting of the American Association of Cancer Research, Bonadonna
presented preliminary data utilizing cytoxan, vincristine, and prednisone alternated
with adriamycin, bleomycin, and prednisone in Stage III and IV non-Hodgkin's lymphoma. With comparable histology, sequential chemotherapy appeared superior to either
regimen used alone (Bonadonna, 1978). In addition to this trial, which continues,
additional studies utilizing this concept are shown in Table 6.

The Contribution of Low-Dose Consolidation Radiation Therapy

Although chemotherapeutic induction is able to be achieved in a high percentage
of cases, it is still not clear whether consolidation with radiation therapy to areas
of bulk disease in advanced lymphoma is valuable. Some of the current protocols
testing this concept are shown in Table 7.

The Role of Nonspecific Immunostimulation or Immune Modulation

Efforts to assess the value of immunotherapy in non-Hodgkin's lymphoma are shown
in Table 8.

The Utility of Total Parenteral Nutrition (TPN)

Recent interest in the use of hyperalimentation in patients with various malignancies has prompted the NCI to investigate the role of TPN versus oral nutrition in
conjunction with its current protocol for diffuse lymphomas. The schema is shown in
Table 9.

The studies represented above attempt to answer some of the major questions in
the current management of non-Hodgkin's lymphoma. As is evident from this review,
some areas are being studied extensively, while others can stand further attention,
either through additional studies or investigations of higher quality. As the data
from these current trials accrue and mature, and as clear answers emerge, new
questions will appear, requiring further well designed clinical trials. Only in this
way can meaningful and consistent progress be maintained in the treatment of the non-
Hodgkin's lymphomas.

REFERENCES

1. Anderson, T., DeVita, V., Bender, R., et al: An important correlation
of survival with complete remission induction. Proc. Amer. Soc. Clin. Oncol.
18: 326, 1977.

2. Bender, R.A., and DeVita, V.T: Non-Hodgkin's lymphoma. In: Randomized
Trials in Cancer: A Critical Review by Sites, Staquet, M.J. (ed.), Raven Press,
New York, 1978, pp. 77-102.

3. Bonadonna, G., Villa, E., Canetta, R., and Monfardini, S: CTX, VCR, PRED
(CVP) alternated with ADM, BLM, PRED (ABP) in advanced non-Hodgkin's lymphomas
(NHL). Proc. Amer. Assoc. Ca. Res., 19: 216, 1978.

4. Carbone, PP., Spurr, C., Schneiderman, M., et al: Management of patients

with malignant lymphoma: a comparative study with cyclophosphamide and vinca alkaloids. Cancer Res. 28: 811-822, 1968.

   5. DeVita, V.T., Canellos, G.P., Chabner, B.A., et al: Advanced diffuse histiocytic lymphoma, a potentially curable disease. Lancet 1: 248-250, 1975.

   6. Hellman, S., Chaffey, J.T., Rosenthal, D.S., et al: The place of radiation therapy in the treatment of non-Hodgkin's lymphomas. Cancer 39: 843-851, 1977.

   7. Johnson, R.E., O'Conor, G.T., and Levin, D: Primary management of advanced lymphosarcoma with radiotherapy. Cancer 25: 787-791, 1970.

   8. Lewis, B.J., and DeVita, V.T: Combination chemotherapy of acute leukemia and lymphoma (in press, 1978).

   9. McKelvey, E.M., Gottlieb, J.A., Wilson, H.E., et al: Hydroxyldaunomycin (adriamycin) combination chemotherapy in malignant lymphoma. Cancer 38: 1484-1493, 1976.

   10. Portlock, C.S., and Rosenberg, S.A: Combination chemotherapy with cyclophosphamide, vincristine, and prednisone in advanced non-Hodgkin's lymphomas. Cancer 37: 1275-1282, 1976.

   11. Portlock, C.S., Rosenberg, S.A., Glatstein, E.J., and Kaplan, H.S: Treatment of advanced non-Hodgkin's lymphomas with favorable histologies: preliminary results of a prospective trial. Blood 47: 747-756, 1976.

   12. Schein, P.S., Chabner, B.A., Canellos, G.P., et al: Potential for prolonged disease-free survival following combination chemotherapy for non-Hodgkin's lymphoma. Blood 43: 181-189, 1974.

   13. Young, R.C., Anderson, T., Bender, R.A., et al: Nodular mixed lymphoma (NML): Another potentially curable non-Hodgkin's lymphoma. Proc. Amer. Soc. Clin. Oncol. 18: 356, 1977.

List of Abbreviations Used

Institutions
  NCI = National Cancer Institute (USA)
 SWOG = Southwest Oncology Group
EROTC = European Organization for the Research and the Treatment of Cancer
 ECOG = Eastern Cooperative Oncology Group
 PAHO = Pan-American Health Organization
  SEG = Southeastern Oncology Group
  INT = Instituto Nationale Tumori (Milan, Italy)

Radiation
   IF = Involved field radiation therapy
   EF = Extended field radiation therapy
  TLI = Total lymphoid irradiation
  TBI = Total body irradiation
  HBI = Hemibody irradiation
  TNI = Total nodal irradiation

Drugs and Combinations
C-MOPP = Cyclophosphamide, Vincristine, Prednisone, Procarbazine
  CHOP = Cyclophosphamide, Adriamycin, Vincristine, Prednisone
   CVP = Cyclophosphamide, Vincristine Prednisone
   VCP = Vincristine, Cyclophosphamide, Prednisone
  CHVP = Cyclophosphamide, Adriamycin, VM26, Prednisone
    CP = Cyclophosphamide, Prednisone
  BCVP = bis-chlorethyl-nitrosylurea-(BCNU), Cyclophosphamide, Vincristine
         Prednisone
  CICS = CHVP with dose and time modification
   CTX = Cyclophosphamide
   COP = Cyclosphosphamide, Vincristine, Prednisone
ProMACE = Cyclophosphamide, Adriamycin, Prednisone, VP-16, High dose
         Methotrexate with Leucovorin rescue
  MOPP = Nitrogen mustard, Vincristine, Prednisone, Procarbazine
 COMLA = Cyclophosphamide, Vincristine, Methotrexate with Leucovorin rescue,
         Cytosine arabinoside
   MTX = Methotrexate
 Adria = Adriamycin
  pred = Prednisone
     L = Leucovorin (Citrovorum factor)
  COPA = Cyclophosphamide, Adriamycin, Vincristine, Prednisone
   CAP = Cyclophosphamide, Adriamycin, Procarbazine
   BOP = Bleomycin, Vincristine, Prednisone
  BCOP = BCNU, Cyclophosphamide, Vincristine, Prednisone
   ABP = Adriamycin, Bleomycin, Prednisone
   Lev = Levamisole
   MER = Methanol extracted residue of bacillus Calmette-Guerin (BCG)

Other
   CR = Complete response
   PR = Partial response
  TPN = Total perenteral nutrition

TABLE 1

THE ROLE OF RADIATION THERAPY IN EARLY (STAGE I AND II) DISEASE

Institution	Prot. #	Patient Population	Schema
NCI	MB-76	II; DH, DM; without abd. involvement	IF + C-MOPP / C-MOPP
Stanford	E1	I, I_E, II, II_E (A&B) NLPD, NML, DLWD	IF / TLI
	E2	I, I_E (A&B) NHL, DLPD, DML, DHL, DUL	EF / TLI
	E3	II, II_E (A&B) NHL, DLP, D, DML, DHL, DUL	TLI / IF + CHOP
SWOG	7433	I, I_E, II, II_E	RT (mantle or whole abd) / RT + CHOP
EORTC	20751	II	local RT (abd or mantle) / abd + mantle RT → CVP / VCP

TABLE 2

THE ROLE OF TBI AND HBI

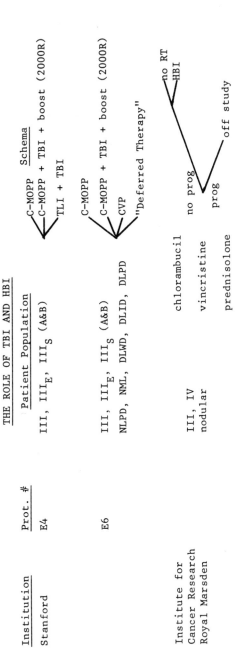

Institution	Prot. #	Patient Population	Schema
Stanford	E4	III, III_E, III_S (A&B)	C-MOPP / C-MOPP + TBI + boost (2000R) / TLI + TBI
	E6	III, III_E, III_S (A&B) NLPD, NML, DLWD, DLID, DLPD	C-MOPP / C-MOPP + TBI + boost (2000R) / CVP / "Deferred Therapy"
Institute for Cancer Research Royal Marsden		III, IV nodular; chlorambucil vincristine prednisolone	no prog; prog → no RT / HBI; off study

TABLE 3

CONSERVATIVE OR DEFERRED THERAPY

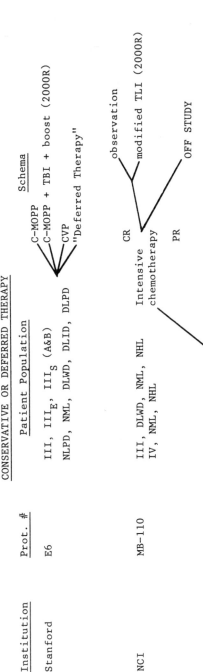

Institution	Prot. #	Patient Population	Schema
Stanford	E6	III, III_E, III_S (A&B) NLPD, NML, DLWD, DLID, DLPD	C-MOPP / C-MOPP + TBI + boost (2000R) / CVP / "Deferred Therapy"
NCI	MB-110	III, DLWD, NML, NHL IV, NML, NHL	Intensive chemotherapy → CR → observation / modified TLI (2000R); PR → OFF STUDY
		IV, DLWD, NLPD	"watch & wait" – palliative RT prn

TABLE 4

MAINTENANCE CHEMOTHERAPY

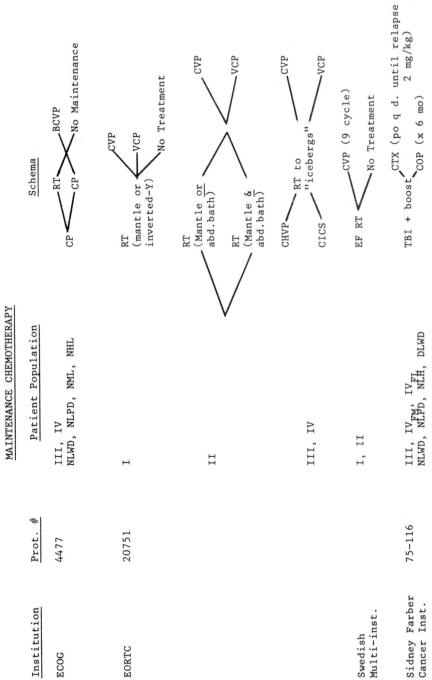

Institution	Prot. #	Patient Population	Schema
ECOG	4477	III, IV NLWD, NLPD, NML, NHL	
EORTC	20751	I	
		II	
Swedish Multi-inst.		III, IV	
		I, II	
Sidney Farber Cancer Inst.	75-116	III, IV$_{FM}$, IV$_{FH}$ NLWD, NLPD, NLH, DLWD	

TABLE 5

CELL CYCLE SPECIFIC CHEMOTHERAPY

Institution	Prot. #	Patient Population	Schema
NCI	MB-98	II, III, IV DLPD, DML, DHL, DUL	ProMACE--MOPP--ProMACE
University of Chicago		III, IV DHL	COMLA
PAHO		III, IV DHL, DLPD	MTX--L --MTX--L < VCR, CTX, Pred. / VCR - CTX, Pred.
		Relapse, all histologies	MTX--L --MTX--L < VCR, CTX, Pred., Adria. / VCR - CTX, Pred., Adria.

TABLE 8

NHL - IMMUNE STIMULATION OR MODULATION

Institution	Prot. #	Patient Population	Schema
SWOG	7713/14	III, IV	CHOP / CHOP + LEV / CHOP + LEV + BCG → CR < No Rx / LEV
NCI	MB-83	NLPD, NHL	CR < MER / NO MER

TABLE 6

SEQUENTIAL, NON-CROSSRESISTANT DRUG COMBINATIONS

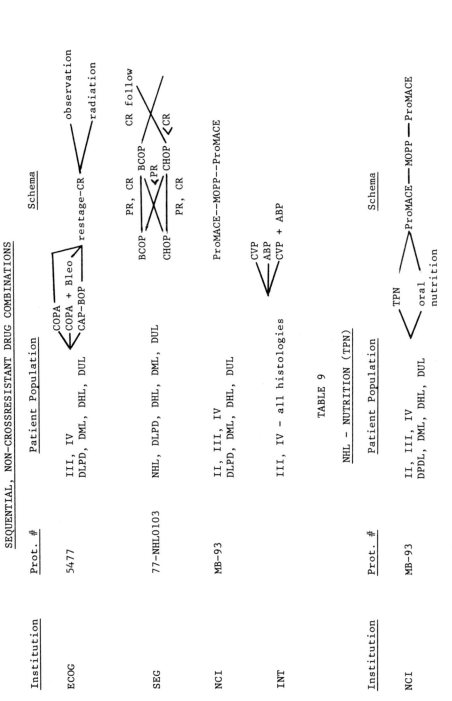

Institution	Prot. #	Patient Population	Schema
ECOG	5477	III, IV DLPD, DML, DHL, DUL	COPA COPA + Bleo CAP-BOP → restage-CR → observation / radiation
SEG	77-NHL0103	NHL, DLPD, DHL, DML, DUL	BCOP, PR, CR → BCOP → CR follow CHOP → PR CHOP → CR / PR, CR
NCI	MB-93	II, III, IV DLPD, DML, DHL, DUL	ProMACE--MOPP--ProMACE
INT		III, IV - all histologies	CVP ABP CVP + ABP

TABLE 9

NHL - NUTRITION (TPN)

Institution	Prot. #	Patient Population	Schema
NCI	MB-93	II, III, IV DPDL, DML, DHL, DUL	TPN oral nutrition → ProMACE—MOPP—ProMACE

TABLE 7

NHL – LOW DOSE CONSOLIDATION RT

Institution	Prot. #	Patient Population	Schema
ECOG	4477	III, IV NLWD, NLPD, NM, NH	CP ⟨ RT → BCVP / CP → No Maintenance ⟩ (crossed)
NCI	MB-93	IV DPDL, DML, DHL, DUL	ProMACE → MOPP → ProMACE consolidation cranial RT
SWOG	7761	III, IV DPDL, DML, DHL, DUL	CHOP/TBI → PR ⟨ CR Follow / boost 2500R off study / <PR ⟩
EORTC	20751	III, IV	CHVP → RT 2 → CVP / "icebergs" / CICS → VCP
Stanford	E7	III, III_E, III_S (A or B) NHL, DML, DNL, DUL	CHOP / CHOP/C-MOPP / CHOP/C-MOPP (split course) + 3000R TNI
NCI	MB-110	III, IV Nodular	aggressive CR chemotherapy ⟨ TLI (2500) / observation ⟩

Radiation Therapy for Patients with Localized Non-Hodgkin's Lymphomas

R. S. Bush*, M. Gospodarowicz*, D. E. Bergsagel* and T. C. Brown

*The Princess Margaret Hospital, Toronto, Ontario, Canada

ABSTRACT

An analysis of the results from treatment of 981 patients seen between 1967 and 1975 is reported. An evaluation of the place of radiation therapy for patients with localized disease is provided. If cure is defined as a normal probability of survival, the overall cure rate is 34%, 2/3 of these cured patients being treated primarily with radiation. The cure rate for the patients with localized disease treated initially with radiation is 60% of that group. Various confounding factors are discussed and the danger of drawing conclusions from the survival within individual stages, rather than the total patient population, is examined.

INTRODUCTION

Before a discussion can be developed to describe the use of radiation therapy for patients with non-Hodgkin's lymphoma, the objectives of treatment have to be defined. In particular, it must be decided whether treatment is being given for palliation or cure. As there is good evidence now that 40% of patients with advanced histiocytic lymphoma have been cured with chemotherapy (Berard et al, 1976), it seems most appropriate to focus the discussion of radiation therapy on its curative capabilities.

Because radiation therapy and chemotherapy, when given with curative intent, are used for patients with different extent of disease, it is difficult to evaluate the contribution of each to the overall curative management of patients with lymphoma. Such an evaluation has been further complicated by the major thrust in many centres towards the aggressive pursuit for evidence of generalized disease to improve the quality of staging. This complication is made greater by the use of stage to define treatment. The results of treatment are then frequently looked at by stage or a group of stages, but not often by survival for the total population of patients with lymphoma. Improved staging of patients increases survival by stage, but of course the overall population survival is not affected unless the effectiveness of therapy has improved. If survival by stage is examined, then the conclusion can be drawn mistakenly that the improvement is due to treatment. Thus, the survival of the total population becomes an important parameter to follow. Because of this, the following discussion of the place of radiation therapy in the treatment of patients with non-Hodgkin's lymphoma will repeatedly return to overall population survival to try to keep the management by one method in perspective.

From an analysis of the experience of The Princess Margaret Hospital, the part that radiation therapy has played in the curative management of patients with non-Hodgkin's lymphoma will be examined. We will also try to formulate a policy for its use based on this experience and pertinent information from the literature.

PATIENTS AND METHODS

Nine hundred and eighty-two (982) patients greater than 16 years of age have been seen at The Princess Margaret Hospital (PMH) between January 1, 1967 and December 31, 1975 for primary evaluation and management of non-Hodgkin's lymphoma. One chart could not be obtained for review. Thus, the remaining 981 patients form the basis for the study. Staging was carried out retrospectively, using the criteria and recommendations for the staging of Hodgkin's Disease derived from the Ann Arbor Conference (1971).

In 963 of the 981 patients available for study the original biopsy material was reviewed by Dr. T.C. Brown, Chief of Pathology at the PMH. Classification was by the criteria of Rappaport et al (1966). The 18 patients in whom no pathology review was possible were kept in the study, but their pathologic classification was listed as 'unclassified'.

Patient follow up was closed at June 30, 1977. Only 3 patients have been lost to continuous follow up. Actuarial survival curves were determined from the date of diagnosis. Failure free survival was also determined from date of diagnosis, although the classification of whether failure had occurred or not was determined from the absence or presence of disease after initial treatment. Kaplan-Meier tests for significance were used for comparisons between survival curves. Standard deviations are also shown in the Figs.

In this discussion the word 'cure' is used when the survival curve for any patient becomes parallel on a semi-logarithmic plot to the expected or normal survival curve. The latter has been obtained from Statistics Canada for a population of people in Ontario of the same age and sex distribution as the patient population being studied in the comparison. To determine whether the study population survival curve was parallel to the normal survival curve, two approaches were followed. Either 'relative' survival curves were calculated, and the survival is considered to represent cure if it remains unchanged with time, or the slope of the survival curve is statistically not significantly different (p $\lesssim$ 0.05) from the normal survival curve slope, with survival plotted logarithmically.

RESULTS

The management methods used for the primary treatment of patients with non-Hodgkin's lymphoma are summarized in Fig. 1. With the staging procedures used between 1967-75, 46% of the patients were classified as being Stage IA or IIA, and 76% of these patients were treated radically (for cure) with radiation. This was, and still is, the policy for management of patients at the PMH who have Stage IA or IIA disease. However, 24% were not treated according to this policy for a variety of reasons which cannot be detailed here, although the major reason for treating palliatively was related to age and lack of symptoms.

The group who were treated radically by radiation will be analysed in more detail later, but two other points need to be made from Fig. 1. First, the cured population is estimated to be 34% of the total population, with approximately 2/3 of these coming from the group whose primary treatment was radical radiation therapy (21% of the total population). Secondly, those with generalized disease can be divided into a potentially curable and an incurable group. The latter appears to be those patients with generalized lymphocytic disease. The justification for this statement is as follows.

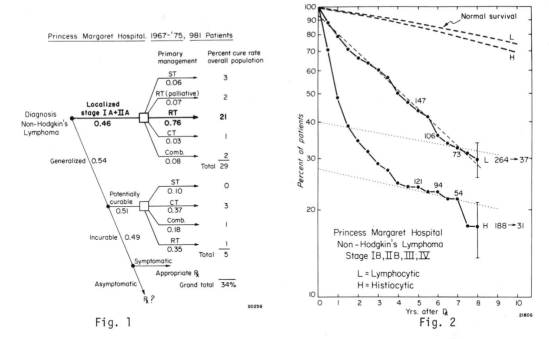

Fig. 1   Fig. 2

In Fig. 2 is shown the survival with time of all those patients with lymphocytic disease and classed as Stage IB, IIB, III or IV. It can be seen that there is a steady
rate of dying over the 8 yrs plotted which is greater than the expected survival for
a normal population. Thus, there is no evidence of cure. This is different to the
survival of those with histiocytic disease. For patients with histiocytic lymphoma
the survival curve is biphasic, indicating two populations with different rates of
dying. The tail of the survival curve is not significantly different from the slope
of the normal survival, indicating that a percentage of patients may be cured. It
should be noted that if the survival of all these patients with advanced disease was
being reported, it would be somewhere between the two curves. So, unless very long
periods of follow up are taken, the cured population will often be smaller than the
total number alive.

Fig. 1 has summarized the methods of management utilized for all patients, the probability of each method being used, and the cure rate as a percentage for the overall
population. The cure rate for any individual method can be obtained by dividing the
cure rate by each of the probabilities along its path. For instance, the 3% cure
rate for chemotherapy (CT) in the potentially curable group with advanced disease
can be shown to be equal to 28% of the subgroup treated with chemotherapy being cured
(0.03/0.37 x 0.51 x 0.56).

As pointed out above, the overall survival of 34% cured is not necessarily the percentage alive at any point after treatment. It is the percentage who no longer have
their lives threatened by disease, but who die from 'normal' causes. For instance,
in Fig. 3 where the actuarial survival curve for all 981 patients out to 9½ yrs is
illustrated, the survival at 9½ yrs is 35%. As the survival curve is still not parallel to the normal curve, cure cannot be demonstrated. The estimated 34% cured in
Fig. 1 will be only 25% at 9½ yrs because of deaths not due to disease. Consequently, the total population survival will have to be followed for a number of years
more before only the cured population remains to form a tail on the survival curve
parallel to the normal survival curve.

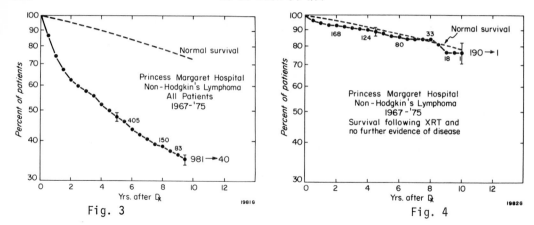

Fig. 3

Fig. 4

That patients without demonstrable disease can have a normal probability of surviving is demonstrated in Fig. 4. In this Fig. is plotted the survival of those patients staged as IA or IIA who at the time of last follow up had never demonstrated
relapse following radical radiation therapy. As can be seen, the survival is not
significantly different than the normal survival curve for that population. Thus,
if the lymphoma is clinically eradicated in those with initially localized disease,
there appears to be no remaining increased threat to life over the period of time
available for follow up.

Before proceeding with the analysis of the effectiveness of radiation therapy in
localized disease, it is necessary to illustrate some of the other factors which
are believed to confound the interpretation of the results of treatment for any
group of patients with lymphoma.

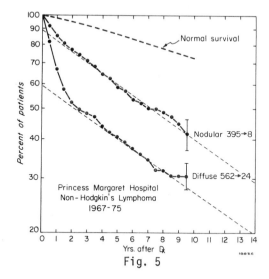

Fig. 5

One potential confounding factor from the pathological classification (lymphocytic
v histiocytic) has already been discussed. Another is the classification of diffuse
v nodular. Chabner et al (1978) report that on the basis of their extensive staging
program, diffuse disease could be localized, but nodular disease only rarely so. If
this statement is true in all pathologies, and this subclassification means an
underlying biological difference between diseases so subclassified, differences in

their survival could be expected. There are indeed differences, and these are illustrated in Fig. 5, where the actuarial survival of all those classified as nodular are compared to diffuse. 'Nodular' appears to describe a single population
whose rate of dying is steady with time out to 9½ yrs. 'Diffuse' describes two populations, one of which dies very quickly, and the other which is similar to those
classed as 'nodular'. If the mean survival of 'diffuse' is compared to 'nodular'
then there is a large difference (2.5 yrs v 7 yrs), but this does not provide the
information which the survival curves present. The survival curves show that there
is a subgroup (40%) of the diffuse pathologies which has a vastly different prognosis with present therapeutic strategies from all remaining patients (nodular and
diffuse), and which is not characterized by the classification used. One further
point should be made, and that is that there is no evidence for cure of either population out to the survival level plotted.

Age is obviously a factor influencing survival, but its effect can be removed by
either comparing survival to the normal, or by determining a relative survival curve.
If there is a difference between ages in the relative survival curves, it suggests
that age is a factor in the lethality of the disease. In Fig. 6(a), the relative
survival curves for patients with histiocytic disease and less than 50 or 50 yrs of
age and greater are shown. There is no significant difference between these curves,
and the conclusion has to be that age is not a confounding factor in the analysis
of survival of patients with histiocytic disease. Note also that the relative survival curve for those less than 50 is clearly parallel to the abscissae, thus indicating a normal probability of survival. The curve for those 50 or greater is not
so clearly parallel to the abscissae, but statistically is not significantly different from that for those less than 50. Thus, patients of all ages with histiocytic
disease can be considered to be potentially curable, and there is no effect of age.

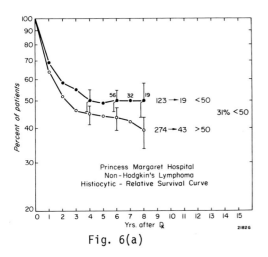

Fig. 6(a)

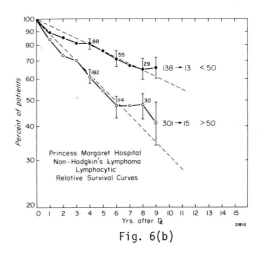

Fig. 6(b)

In Fig. 6(b) is shown the relative survival curves for those patients less than 50,
or 50 yrs or greater with lymphocytic disease. Neither curve shows any significant
break from a straight line exponential type of survival, but there is a clear separation of the two curves. Note that these are relative survival curves and so the
normal threats to life from age have been removed. Consequently, the conclusion
must be that age is a confounding factor because those 50 yrs and greater die more
rapidly from disease than those less than 50. It should be recorded that there is
no difference in the distribution of nodular and diffuse pathologies in the two age
groups compared. As noted earlier, no evidence for cure can be demonstrated out to
the survival level plotted for these patients with lymphocytic disease. However,
in this Fig. patients with all stages are included. Does the lack of any suggestion

of cure in the analysis of the survival of patients with lymphocytic disease indicate that the disease is incurable in all stages of the disease?

To respond to the last question, survival by stage has been examined for all histologies and some of the data is shown in Fig. 7. The survival of patients classed as
having B symptoms has not been plotted, but for all A patients it can be seen that
Stages I & II signify a clearly better survival than Stages III & IV. A second
point is that there is little difference in survival between Stages IA & IIA, and
they appear to be approaching the same slope as the normal survival curve. As all
pathologies are represented in these two stages, it suggests that patients with
localized lymphocytic disease may be curable. This will be examined further as we
examine the results from the use of radiation therapy in patients with Stage IA &
IIA lymphoma.

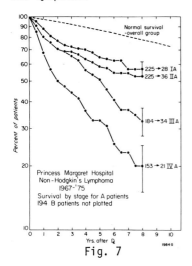

Fig. 7

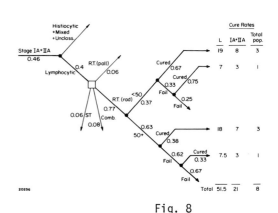

Fig. 8

With the Stage IA & IIA categories radiation was used as a primary modality in 83%,
but radically only in 76%. The results of this primary management for cure are
shown in the following decision trees, one for patients with lymphocytic disease and
one for all the remaining pathologies, the majority of which are histiocytic.

In Fig. 8 the results of management of patients with lymphocytic disease is shown.
Patients with this pathology comprise 40% of the Stage IA & IIA patients, and 77%
were treated radically with radiation. Thirty-seven percent (37%) were less than
50 yrs of age, and of these 67% were cured. This is 25% of the patients treated
radically with radiation, but is only 19% of all Stage IA & IIA patients with lymphocytic disease. For the 63% of patients who were 50 yrs or more, the failure
free survival rate was only 38%. This 38% is 24% of the patients with lymphocytic
disease radically treated, 18% of the overall group of Stage IA & IIA patients classed as having lymphocytic lymphoma.

In those less than 50, treatment of failure resulted in 2/3 having a long term survival compatible with cure, but in those over 50 only 1/3 of the failures were so
benefited. This results in 67% of patients treated radically by radiation being
cured, 57% of the overall group of Stage IA & IIA lymphocytic patients. This is 21%
of all Stage IA & IIA patients, 8% of the overall group of non-Hodgkin's lymphoma
patients. Thus, this analysis has shown that some patients with lymphocytic disease
are cured.

A similar analysis has been done for all those with histiocytic, mixed and undiffer-

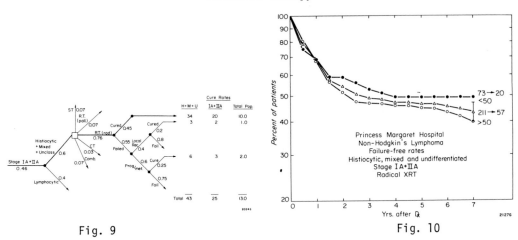

Fig. 9   Fig. 10

entiated pathologies, and is shown in Fig. 9. These patients make up the remaining
60% of the localized group, and 76% were treated radically with radiation. Forty-
five percent (45%) were cured by their initial treatment. The data for this probability is shown in Fig. 10. In this Fig. the failure free rate is plotted. The
tail of the biphasic curve can be seen to be not significantly different from a
line parallel to the abscissae. This appears to be true for both those less than
50 or 50 yrs and over, as in the data for all patients with histiocytic lymphoma
shown earlier in Fig. 6(a).

For the 55% who failed, two general classifications have been made for this discussion. One is for local recurrence, which is failure within the treatment volume.
The other is for those who failed outside the volume irradiated and classed as pro-
gression/metastases. In each subgroup between 20-25% of patients are cured following further therapy for failure. An example of the data used to obtain such probabilities will be shown next.

In Fig. 11 the progression/metastases rate and survival rate is shown. The separation of the two curves shows that death does not occur immediately as a result of
progression/metastases, and as the tails of the two curves are parallel the conclusion must mean that a fraction of the patients who relapse do not die as a result.
This fraction is estimated from the separation of the curves to be 26%.

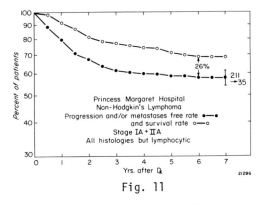

Fig. 11

Thus, using analyses such as have just been described, the results of primary management by radiation therapy for this group of patients results in 57% having a long

term survival compatible with cure. This 57% is 43% of the whole group of histiocytic, mixed and undifferentiated lymphomas, 25% of all localized, and 13% of the
total lymphoma population.

Having completed the analysis of all patients with localized disease treated by radiation therapy, the basis for the probabilities for cure shown in Fig. 1 can now be
appreciated. It can be realized now that although primary management by radiation
therapy results in 21% of the total population being cured, only 16% (80% of the
21%) can be credited to the initial treatment, 5% resulting from the treatment of
failure.

DISCUSSION

The analysis reported above was done in order to try to define the role of radiation
therapy in the management of patients with localized non-Hodgkin's lymphoma. As was
pointed out in the Introduction, if the effect of therapy is examined only for a
subgroup of the total population, it is easy to be misled about the effectiveness of
that therapy. This is because of uncertainty about the natural history of the disease, particularly in any subgroup, and because confounding factors which influence
prognosis are numerous and powerful in non-Hodgkin's lymphoma. Thus the reported
analysis first encompassed the total patient population, then some of the confounding factors, before finally examining the results of radiation therapy for patients
with localized disease.

By considering the total population survival, it becomes obvious how this can prevent deception from the improvement which occurs by simply changing the criteria
for entry into any subgroup. This is illustrated very simply in Fig. 12 where a
population which can be divided into 6 clearly demarcated groups is represented by
the divisions in the Fig.

The numbers represent the cure rates for each subgroup, and the overall cure rate
is 50%. One stage grouping, shown on the upper margin of Fig. 12 results in the
following: Stage I - 90%, Stage II - 50%, Stage III - 10%. However, by changing
the criteria for staging, and therefore the distribution of the subgroups, a new arrangement occurs for each stage. In each case the results by stage are improved.
However, because the population is the same, the overall results cannot change, and
stay at 50%. Consequently, because the results of radiation therapy will depend on
the criteria used for choosing the patients for treatment, the results of treatment
have been presented always both in terms of the total population as well as the subgroup. As the PMH is a general referral centre for patients with malignancy, it is
to be expected that the total population survival is reasonably representative of
an unselected lymphoma population.

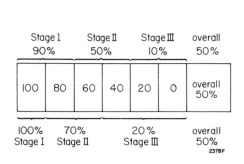

Fig. 12

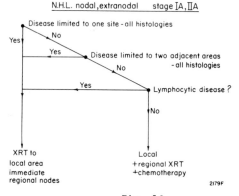

Fig. 13

Evidence has been presented that radiation therapy can provide cure for approximately 16% of the total population, or 35% of those classed as Stage IA, IIA. This is 46% of those treated radically with radiation. Because patients who fail following initial radiation therapy can still be cured by further treatment, the overall percentage who achieve a normal survival after being selected for initial treatment by radical radiation therapy is 21% of the total population, 60% of the group so treated.

What recommendations for therapy, particularly radiation, can be made as a result of the analysis? We have previously reported that localized lymphoma is best defined as involvement of the primary site (nodal or extra-nodal) with or without involvement of the immediate regional nodes only (Bush, R.S. et al, 1977). Extension beyond the immediate regional nodes indicates a high risk of disease elsewhere in the body and thus, a significant risk of early failure after loco-regional radiation therapy in a majority of those with extensive disease. For those with localized disease, loco-regional radiation is appropriate because a majority will not fail, and they receive local treatment only (Fig. 13). Further management can still cure approximately 25% of those that do fail. Those with extensive Stage IIA disease are divided into two groups. First, patients with histiocytic, mixed or undifferentiated lymphomas would be treated with a combination of chemotherapy and radiation. As pointed out above, most of these patients have unrecognized generalized disease and thus will fail loco-regional treatment. Whether radiation is necessary is still not known, but without information to show that the response to drugs and radiation is the same for each individual patient, for this group of patients it is most likely wisest to use a combination of methods. For those with lymphocytic disease, the majority of those who fail are those with generalized disease. As such patients may be incurable by present methods, unless specific studies are being carried out, treatment should be individualized.

What recommendations can be made for those who practice in centres where detailed investigation can be undertaken? Should the thrust of investigation be aimed at refining the present staging criteria and thus, more carefully define the population to be treated by radiation? Recently Chabner et al (1978) have reported the stage changes which occur from extensive investigation for generalized disease. The report demonstrated that in the 170 patients investigated, only 14% were finally found to be Stage I or II. Interestingly, this figure is close to the 16% controlled by the initial course of radiation therapy in the PMH patients. However, because of some local failures, it would be unlikely that the 14% would have a 100% chance of being cured by radiation alone. In fact, our estimate from the PMH experience is that it is more likely to be only 11% of the total population, which is approximately 1/3 lower than our cure rate with radiation alone. Another consideration is what fraction of the 14% are falsely classified as Stage I or II, because no medical investigation has an accuracy of 100%.

The sequential testing of patients who have previously been negative for generalized disease increases the specificity of the evaluation, but decreases the sensitivity (Galen & Gambino, 1975). Thus, the number of false positives increases with the decrease in false negatives. The size of the false positive population is not clear but that it will be present is sure. However, all the emphasis has been on the false negative population with the belief that failure to treat systemically at the earliest point in time will be detrimental to the patient. This is a good dictum in general oncological practice, but may not be true in the management of patients with lymphomas. Rosenberg has addressed himself to this problem in the management of patients with Hodgkin's Disease (1978), and his data would suggest that the treatment of failure after local treatment is so successful that adjuvant chemotherapy for radiation therapy appears to be no more successful for cure than treatment of those who fail. Treatment of failure in the non-Hodgkin's lymphoma group is also successful, and indeed in the series from the PMH the treatment of failure outside the treatment volume appeared to be similar to the results for the management of advanced disease (26% v 28%). However, whether the systemic treatment of patients who are falsely staged as III & IV, or IB & IIB will provide the same chance of cure as appropriate localized radiation therapy is not at all clear. We know of no data to use.

We believe that confounding factors, apart from stage, are such in number and in strength of effect that it is not possible to be specific about treatment recommendations at this time. Studies of treatment comparisons need to stratify confounding factors such as site, bulk of disease, age, etc., otherwise the comparisons can be very misleading. If the population of patients who have a very poor prognosis with any of the current therapies can be clearly identified, and we anticipate we will be able to do this, then the place of radiation and chemotherapy can more clearly be compared in the remainder. Until that time, we would have to recommend our policy summarized in Fig. 13, and warn the reader to beware of sequential staging procedures if stage is going to be used to define therapy.

REFERENCES

Bush, R.S., Gospodarowicz, M., Sturgeon, J., Alison, R. (1977). Radiation therapy of localized non-Hodgkin's lymphoma. Cancer Treat. Rep., 61, 1129-1136.

Chabner, B.A., Johnson, R.E., Young, R.C., Canellos, G.P., Hubbard, S.P., Johnson, S.K., and DeVita, V.T. (1978). Sequential nonsurgical and surgical staging of non-Hodgkin's lymphoma. Cancer, 42, 922-925.

Galen, R.S., and Gambino, S.R. (1975). Beyond normality: the predictive value and efficiency of medical diagnoses. John Wiley & Sons, New York.

Rosenberg, S.A., Kaplan, H.S., Glatstein, E.J., and Portlock, C.S. (1978). Combined modality therapy of Hodgkin's Disease: a report on the Stanford trials. Cancer, 42, 991-1000.

ACKNOWLEDGEMENTS

The authors wish to acknowledge the contribution of the rest of the staff at the PMH in agreeing to the inclusion of all patients seen and treated at the Hospital. Also, the contribution from the Biostatistics Department, particularly Mrs. Joan Reid and Miss Theresa Chua must be recognized and particular thanks go to Miss Dyanne Attlewhyte for her secretarial assistance.

Combined Modality Treatment in New Approaches to the Management of Non-Hodgkin's Lymphomas

L. M. Fuller*, W. S. Velasquez**, J. F. Gamble**, J. J. Butler***,
R. G. Martin****, and C. C. Shullenberger**

*Departments of Radiotherapy, **Medicine, ***Pathology and ****Surgery
The University of Texas System Cancer Center,
M.D. Anderson Hospital and Tumor Institute, Texas Medical Center,
Houston, Texas 77030, U.S.A.

ABSTRACT

On the basis of inferior results for stages I and II non-Hodgkin's lymphoma patients treated with involved field radiotherapy and for stage III patients treated with chemotherapy, the Departments of Radiotherapy, Medicine, Surgery and Pathology at the M.D. Anderson Hospital decided that a concerted multimodality program was indicated for all three stages of these diseases. All medically fit patients with stage III disease and those patients with abdominal presentations of diffuse histiocytic lymphoma have been treated with alternating courses of a multiple agent regimen of cytoxan, adriamycin, vincristine, prednisone and bleomycin (CHOP-Bleo) and involved field (IF) radiotherapy. All other stages I and II patients were treated initially with IF radiotherapy. Thereafter, lymphangiogram staged patients received 12 courses of CHOP-Bleo. Since 1975, laparotomy staged I and II patients were randomized to receive no further treatment vs. CHOP-Bleo. For the nodular lymphomas, insufficient time has elapsed to determine the effect of a multimodality approach on survival with any degree of certainty. Similarly in the laparotomy staged I and II diffuse histiocytic lymphoma patients, no significant difference could be detected for patients treated with or without adjunctive chemotherapy. Projected 5 year survival figures of 78% for lymphangiogram staged I and II patients and 74% for stage III disease have been gratifying.

Keywords: Lymphomas, Non-Hodgkin's, Radiotherapy, Chemotherapy, Survival

INTRODUCTION

Patterns of progression in lymphangiogram staged I and II non-Hodgkin's lymphoma patients treated with involved field (IF) radiotherapy have shown that the majority of such patients had systemic disease on admission regardless of the histologic subtype (Fuller, 1975). In 1973, at the London Symposium on the Non-Hodgkin's Lymphomas, we presented results for the Rappaport classification (1956) for patients with localized presentations. More than half of those patients were staged by lymphangiography. Since that time, we have calculated separate survival and disease free survival curves for the lymphangiogram studied patients in this series using our original data. For the nodular group, the 5 year survival and disease free survival figures were 67% and 38% respectively. The corresponding 5 year survival figure for the diffuse histiocytic group which constituted the majority of the diffuse lymphomas was only 26%.

In the nodular group, patients with abodminal presentations had a 5 year survival
figure of 70%, with a corresponding disease free figure of 39%. These results compared very favorably with those for upper torso presentations which were 58% and
37% respectively (Fig. 1). Positive laparotomy findings of 61% in a subsequent
study of lymphangiogram staged I and II patients with upper torso disease were consistent with this experience (Heifetz, in press).

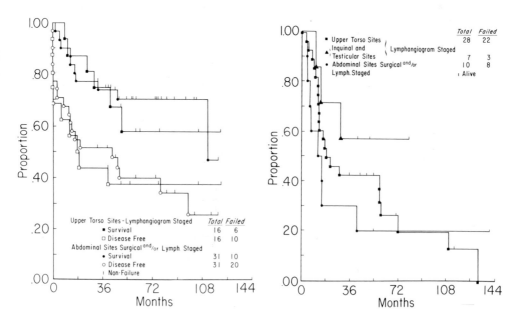

Fig. 1.   Nodular lymphomas,   Fig. 2.   Diffuse histiocytic lymphomas,
          past experience.   past experience.

Results for stages I and II diffuse histiocytic lymphomas treated with radiotherapy
only were poor except for patients with stage I inguinal and stage IE testicular
disease for whom the 5 year survival figure was 57% (Fig. 2). These results for
diffuse histiocytic lymphomas have not been entirely substantiated by staging laparotomy findings in which the incidence of postive abdominal disease was only 29% for
nodal and 11% for extranodal presentations. This may possibly be explained in part
by the fact that patterns of spread in lymphangiogram staged patients have been
largely extranodal.

Extended field radiotherapy has not been entirely satisfactory in the treatment of
non-Hodgkin's lymphomas and particularly in the diffuse histiocytic lymphomas
(Jones, 1973). In stages III and IV disease gradual improvement in survival has
followed the development of multiple agent chemotherapy programs. The addition of
adriamycin and bleomycin to the conventional regimen of cytoxan, vincristine and
prednisone (COP) has been found to be highly effective in the treatment of diffuse
histiocytic lymphoma, and this combination of CHOP-Bleo compares very favorably with
other programs in the treatment of generalized nodular lymphoma (Rodriguez, 1977).
However, a limiting factor in the effectiveness of chemotherapy alone has been a
relatively high incidence of relapse in initially involved sites either during or
after completion of chemotherapy.

In 1966, we initiated a multimodality program for abdominal and stage III presentations of diffuse histiocytic lymphoma (Gamble, 1966). Encouraged by results for a combination of COP chemotherapy and radiotherapy, this program was expanded to include all three stages of nodular as well as diffuse lymphomas. In our current studies, the chemotherapy combination was modified to include adriamycin and bleomycin. In view of the possible long term effects of multimodality treatment, including second malignancies and acute leukemia (Arseneau, 1972; Einhorn, 1978), we felt that it was important to identify by laparotomy those few patients who may have truly localized disease and to randomize them to treatment with IF radiotherapy alone vs. IF radiotherapy and CHOP-Bleo chemotherapy. Preliminary results from these trials are the basis of this report.

Table 1 Nodular Lymphomas

Stage (incl. E)	Number*	Staging Method		
		Clin	Lymph	Lap
I+	19-11%	1	10	8
II+	22-13%	1	13	8
III	63- 37%	5	45	13
IV	67-39%			
TOTAL	171-100%			

*54% of stages I, IE, II, IIE were abdominal presentations

Table 2 Diffuse Lymphomas

Stage (incl. E)	Number*	Staging Method		
		Clin	Lymph	Lap
I+	54-26%	5	28	21
II+	65-31%	5	41	19
III	38-18%	7	28	3
IV	52-25%			
TOTAL	209-100%			

*Of the 209 patients, 183 were diffuse histiocytic cases.
+38% of stages I, IE, II, IIE were abdominal presentations.

MATERIALS AND METHODS

In 1974, members of the Departments of Radiotherapy, Medicine, Surgery and Pathology established a weekly planning clinic to review the case material and plan the treatment for all adult lymphoma patients. During the ensuing four years, 436 previously untreated patients were admitted with a diagnosis of non-Hodgkin's lymphoma. The proportion of nodular and diffuse lymphoma cases was approximately equal. The initial investigation of these patients included bilateral bone marrow biopsies, lymphangiography and staging laparotomy in medically fit lymphangiogram negative stages I and II patients. The distributions for the nodular and diffuse lymphoma patients are shown in Tables 1 and 2. It is to be noted that 54% of stages I and II patients with nodular lymphomas had abdominal presentations; the corresponding figure for diffuse lymphomas was 38%. It was from this population that the case material for our multimodality protocols was obtained.

Treatment

The chemotherapy and radiotherapy sections of our current protocols are similar for all three stages of disease; modifications in scheduling and dosages are based on histopathology and stage of disease (Tables 3, 4 and 5).

---

[1]Cytoxan is the trademark of cyclophosphamide and is produced by Mead-Johnson Laboratories of Evansville, Indiana.

Table 3 Schedule for CHOP-Bleo

Drug	Mg/M^2	Schedule
Cytoxan[1]	750 IV	Day 1
Adriamycin	50 IV	Day 1
Vincristine	1.4 IV	Day 1
Prednisone	40 PO	Days 1-5
Bleomycin	5 IV	Day 1

Courses repeated at 3-4 week intervals

222   L. M. Fuller *et al.*

Chemotherapy. Unless medically contraindicated, the combination of chemotherapeutic
agents used in all of our multimodality studies consisted of cytoxan, adriamycin,
vincristine, prednisone and bleomycin (CHOP-Bleo) (Table 3). Side effects, complications and limitations of the total dosage of adriamycin and bleomycin have been
previously described (Rodriguez, 1977). After a total dose of 450 mg/M^2, adriamycin
was deleted from the chemotherapy regimen. Bleomycin was deleted after a total dose
of approximately 180 mg.

Radiotherapy. In all three stages of disease, radiotherapy was administered to the
initially involved regions. In abdominal presentations of nodular lymphoma, the
entire abdomen was irradiated. In most cases, the upper two-thirds of the abdomen
and pelvis were treated in series. In the diffuse histiocytic lymphomas, abdominal
fields were limited to known disease.

The radiotherapy dose was based on the histopathology and the involved regions.
Peripheral and mediastinal presentations of nodular lymphoma were treated with 4000
rad tumor dose in 4 weeks. Residual disease in peripheral regions was given additional treatment through reduced fields. Because of the dose limitations of the
heart and spinal cord, treatment to the mediastinum was limited to 4000 rad. The
tumor dose delivered to the entire abdomen in nodular lymphomas was 3000 rad administered through parallel opposed anterior and posterior fields at a rate of 750
rad per week. During this treatment, the right lobe of the liver was shielded an-
teriorly with 1 HVL of lead. The kidneys were shielded posteriorly with 2 HVL.
When feasible, additional treatment was given for residual disease.

Because the diffuse histiocytic lymphomas are generally less radiosensitive, peripheral regions were treated with a basic tumor dose of 5000 rad and additional
treatment was given for residual disease. Abdominal disease was treated to limited
fields to a tumor dose of 4000 rad or more when indicated.

Table 4   Treatment Plan: Stages I, IE, II, IIE Nodular and Diffuse Lymphomas

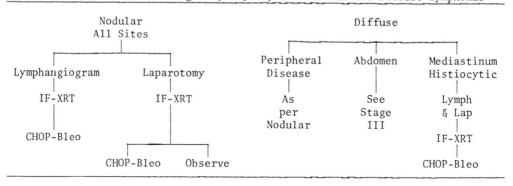

Stages I and II disease. To reiterate, except for diffuse histiocytic lymphomas
involving the abdomen, stages I and II disease including extranodal presentations
were treated initially with involved field radiotherapy (Table 4). All patients who
were not staged by laparotomy received CHOP-Bleo following radiotherapy for one year
unless medically contraindicated. In patients with cardiac or pulmonary disease,
adriamycin and/or bleomycin was deleted from the chemotherapy regimen. Since 1975,
laparotomy staged patients who were willing to participate on a protocol study were
randomized to receive no further treatment vs. CHOP-Bleo. Stages I and II patients
with diffuse histiocytic lymphoma of the abdomen were given CHOP-Bleo prior to radiotherapy according to our stage III protocol to reduce bulk disease. The rationale
for preliminary chemotherapy was based on our previous experience that local control

was seldom achieved with radiotherapy alone (Fuller, 1975).

Stage III disease. Patients with stage III disease were treated with alternating
courses of CHOP-Bleo chemotherapy and radiotherapy to the involved regions (Table 5).

Table 5   Basic Design for Management of Stage III and IIIE Non-Hodgkin's
          Lymphomas (including Stage II Abdominal Diffuse Histiocytic)

Nodular		Diffuse	
↓ CHOP-Bleo (R)	2 courses	↓ CHOP-Bleo (F)	4 courses
↓ XRT Abdomen, upper 2/3		↓ XRT Abdomen	Limited fields
↓ CHOP-Bleo (R)	2 courses	↓ CHOP-Bleo (F)	4 courses
↓ XRT Pelvis		↓ XRT Head & Neck and/or Axilla(e)	
↓ CHOP-Bleo (R)	2 courses	↓ COP* (F)	4 courses
↓ XRT Neck and/or Axilla(e)			
↓ CHOP-Bleo (R)	4 courses		

R=Reduced dose (see text); F=Full dose   *See text

In the nodular lymphomas, emphasis was placed on radiotherapy. To ensure completion
of treatment to the entire abdomen, the dosages of cytoxan and adriamycin were reduced by approximately 25% for each course of CHOP-Bleo. Two courses of CHOP-Bleo
were given between each course of radiotherapy. The total number of courses of
chemotherapy was limited to 10.

In the diffuse lymphomas, emphasis was placed on chemotherapy. Treatment was initiated with 4 courses of full dose CHOP-Bleo, which was subsequently alternated with
IF radiotherapy. The number of courses of chemotherapy was limited to 12.

Analysis of the Data

Survival and disease free survival curves were calculated according to the method
of Kaplan and Meier (1958). Gehan's modification of the generalized Wilcoxon test
(1965) was employed to evaluate differences in survival. Patients lost to follow
up and those who died of complications were considered dead of disease. Those patients in complete remission who died of other causes were carried as alive and
free of disease at the time of last follow up.

RESULTS

Laparotomy Stages I and II

Fifty-three laparotomy stages I and II patients have been followed 6-66 months from
admission.

Nodular lymphomas. The projected 5 year survival figure for 14 nodular lymphoma
patients was 87% (Fig. 3). No difference was detected in results for lymphocytic,
mixed or histiocytic cell types. Of the surviving patients, 3 have relapsed at 19,
21 and 36 months. One of 3 patients treated with a combination of chemotherapy and
radiotherapy has had progression.

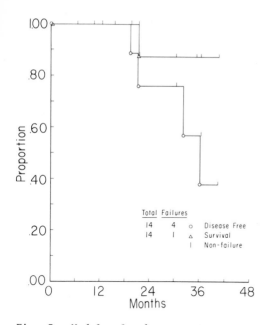

Fig. 3. Nodular lymphomas,
laparotomy staged I and II;
survival and disease free.

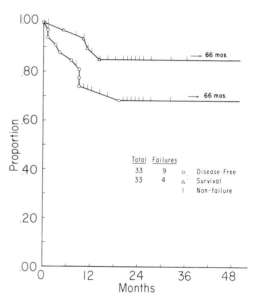

Fig. 4. All diffuse histiocytic,
laparotomy staged I and II;
survival and disease free.

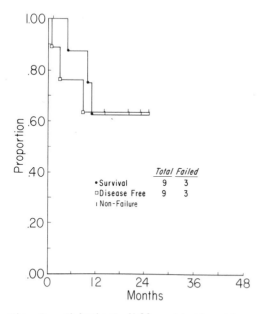

Fig. 5. Abdominal diffuse histiocytic,
chemotherapy and radiotherapy;
survival and disease free.

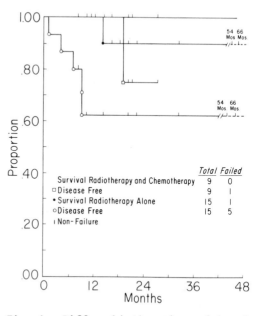

Fig. 6. Diffuse histiocytic peripheral
and mediastinal presentations,
laparotomy staged I and II;
radiotherapy vs. radiotherapy
and CHOP-Bleo chemotherapy.

Diffuse lymphomas. Of 39 patients with diffuse lymphomas, 33 had diffuse histiocytic lymphoma. The projected 5 year survival figure for the entire group of diffuse
histiocytic lymphoma patients was 85% (Fig. 4); the corresponding disease free survival figure was 69%. There was no statistical difference in results for extranodal
disease of 87% vs. 83% for nodal presentations. However, the corresponding disease
free survival figures were 76% and 56%. No patient with diffuse histiocytic lymphoma relapsed after 20 months. The effect of chemotherapy on results for the entire group of diffuse histiocytic lymphoma patients could not be ascertained because
abdominal presentations, which were considered unfavorable, were all treated with
chemotherapy and radiotherapy. This group of abdominal cases has been analyzed
separately; the projected 5 year survival and disease free survival figures were
64% and 63% (Fig. 5).

For patients with peripheral presentations of diffuse histiocytic lymphoma, no significant difference in survival was found for treatment with radiotherapy alone vs.
radiotherapy and chemotherapy. Of 15 patients treated with radiotherapy only, one
is deceased and 4 others have relapsed. Only one of 9 patients on the combined
program has had progression (Fig. 6).

Miscellaneous lymphomas. Six laparotomy staged patients with various diagnoses of
non-Hodgkin's lymphoma were analyzed separately. These included diffuse lymphocytic
lymphomas of the well, intermediate and poorly differentiated subtypes, including
the convoluted cell type, undifferentiated lymphoma and Lennert's lymphoma. Of
these patients, 4 were treated with radiotherapy alone; 2 received multiple agent
chemotherapy in addition to radiotherapy. To date, 4 of these patients have experienced progression; of these, 2 are dead.

Information on patterns of spread and response to subsequent management of laparotomy stages I and II nodular and diffuse lymphoma patients has been reported elsewhere and is not, therefore, included in this report (Toonkel, in press).

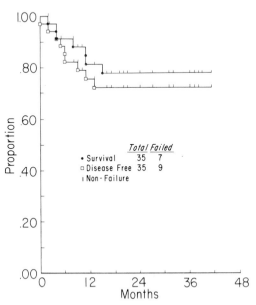

Fig. 7. Diffuse histiocytic lymphomas,
lymphangiogram staged I and II;
chemotherapy and radiotherapy.

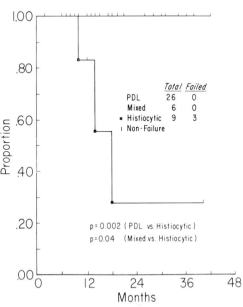

Fig. 8. Nodular lymphomas, stage III;
survival, combined program of
chemotherapy and radiotherapy.

Lymphangiogram Stage I and II

Insufficient numbers of nodular lymphoma patients were entered into this project for analysis. Thirty-five diffuse histiocytic lymphoma patients treated with radiotherapy and chemotherapy have been followed a maximum of 42 months. The projected 5 year survival and disease free survival figures for this group were 78% and 73% respectively (Fig. 7). To date, 26 patients are free of disease; no patient developed new disease after 15 months. One patient in complete remission died of pneumocystic carinii at 11 months. Of the 8 patients who relapsed, 6 had wide spread disseminated disease and 2 patients had spread to lymph nodes. All but one of these 8 patients are deceased.

Stage III Disease

Non-Hodgkin's lymphoma patients with stage III disease have been followed a maximum of 45 months from admission.

Nodular lymphomas. Forty-one patients have been entered in this study. The distribution by cell type was as follows: poorly differentiated lymphocytic 26; mixed 6; histiocytic 9. To determine whether cell type influenced results, separate survival and disease free survival curves were calculated for these 3 groups (Figs. 8 and 9). To date, no patient with poorly differentiated lymphocytic or mixed cell disease has died of lymphoma, whereas 3 of 9 patients of the histiocytic variety are dead.

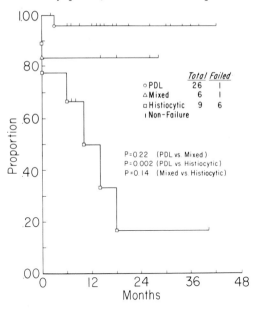

Fig. 9. Nodular lymphomas, stage III;   Fig. 10. Diffuse histiocytic lymphoma,
         chemotherapy and radiotherapy,   chemotherapy and radiotherapy.
         disease free survival.   Stage III.

Progression of disease during treatment occurred in one patient with poorly differentiated lymphocytic lymphoma, one patient with mixed cell disease and 6 patients with histiocytic disease.

Diffuse lymphomas. All 21 patients entered in this study had diffuse histiocytic lymphoma. The projected 5 year survival figure for this group was 74% (Fig. 10).

Of 6 patients who failed, all but one had progression within the first 15 months; 4 of these patients are dead.

DISCUSSION AND CONCLUSIONS

In non-Hodgkin's lymphomas, assessment of the influence on results of surgical staging in stages I and II patients and multiple agent chemotherapy in all 3 stages of disease is dependent on the histologic subtype. In the nodular lymphomas which tend to have an indolent course regardless of the stage when the patient is first seen, insufficient time has elapsed to determine the influence of either surgical staging or multiple agent chemotherapy in stages I and II disease. In stage III disease treated with CHOP-Bleo and radiotherapy, results were satisfactory for the poorly differentiated lymphocytic and mixed cell types, but not for the histiocytic variety. In the future, our plan is to treat stage III nodular histiocytic lymphoma patients according to our stage III protocol for diffuse disease which has been very effective.

In the diffuse histiocytic lymphomas, results for abdominal presentations treated with chemotherapy and radiotherapy were dramatically improved over previous results for radiotherapy alone. At the present time, it is still too early to determine whether adjunctive chemotherapy will influence results for laparotomy staged I and II patients with peripheral presentations. For stage III diffuse histiocytic lymphomas treated with CHOP-Bleo and radiotherapy, our projected 5 year survival figure of 74% compares very favorably with 65% for 12 stage III patients treated with combination chemotherapy (Fisher, 1977).

SUMMARY

Preliminary results of the M.D. Anderson team and those of other centers (Glatstein, 1977) indicate that the combined use of chemotherapy and radiotherapy is more effective than either modality alone for most categories of non-Hodgkin's lymphomas. In view of the increased risk of a second malignancy, including acute leukemia, associated with multimodality therapy, it is our opinion that trials to determine whether adjunctive chemotherapy is needed in laparotomy staged patients should be continued.

ACKNOWLEDGMENTS

This research has been supported in part by U.S. Public Health Service Grant number CA-06294.

The authors wish to thank Jane A. Sullivan, B.S., for her assistance in compiling and analyzing the data and Ruth Roberts, B.A., for her editorial assistance.

REFERENCES

Arseneau, J.C., R.W. Sponzo, D.L. Levin, L.E. Schnipper, H. Bonner, R.C. Young, G.P. Canellos, R.E. Johnson and V.T. DeVita (1972). Nonlymphomatous malignant tumors complicating Hodgkin's disease. Possible association with intensive therapy. N. Engl. J. Med., 287, 1119-1122.
Einhorn, N. (1978). Acute leukemia after chemotherapy (Melphalan). Cancer, 41, 444-447.
Fisher, R.I., V.T. DeVita, B.L. Johnson, R. Simon and R.C. Young (1977). Prognostic factors for advanced diffuse histiocytic lymphoma following treatment with combination chemotherapy. Am. J. Med., 63, 177-182.

Fuller, L.M., F.L. Banker, J.J. Butler, J.F. Gamble and M.P. Sullivan (1975). The natural history of non-Hodgkin's lymphomata stages I and II. Br. J. Cancer, 31, Suppl. II, 270-285.

Gamble, J.F., L.M. Fuller, J.J. Butler and C.C. Shullenberger (1971). Combined chemotherapy and radiotherapy for advanced Hodgkin's disease and reticulum cell sarcoma. South. Med. J., 64, 775-783.

Gehan, E.A. (1965). A generalized Wilcoxon test for comparing arbitrarily singly-censored samples. Biometrika, 52, 203-223.

Glatstein, E., S.S. Donaldson, S.A. Rosenberg and H.S. Kaplan (1977). Combined modality therapy in malignant lymphomas. Cancer Treat. Rep., 61, 1199-1207.

Heifetz, L.J., L.M. Fuller, J.F. Gamble, R.G. Martin and J.J. Butler (in press). Findings of staging laparotomy in lymphangiogram staged I and II non-Hodgkin's lymphomas.

Jones, S.E., Z. Fuks, H.S. Kaplan and S.A. Rosenberg (1973). Non-Hodgkin's lymphoma. V. Results of radiotherapy. Cancer, 32, 682-691.

Kaplan, E.L. and P. Meier (1958). Non-parametric estimation from incomplete observations. J. Am. Stat. Assoc., 53, 457-481.

Rappaport, H., W.J. Winter and E.B. Hicks (1956). Follicular lymphoma. A re-evaluation of its position in the scheme of malignant lymphoma, based on a survey of 253 cases. Cancer, 9, 792-821.

Rodriguez, V., F. Cabanillas, M.A. Burgess, E.M. McKelvey, M. Valdivieso, G.P. Bodey and E.J. Freireich (1977). Combination chemotherapy ("CHOP-Bleo") in advanced (non-Hodgkin) malignant lymphoma. Blood, 49, 325-333.

Toonkel, L.M., L.M. Fuller, J.F. Gamble, J.J. Butler, R.G. Martin and C.C. Shullenberger (in press). Laparotomy stage I and II non-Hodgkin's lymphomas: Preliminary results of radiotherapy and adjunctive chemotherapy.

Chemotherapy of Non-Hodgkin's Lymphomas — Indications and Results*

G. Brittinger**, **U. Schmalhorst** (Essen), **H. Bartels** (Lübeck),
K. Bremer (Essen), **F. Brunswicker, A. Burger** (München),
H. Common (Freiburg), **E. Dühmke** (Kiel), **H. H. Fülle** (Berlin),
R. Heinz (Wien), **H. Huber** (Linz), **E. König** (Essen), **K.-M. Koeppen**
(Berlin), **H. Leopold** (Freiburg), **P. Meusers** (Essen), **L. Nowicki**
(Flensburg), **R. Nürnberger** (Würzburg), **J. Oertel** (Berlin),
H. W. Pees (Homburg/Saar), **M. Pfoch** (Berlin), **H. Pralle** (Giessen)
and M. Schmidt (Bremen) (Kiel Lymphoma Study Group)

***Division of Hematology, Department of Medicine, University of Essen,
4300 Essen 1, Germany*

ABSTRACT

Chemotherapy is indicated as treatment of choice in advanced non-Hodgkin's lymphomas (NHL). Benefit of adjuvant chemotherapy in stage I and II disease to eradicate microfoci of tumor not controlled by radiotherapy yet remains to be established. Among stage III and IV NHL with favorable histologies according to the Rappaport classification (diffuse well-differentiated lymphocytic, DWDL; nodular well-differentiated lymphocytic, NWDL; nodular poorly differentiated lymphocytic, NPDL; nodular mixed histiocytic-lymphocytic, NM) in DWDL, NWDL and NPDL long survival has been observed after single-agent or mild combination chemotherapy and even after prolonged periods of no treatment in asymptomatic patients. It is suggested, however, that in NPDL and NM survival is improved if complete remission is attained. In stage III and IV NHL with unfavorable histologies (diffuse poorly differentiated lymphocytic, DPDL; diffuse histiocytic, DH; nodular histiocytic, NH; diffuse mixed histiocytic-lymphocytic, DM; diffuse undifferentiated, DU) complete remission which has prognostic significance is only achieved at high rates with aggressive chemotherapy. In DH long relapse-free survival in a high percentage of complete responders suggests that cure might be possible by chemotherapy alone.

Preliminary data of a prospective multicentric study (still in progress) on patients with NHL diagnosed according to the Kiel classification show that survival of patients with low-grade malignant lymphomas (LGML) significantly exceeds that of patients with high-grade malignant lymphomas (HGML). Responders (patients attaining complete or partial remission) with stage III and IV lymphomas usually had a significantly longer survival than nonresponders. Among LGML probability of survival of responders to mild chemotherapy was different (chronic lymphocytic leukemia, centroblastic-centrocytic, and centrocytic > immunocytic lymphoma). In HGML treated with relatively mild regimens or drug combinations of intermediate intensity, rates of response were unsatisfactory and probability of survival of nonresponders was very poor. Therefore, more aggressive chemotherapy is now used for initial remission induction.

*Supported by the Deutsche Krebshilfe e.V., Bonn, Germany

KEYWORDS

Non-Hodgkin's lymphomas, Rappaport classification, favorable histology, unfavorable
histology, Kiel classification, low-grade malignant non-Hodgkin's lymphomas, high-
grade malignant non-Hodgkin's lymphomas, chemotherapy, adjuvant chemotherapy

INTRODUCTION

During recent years approaches to the treatment of non-Hodgkin's lymphomas (NHL)
were much influenced by the now well-established correlations between certain histopathologic patterns and prognosis and, in addition, by the impressing long-term
results of a stage - related treatment of patients with Hodgkin's disease. Thus,
the Ann Arbor classification originally designed for Hodgkin's disease (12) is widely used also for staging of patients with NHL although it has certain limitations
due to well-known differences between the natural history of these disorders and
that of Hodgkin's disease (11, 36).

HISTOPATHOLOGIC CLASSIFICATIONS

For most therapeutic studies performed during the last decade the histopathologic
classification proposed by Rappaport in 1966 on purely morphologic grounds was used
which has been shown to be of clinical relevance, especially in distinguishing NHL
of *favorable* prognosis (in most instances lymphomas with "nodular" histologic structure, i.e. NWDL[1], NPDL[1], NM[1]) from NHL of *unfavorable* prognosis (mainly lymphomas
with "diffuse" histologic structure, i.e. DH[1], DM[1], DU[1]); DPDL[1] is also attributed
to the latter group by most authors (1, 11, 32). However, there are exceptions from
this rule in that DWDL[1] has a good prognosis whereas NH[1] behaves much like diffuse
lymphomas (1, 11, 32). More recently, new histopathologic schemes such as the Kiel
classification based both on functional, predominantly immunologic, and morphologic
criteria (20, 27) have been developed and have caused modifications of the Rappaport classification (34). This paper will first review treatment results obtained
by authors using the original Rappaport classification, and then present preliminary data of a prospective multicentric study performed by the Kiel Lymphoma Study
Group on patients diagnosed according to the Kiel classification.

RESULTS OF THERAPEUTIC STUDIES USING THE RAPPAPORT CLASSIFICATION

Several authors were able to demonstrate that a high percentage of patients with
localized (stage I) NHL of various histologies can be controlled by radiotherapy
alone (23, 30, 41). In DH which is considered to be one of the most malignant NHL
entities 65 % of patients presenting with stage I attained a five-years survival
(24). Similar or even better data were obtained in stage I patients with other,
more favorable histologies (9, 23, 24, 30). Results of radiotherapy in patients with
DH and other NHL entities diagnosed at stage II are more variable. Whereas some authors reported that 59 to 70 % of patients, especially with nodular histologies
(NPDL, NML), survived five years (3, 23) other data are less promising (five-years
survival in only 0 to 30 % of patients) (24, 30). Thus, if failure occurs despite
pathologic staging and extended radiotherapy with sufficient doses it must be assu-
med that microscopic disease outside the radiation field was already present at
diagnosis or developed during the radiotherapy period. Since early dissemination
seems to be a feature more characteristic for NHL of favorable than of unfavorable
histologies (11) adjuvant chemotherapy would be expected to predominantly increase
the chance of complete control of stage I and II disease in patients with NHL of
favorable histologies. However, no data of careful prospective trials are available
as yet to definitely support this hypothesis. Randomized studies by Glatstein and
others (22) and Bonadonna and Monfardini (4) have only shown that stage I and II

---

[1]NWDL = nodular well-differentiated lymphocytic lymphoma; NPDL = nodular poorly differentiated lymphoma; NH = nodular histiocytic lymphoma; NM = nodular mixed histiocytic-lymphocytic lymphoma; DWDL = diffuse well-differentiated lymphocytic lympho-
ma; DPDL = diffuse poorly differentiated lymphocytic lymphoma; DH = diffuse histiocytic lymphoma; DM = diffuse mixed histiocytic-lymphocytic lymphoma; and DU = diffuse undifferentiated lymphoma.

patients with NHL of unfavorable histologies (NH, DPDL, DH, DU) and histiocytic and lymphocytic lymphomas, respectively, did not benefit from such a combined modality approach.

It is generally accepted that chemotherapy is the initial treatment of choice in the more generalized stages III and IV of NHL even though total lymphoid irradiation of stage III disease of favorable histology has been performed by some authors resulting in high remission rates of long duration (21, 24). Combination chemotherapy with relatively mild (e.g. COP[2],[3]), intermediate (e.g. COM[2], MOPP[2], C-MOPP[2]) or aggressive (e.g. BACOP[2],[3], HOP[2], CHOP[2], CHOP + bleomycin, COMLA[2]) regimens is usually administered. However, single-agent treatment is also performed in NHL with favorable histologies (32). Although it is difficult to compare many results published in the literature due to differences in the design of the therapeutic trials and in the evaluation criteria, synopsis of the majority of data (Table 1 and Table 2) shows that the aforementioned chemotherapeutic combination regimens are able to induce a significant percentage of complete and partial remissions in patients with all NHL entities. It becomes evident that the percentage of responders to relatively mild or intermediate drug combinations is higher among patients with favorable histologies than among those with unfavorable histologies. However, more aggressive chemotherapy increases the rate of response in both groups of patients. As discussed below, in many NHL entities a clear-cut correlation between complete response to chemotherapy and probability of survival could be demonstrated.

Considering the various NHL entities with *favorable* histology (Table 1) it can be shown that in DWDL single-agent treatment, e.g. with chlorambucil, or mild combination chemotherapy or even no treatment for prolonged periods of time in asymptomatic patients is accompanied by long median survival times of up to 7 years (32). There are no data which convincingly indicate a longer survival of patients attaining complete remission as compared to patients who do not. Apparently, there are similarities between DWDL and chronic lymphocytic leukemia (CLL) or Waldenström's macroglobulinemia (which, according to the Kiel classification, is categorized under the immunocytic lymphoma) both from histopathologic and clinical points of view (31). Therefore, therapeutic strategy should be analogous to that performed in patients with CLL and Waldenström's macroglobulinemia.

NPDL represents one of the most frequent NHL entities observed in the U.S.A. It behaves much like DWDL in that it responds well to mild combination or single-agent chemotherapy which only rarely leads to complete remission and, according to Portlock and Rosenberg (32), can be started in asymptomatic patients several months or years after diagnosis without deteriorating prognosis. However, it is remarkable that there are some data suggesting that patients achieving complete remission do prognostically better than partial responders (1, 17). If this dependency of prognosis on optimal response to chemotherapy holds true in further trials administration of more aggressive drug regimens inducing higher complete remission rates must be considered in this disease.

Survival of patients with the more rarely observed NHL entities NWDL and NM is comparable to that described for patients with NPDL. So far, there is no evidence indicating that in NWDL prognosis might be improved by aggressive chemotherapy whereas this has been observed in patients with NM (1, 28).

---

[2]COP = cyclophosphamide, vincristine, and prednisone; COM = cyclophosphamide, vincristine, and methotrexate; MOPP = mechlorethamine, vincristine, procarbazine, and prednisone; C-MOPP = MOPP with cyclophosphamide instead of mechlorethamine; BACOP = bleomycin, adriamycin, cyclophosphamide, vincristine, and prednisone; HOP = hydroxyldaunomycin (adriamycin), vincristine, and prednisone; CHOP = cyclophosphamide, hydroxyldaunomycin (adriamycin), vincristine, and prednisone; COMLA = cyclophosphamide, vincristine, methotrexate, leucovorin (citrovorum factor), and cytosine arabinoside.
[3]Different dosages and schedules are used.

G. Brittinger *et al.*

TABLE 1 Synopsis of Results of Chemotherapy in Patients with Advanced Non-Hodgkin's Lymphomas Diagnosed According to the Rappaport Classification: Favorable Histologies

Histo-logy	Therapy	n	CR	Duration (m=Median)	Survival (m=Median)	PR	Survival (m=Median)	NR	Survival (m=Median)	Entire Group Survival (m=Median)	Reference
DWDL	COP	11	64%	23 (4-107+)mos	m: 84 mos	36%	1-81+mos			m: 78.2 mos	Anderson and others, 1977
	HOP CHOP	45	58%	2 yrs: 83%						m: n.r. 2 yrs: 55%	McKelvey and others, 1976
NWDL	HOP CHOP	43	72%	2 yrs: 92%						m: n.r. 2 yrs: 95 %	McKelvey and others, 1976
NPDL	COP, C-MOPP	49	67%	16 mos	m: 95 mos 2 yrs: 92%	PR+NR: 16%			m: 35 mos 2 yrs: 56%	m: 83.3 mos 2 yrs: 73%	Anderson and others, 1977
	COP COP+Bleo CHOP	17 15 62	53% 67% 77%	m: n.r. m: 33 mos m: n.r.						m: 36 mos m: 44 mos m: n.r. 2 yrs: 82%	Coltman and others, 1977
	HOP	54	59%	m: n.r.						m: n.r. 2 yrs: 87%	
	C+P BCNU+P	97	47%	9.5 mos	m: n.r. 3 yrs: 79%	34%	m: n.r. 3 yrs: 64%	19%	m: n.r. 3 yrs: 55%	m: n.r. 3 yrs: 70%	Ezdinli and others, 1978
	HOP CHOP	68	74%	2 yrs: 87%						m: n.r. 2 yrs: 85%	McKelvey and others, 1976
	CHOP + Bleo	13	62%	2 yrs: 86%		38%				m: n.r. 2 yrs: 84%	Rodriguez and others, 1977
NM	C-MOPP, COP, BACOP	31	77%	2 yrs: 82%	m: n.r. 2 yrs: 92%	23%	m: 13 mos 2 yrs: 8%			m: n.r. 2 yrs: 83%	Anderson and others, 1977
	HOP CHOP	20	70%	2yrs: 71%						m: 24 mos 2 yrs: 50%	McKelvey and others, 1976

For abbreviations see footnotes 1 and 2. n.r. = not reached; CR = complete remission; PR = partial remission; NR = no response.

DH, the most common NHL with *unfavorable* histology (Table 2), deserves great interest since recent experience has shown that in patients with advanced disease chemotherapy is able to induce complete remission rates in the range of 40 to 56 % using COP, MOPP, C-MOPP, COMLA or BACOP (1, 10, 13, 15, 17, 37, 39), and up to 80 % using COM, HOP, CHOP or CHOP + bleomycin (13, 26, 28, 35). In a considerable percentage of patients relapse-free survival was found to last 10 years or longer (15, 16). Analysis of remission duration curve by McKelvey and Moon (29) has demonstrated that patients with DH initially have the greatest risk of disease recurrence (42 %) and subsequently show a significant fall in their rate of relapse. The slope of the curve indicates a marked change which becomes maximal about 17 months following the onset of therapy. Then, the curve begins to plateau suggesting that a cure may have been achieved in as many as 50 % of patients attaining a complete remission.

Results of treatment of patients with advanced DPDL are still more unsatisfactory. As pointed out by Anderson and others (1) and Ezdinli and others (17) correlation between complete response to chemotherapy and time of survival exists in this disease as in DH and other NHL entities. However, rates of complete remissions obtained by administration of mild chemotherapy (COP, BCNU + prednisone) are low (25 to 32 %) (1, 17) so that more aggressive regimens (BACOP, HOP, CHOP) have been used leading to better results (rates of complete remissions 62 to 80 %) (28, 39). According to McKelvey and Moon (29) extrapolation from the remission duration curve of patients with DPDL suggests a plateau after 69 months with only 15 % of patients remaining in complete remission.

Patients with NH experienced a high rate of complete remissions (71 %) after ag-

TABLE 2 Synopsis of Results of Chemotherapy in Patients with Advanced Non-Hodgkin's Lymphomas Diagnosed According to the Rappaport Classification: Unfavorable Histologies

Histology	Therapy	n	CR	Duration (m=Median)	Survival (m=Median)	PR	Survival (m=Median)	NR	Survival (m=Median)	Entire Group Survival (m=Median)	Reference
NH	HOP, CHOP	17	71%	2 yrs: 91%						m: n.r. 2 yrs: 68%	McKelvey and others, 1976
DPDL	COP	25	32%	m: 8 (3-72+)mos	m: n.r. 3 yrs: 72%	68%	m: 10.4 mos 3 yrs: 19%	0		m: 23.2 mos 3 yrs: 40%	Anderson and others, 1977
	BACOP	15	80%			13%		7%		m: n.r. 2 yrs: 58%	Skarin and others, 1977
	C+P, BCNU+P	77	25%	m: 8 mos	m: n.r. 2 yrs: 84%	34%	m: n.r. 2 yrs: 58%	41%	m: 13 mos 2 yrs: 17%	m: 23 mos 2 yrs: 47%	Ezdinli and others, 1978
	HOP, CHOP	76	62%	2 yrs: 60%						m: n.r. 2 yrs: 74%	McKelvey and others, 1976
DH	COP	49	49%	m: 14 mos						m: 16 mos 2 yrs: 38%	Coltman and others, 1977
	BCNU + COP	28	50%	8 mos	m: 23 mos 2 yrs: 48%	25%		25%		m: 15 mos 2 yrs: 36%	Durant and others, 1975
	C-MOPP, MOPP	27	41%	m: 42 mos	m: n.r. 1 yr: 100%	PR+NR:		59%	m: 5 mos 1 yr: 62%	m: 8 mos 1 yr: 45%	DeVita and others, 1975
	BACOP, C-MOPP, MOPP, COP	62	47%	74%: 111+ mos	m: n.r. 1 yr: 92%	53%	m: 7 mos 1 yr: 9%	0		m: 11 mos 1 yr: 48%	Anderson and others, 1977
	C-MOPP, BACOP	56	46%		m: n.r. 1 yr: 94%	38%	m: 7.6 mos 1 yr: 10%	16%	m: 3.2 mos 1 yr: 0	m: 11.4 mos 1 yr: 49%	Fisher and others, 1977
	BACOP	25	48%	m: 12+ mos	m: n.r. 1 yr: 100%	PR+NR:		52%	m: 7 mos 1 yr: 22%	m: 14 mos 1 yr: 57%	Schein and others, 1976
	BACOP	18	56%			16%		28%		m: 9 mos 1 yr: 38%	Skarin and others, 1977
	COMLA	30	40%	m: 48+mos		36%	m: 18 mos	24%	m: 6 mos		Cadman and others, 1977
	HOP, CHOP	115	67%	1 yr: 72 %						m: 22 mos 1 yr: 66%	McKelvey and others, 1976
	CHOP + Bleo	26	69%	1 yr: 88%		31%				m: n.r. 1 yr: 76 %	Rodriguez and others, 1977
	CHOP	68	47%	m: 23 mos						m: 11 mos 2 yrs: 43 %	Coltman and others, 1977
	HOP	69	55%	m: 22 mos						m: 2o mos 2 yrs: 43%	
	COP + Bleo	16	63%	m: 25 mos						m: 10 mos 2 yrs: 41%	
	COM	27	81%	41%: 36-60 mos							Lauria and others, 1978
DM	COP, C-MOPP, BACOP	10	10%	44 + mos	51+ mos	90%	m: 4 mos 2 yrs: 12%	0		m: 4 mos 2 yrs: 23%	Anderson and others, 1977
	BACOP	6	67%			33%				m: 9 mos 2 yrs: 35%	Skarin and others, 1977
	HOP, CHOP	26	62%	1 yr: 70%						m: n.r. 1 yr: 64%	McKelvey and others, 1976

For abbreviations see footnotes 1 and 2 and Table 1.

gressive chemotherapy (HOP or CHOP) with 91 % still relapse-free after a follow-up period of two years (28). In DM chemotherapy with COP, C-MOPP or BACOP led to a complete remission in only 1 out of 10 patients (1). However, other authors using HOP, CHOP and BACOP report higher rates of complete responders (62 to 67 %)(28, 39). Seventy percent of the patients treated with HOP or CHOP were still in complete remission after 1 year and at this time the entire group had a probability of survival of 64 % (28).

The exact role of adjuvant radiotherapy in the treatment of advanced NHL is still ill-defined. Glatstein and others (22) observed some improvement in stage III and

IV disease with unfavorable histologies (DPDL, DH, DM, DU, NH).

RESULTS OF THERAPEUTIC STUDIES USING THE KIEL CLASSIFICA-
TION (PROSPECTIVE STUDY OF THE KIEL LYMPHOMA STUDY GROUP)

With regard to the Kiel classification a retrospective study on 405 patients performed by the Kiel Lymphoma Study Group, comprising several clinicians at different
institutions in Germany and Austria, has demonstrated the prognostic relevance of
the histologic subdivision into lymphomas of *low-grade* (malignant lymphoma, M.L.,
lymphocytic, mainly CLL; M.L. immunocytic; M.L. centrocytic; M.L. centroblastic-
centrocytic) and *high-grade* (M.L. centroblastic; M.L. immunoblastic; M.L. lymphoblastic) malignancy and, in addition, differences of survival between entities belonging to the group of malignant lymphomas of low-grade malignancy. Furthermore,
clinical features characteristic for certain NHL entities could be evidenced (5,
8, 40). However, since in these patients the diagnostic and therapeutic procedures
as well as the follow-up had not been performed according to a single protocol, data regarding several clinical and therapeutic features were not available. Therefore, in October 1975 a prospective multicentric study was started (6). The diagnostic protocol requires staging of all consecutive, previously untreated patients
admitted to the various institutions according to a modification by Musshoff (30)
of the Ann Arbor classification. With respect to treatment no randomization is made since it is the major goal of the study to evaluate the clinical relevance of
the Kiel classification rather than to answer specific therapeutic questions. The
treatment protocol is largely based on the data obtained in patients classified
according to Rappaport. Thus, in patients with stages I and II of all NHL entities
extended field irradiation without adjuvant chemotherapy is performed, however,
lower doses are used in NHL of low-grade malignancy (36 - 44 Gy) than in NHL of
high-grade malignancy (at least 45 Gy)[4]. Patients with the more advanced stages III
and IV receive chemotherapy and additional radiotherapy applied at least to the
regions with remnant manifestations of lymphoma. As exception differing from the
general therapeutic concept the very radiosensitive centroblastic-centrocytic
lymphoma is considered which is tentatively treated in stage III patients with total lymphoid irradiation alone[4]. Furthermore, in children and young adults with
all stages of lymphoblastic lymphoma which apparently has a high tendency to generalize early during course of the disease chemotherapy plus radiotherapy of the
involved regions plus CNS prophylaxis are performed. In adult patients over 30 years
of age with this disease the chemotherapeutic regimen is identical with that used
in other lymphomas of high-grade malignancy.

Extrapolating from the relatively good results of a mild chemotherapy obtained in
NHL with favorable histologies according to Rappaport, NHL of *low-grade* malignancy
are first treated with intermittent chlorambucil + prednisone as proposed by Knospe
and others (25) which is substituted by COP (2) if response is not sufficient. Chemotherapy is not started before certain criteria such as marked anemia (hemoglobin < 10 g/dl in females and < 11 g/dl in males) and/or thrombocytopenia
(< 100 000/µl) and/or significant increase in size of lymph nodes within 3 months
are fulfilled. This tentatively expectative approach to patients with advanced NHL
of low-grade malignancy seems to be justified by the good prognosis observed in patients with favorable histologies who did not receive any specific therapy as long
as they remained asymptomatic (32).

In the early phase of the study patients with NHL of the *high-grade* malignant centroblastic and immunoblastic varieties were first treated with COP and, in case of
failure, with COP + MTX and with ABP[5] if this second regimen remained unsuccessful.

---

[4]For clinical reasons, in single patients with centroblastic and centroblastic-centrocytic lymphoma radiotherapy was substituted by chemotherapy of the type applied
to patients with stages III and IV and stage IV, respectively.

[5]ABP = adriamycin, bleomycin, and prednisone.

TABLE 3 Preliminary Results of Therapy in Patients with Non-Hodgkin's Lymphomas Diagnosed According to the Kiel Classification

Histology	Stage	Therapy	n	Responders	Duration (Range) Months	Survival (Responders) Median	Survival (Responders) 1 Year (2 Years)	Non-responders	Survival (Non-resp.) Median	Survival (Non-resp.) 1 Year (2 Years)	Entire Group Survival Median	Entire Group Survival 1 Year (2 Years)	Interval from Diagnosis to Onset of Therapy
CLL	IV	CT	19	74%	10+ (2-29+)	n.r.	100% (100%)	26%	21 mos	100% (47%)	n.r.	100% (91%)	12+(3-33+) mos
		No therapy	18		14+ (8-33+)	n.r.	100% (100%)						
M.L. Immunocytic	IV	CT	44	61%	5+ (2-12+)	29 mos	92% (70%)	39%	12.5 mos	52% (38%)	27 mos	80% (64%)	8+ (1-28+) mos
	I + IV	Splen-ectomy	4	100%	13+ (6+-30+)	n.r.	100% (100%)	0					
	IV	No therapy	10		10+ (5+-28+)	n.r.	100% (100%)						
M.L. Centro-blastic-centro-cytic	III + IV	CT	15	60%	5+ (4-12+)	n.r.	100% (83%)	40%	14 mos	64% (42%)	n.r.	78% (61%)	6 (2-9) mos
	I - III	RT	12	100%	2+ (1-5+)	n.r.	79% (79%)	0					
M.L. Centro-cytic	III + IV	CT	19	63%	12+ (2-27+)	n.r.	100% (90%)	37%	12.5 mos	56% (0)	n.r.	88% (65%)	3 (3-6) mos
	I + II	RT	5	100%	17+ (1-27+)	n.r.	100% (83%)	0					
M.L. Centro-blastic	II - IV	CT	10	50%	5+ (2-18+)	n.r.	80%	50%	7 mos	0	n.r.	64%	
	I + II	RT	11	100%	4+ (1-10+)	n.r.	90%	0					
M.L. Immuno-blastic	III - IV	CT	10	30%	2+,3,6	n.r.	67%	70%	10 mos	32%	12.5 mos	52% (34%)	
	I + II	RT	9	100%	8+ (2-30+)	19 mos	65% (47%)						
M.L. Lympho-blastic	III + IV	CT	16	CR 44%	2+ (1-30+)	n.r.	80%	PR + NR 54%	5 mos	16%	11 mos	32%	

M.L. = malignant lymphoma; CT = chemotherapy; RT = radiotherapy; n.r. = not reached; CR = complete remission; PR = partial remission; NR = no response.

However, more recently unsatisfactory results of this approach and the promising experience of other authors with intensive chemotherapy in patients with unfavorable histologies gave rise to substitution of COP by the more aggressive regimen C-MOPP as treatment of first choice. Chemotherapy of children and young adults with lympho-blastic lymphoma consists of a modification of a three-phase program originally designed for childhood acute lymphoblastic leukemia (phase I: remission induction with adriamycin, vincristine, and prednisone; phase II: 6-thioguanine, prednisone, and cytosine arabinoside, CNS prophylaxis with intrathecal methotrexate and cranial irradiation, involved field irradiation; phase III: maintenance with 6-thioguanine and methotrexate, and alternate pulses with vincristine and prednisone, and COP, respectively) (6).

Preliminary results of this prospective study (7)[6], still in progress, obtained after a follow-up period of only 20 to 33 months show that the overall probability of survival of patients with low-grade malignant lymphomas is much exceeding that found in patients with NHL of high-grade malignancy (Fig. 1). Statistical analysis showed that *responders* with both low-grade and high-grade malignant lymphomas (except for immunoblastic lymphoma) had a significantly higher probability of survival than *non-responders* (Fig. 2-8, Table 3). With regard to the various entities of low-grade ma-

_____
[6]see next page

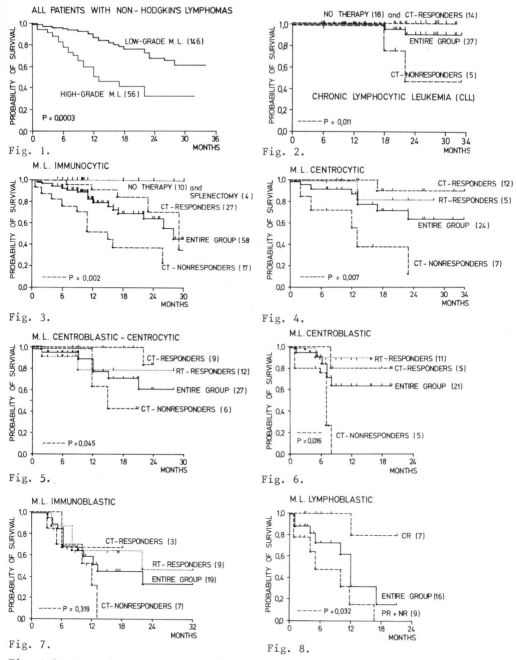

Fig. 1-8. Actuarial survival curves for the evaluated patients (n= 202) with non-Hodgkin's lymphomas (NHL) diagnosed according to the Kiel classification. Fig. 1. Patients with low-grade malignant vs. patients with high-grade malignant NHL. Fig. 2-8. Patients with the various entities of low-grade and high-grade malignant NHL treated with chemotherapy (CT) or radiotherapy (RT). Statistical analysis: CT-responders vs. CT-nonresponders; in lymphoblastic lymphoma: complete responders (CR) vs. partial (PR) and nonresponders (NR).

lignancy patients with the lymphocytic lymphoma CLL (Fig. 2, Table 3) had a 2-years survival probability of 91 %. Using the criteria mentioned above only about 50 % of these patients required treatment within the follow-up period with 2 deaths 18 and 22 months after diagnosis. Overall survival of patients with immunocytic lymphoma (Fig. 3, Table 3) was considerably shorter than that of patients with CLL, and response to therapy which was observed in 61 % of patients was correlated with an increase of the 2-years survival probability as compared to the 39 % of nonresponders. These data clearly demonstrate the clinical relevance of the histopathologic differentiation between CLL and immunocytic lymphoma. Only a small group of patients with immunocytic lymphoma predominantly localized in an enlarged spleen, who were treated exclusively by splenectomy, had the same good prognosis as asymptomatic untreated patients with CLL and immunocytic lymphoma. The 63 % of patients with stages III and IV of centrocytic lymphoma (Fig. 4, Table 3) responding to chemotherapy did apparently better than corresponding patients with immunocytic lymphoma and exhibited survival probabilities similar to those observed in stage I and II patients with centrocytic lymphoma treated by radiotherapy alone. Patients with stages III and IV of centroblastic-centrocytic lymphoma (Fig. 5, Table 3) responding to chemotherapy (60 %) also showed a high 2-years survival probability which approached that of the irradiated patients with stages I to III who all responded to radiotherapy.

In the group of high-grade malignant lymphomas patients with the centroblastic variety (Fig. 6, Table 3) responding to chemotherapy (50 %) and radiotherapy (100 %) had a higher survival probability than the responders among patients with immunoblastic lymphoma (Fig. 7, Table 3) (30 % responders to chemotherapy, 100 % responders to radiotherapy). Patients with lymphoblastic lymphoma (Fig. 8, Table 3) achieving complete remission after chemotherapy (44 %) behaved as patients with centroblastic lymphoma responding to chemotherapy. Prognosis of nonresponders with centroblastic (50 %) and immunoblastic lymphomas (70 %) as well as of partial and nonresponders with lymphoblastic lymphoma (56 %) was strikingly worse than that of nonresponding patients with the low-grade malignant immunocytic, centrocytic and centroblastic-centrocytic lymphomas.

CONCLUSIONS
Because data of studies correlating on a large-scale basis the histopathologic and clinical features of the Rappaport and the Kiel classifications of NHL are not available as yet, results of chemotherapy obtained in patients diagnosed according to these different schemes can only be compared in a tentative way. However, it is justified to assume that the majority of patients with neoplasias defined as lymphomas of *favorable* histologies or as lymphomas of *low-grade* malignancy suffers from the same diseases as suggested by the relatively long survival times and a good response to mild chemotherapy documented for both groups. Histopathologic heterogeneity of NHL entities subsumed under these headings is reflected by variations in

---

⁶Out of a total of more than 500 patients who had entered the study until Juli 1978 202 patients were evaluated in whom therapy had been performed without major deviations from the aforementioned protocol and at least 2 cycles of a given chemotherapeutic regimen had been administered. All deaths occurring after initiation of therapy were considered. With the exception of lymphoblastic lymphoma, patients achieving complete and partial remissions (complete remission = complete disappearance of all previous disease, verified by appropriate restaging procedures, and a return to normal performance status; partial remission => 50 % reduction in all evidence of disease) were categorized under the heading "responders" since at the time of evaluation too few complete remissions had been documented. Actuarial survival curves were calculated from the date of diagnosis using the method of Cutler and Ederer (14). Statistical significance of differences between the curves was tested by Gehan's generalized Wilcoxon test (19).

terms of need for and response to therapy. Thus, long asymptomatic periods not ne-
cessitating treatment have been observed in patients with both DWDL and CLL, two
histologically similar lymphoma entities. In advanced NPDL which seems to correspond predominantly to the centroblastic-centrocytic lymphoma of the Kiel classification (27) analogous observations have been published. However, other studies show
that in NPDL probability of survival can be increased by aggressive combination
chemotherapy early after diagnosis, leading to higher complete remission rates as
compared to those obtained after administration of only mild regimens (13, 28, 35).
In most patients with advanced centroblastic-centrocytic lymphoma the course of
the disease did not allow to leave patients untreated for more than several months
after diagnosis. It can be hypothesized that in immunocytic lymphoma which belongs
to the lymphocytic lymphomas of the Rappaport classification prognostic features
depend on the histopathologic subtype present. Since Silvestrini and others (38)
have demonstrated that neoplastic cells of the polymorphic subtype possess a higher
proliferative activity in vitro than lymphoid cells of the lymphoplasmacytoid and
the lymphoplasmacytic varieties, malignancy of polymorphic immunocytic lymphoma
might be intermediate between typical low-grade and typical high-grade malignant
lymphomas. Similar high ^{3}H-thymidine labeling index data have been reported for the
centrocytic lymphoma. These kinetic features of the centrocytic lymphoma cell could
be the basis for the rapid tumor progression seen in the evaluated patients with
this lymphoma entity who showed the shortest asymptomatic interval between diagnosis and onset of therapy observed among patients with NHL of low-grade malignancy.
It is of interest that most authors consider DPDL of the Rappaport classification,
which is related to centrocytic lymphoma, a lymphoma entity with unfavorable prognosis. Heterogeneity of *low-grade* malignant lymphomas and of NHL with *favorable*
histologies, respectively, necessitates further attempts to better define the efficiency of various chemotherapeutic approaches to the main entities and their subtypes so that more specific treatment protocols can be developed. In particular, it
is relevant to find out those lymphomas in which improvement of prognosis can only
be reached by the induction of higher rates of complete remissions, and to distinguish them from disorders which show a high benefit also from a good partial response to induction and maintenance therapy. This differentiation seems to be essential since more aggressive regimens are only justified if their beneficial effects
significantly exceed the risks of their higher toxicity. The well-known tendency of
NHL with favorable histologies to early disseminate, questioning the therapeutic
impact of initial staging procedures (11), implies the need for careful investigation of the possible prognostic relevance of adjuvant chemotherapy in irradiated
stage I and II patients.

It is generally accepted that patients with advanced lymphomas of *unfavorable* histologies should be treated with intensive chemotherapy in order to obtain high complete remission rates. This is documented by several authors for patients with DH who,
after reaching complete remission, apparently have a good chance to be cured (15,
28). Even though immunoblastic lymphoma of the Kiel classification might be best
compared to DH, it cannot be excluded that DH, as defined by the Rappaport classification, is morphologically more heterogeneous. Therefore, histologies might be
subsumed under this term which, according to the Kiel classification, would not be
classified as immunoblastic lymphoma (centroblastic-centrocytic or centroblastic
lymphomas?) (27). This problem is linked to the question whether or not DH patients
attaining durable remissions differ from the rest of the population in terms of both
histopathologic and clinical parameters. If such differences could be evidenced individual course and/or response to chemotherapy might be predictable at diagnosis.
As for NHL of low-grade malignancy, preliminary data of the prospective study using
the Kiel classification also suggest some heterogeneity of *high-grade* malignant
lymphomas. Thus, patients with centroblastic lymphoma seemed to respond best to the
chemotherapeutic programs used whereas patients with lymphoblastic lymphoma exhibited poorest prognosis. The considerable percentage of nonresponders among patients
with high-grade malignant lymphomas and the low survival probability of this group

clearly demonstrate the need for more aggressive chemotherapy. Since the C-MOPP program combines high efficiency with only moderate toxicity (11, 15, 18) it has been recently selected by the Kiel Lymphoma Study Group to improve treatment results in advanced high-grade malignant NHL.

REFERENCES

1. Anderson, T., R.A. Bender, R.I. Fisher, V.T. DeVita, B.A. Chabner, C.W. Berard, L. Norton, and R.C. Young (1977). Combination chemotherapy in non-Hodgkin's lymphoma: Results of long-term followup. Cancer Treat. Rep., 61, 1057-1066.

2. Bagley, C.M., V.T. DeVita, C.W. Berard, and G.P. Canellos (1972). Advanced lymphosarcoma: Intensive cyclical combination chemotherapy with cyclophosphamide, vincristine and prednisone. Ann. Intern. Med., 76, 227-234.

3. Bitran, J.D., J. Kinzie, D.L. Sweet, D. Variakojis, M.L. Griem, H.M. Golomb, J.B. Miller, N. Oetzel, and J.E. Ultmann (1977). Survival of patients with localized histiocytic lymphoma. Cancer, 39, 342-346.

4. Bonadonna, G., and S. Monfardini (1974). Chemotherapy of non-Hodgkin's lymphomas. Cancer Treat. Reviews, 1, 167-181.

5. Bremer, K., H. Bartels, G. Brittinger, A. Burger, E. Dühmke, U. Gunzer, E. König, A. Stacher, H. Theml, and R. Waldner (Kiel Lymphoma Group) (1977). Clinical significance of the Kiel classification of non-Hodgkin's lymphomas (NHL). In S. Seno, F. Takaku, and S. Irino (Eds.), Topics in Hematology, Intern. Congress Series, No. 415, Excerpta Medica, Amsterdam, pp. 352-355.

6. Brittinger, G. (for the Kiel Lymphoma Study Group) (1978). Outline of a prospective multicentric study on the clinical significance of the Kiel classification of non-Hodgkin's lymphomas. In G. Mathé, M. Seligmann, and M. Tubiana (Eds.), Lymphoid Neoplasias: Clinical and Therapeutic Aspects. Recent Results in Cancer Research, 65, Springer, Berlin-Heidelberg-New York, pp. 195-199.

7. Brittinger, G., H. Bartels, A. Burger, E. Dühmke, H.H. Fülle, U. Gunzer, R. Heinz, D. Huhn, G.W. Löhr, K. Musshoff, L. Nowicki, M. Pfoch, H. Pralle, and U. Schmalhorst (Kieler Lymphomgruppe) (1978). Grundlagen und bisherige Ergebnisse der prospektiven Studie der Kieler Lymphomgruppe über Non-Hodgkin-Lymphome. In A. Stacher, and P. Höcker (Eds.), Lymphknotentumore. Urban und Schwarzenberg, München, pp. 193-200.

8. Brittinger, G., H. Bartels, K. Bremer, E. Dühmke, U. Gunzer, E. König, and H. Stein (Kieler Lymphomgruppe) (1976). Klinik der malignen Non-Hodgkin-Lymphome entsprechend der Kiel-Klassifikation: Centrocytisches Lymphom, centroblastisch-centrocytisches Lymphom, lymphoblastisches Lymphom, immunoblastisches Lymphom. In H. Löffler (Ed.), Maligne Lymphome und monoklonale Gammopathien. Hämatologie und Bluttransfusion, Vol. 18, Lehmann, München, pp. 211-223.

9. Bush, R.S., M. Gospodarowicz, J. Sturgeon, and R. Alison (1977). Radiation therapy of localized non-Hodgkin's lymphoma. Cancer Treat. Rep., 61, 1129-1136.

10. Cadman, E., L. Farber, D. Berd, and J. Bertino (1977). Combination therapy for diffuse histiocytic lymphoma that includes antimetabolites. Cancer Treat. Rep., 61, 1109-1116.

11. Canellos, G.P., T.A. Lister, and A.T. Skarin (1978). Chemotherapy of the non-Hodgkin's lymphomas. Cancer, 42, 932-940.

12. Carbone, P.P., H.S. Kaplan, K. Musshoff, D.W. Smithers, and M. Tubiana (1971). Report of the committee on Hodgkin's disease staging classification. Cancer Res., 31, 1860-1861.

13. Coltman, C.A., J.K. Luce, E.M. McKelvey, S.E. Jones, and T.E. Moon (1977). Chemotherapy of non-Hodgkin's lymphoma: 10 years-experience in the Southwest Oncology Group. Cancer Treat. Rep., 61, 1067-1078.

14. Cutler, S.J., and F. Ederer (1958). Maximum utilization of the life table method in analyzing survival. J. Chron. Dis. 699-712.

15. DeVita, V.T., G.P. Canellos, B. Chabner, P. Schein, S.P. Hubbard, and R.C. Young (1975). Advanced diffuse histiocytic lymphoma, a potentially curable disease. Lancet, i, 248-250.

16. DeVita, V.T. (1977). Summary of symposium. Cancer Treat. Rep., 61, 1223-1227.

17. Ezdinli, E.Z., W. Costello, R.E. Lenhard, R. Bakemeier, J.M. Bennett,C.W.Berard, and P.P. Carbone (1978). Survival of nodular versus diffuse pattern lymphocytic poorly differentiated lymphoma. Cancer, 41, 1990-1996.

18. Fisher, R.I., V.T. DeVita, B.L. Johnson, R. Simon, and R.C. Young (1977). Prognostic factors for advanced diffuse histiocytic lymphoma following treatment with combination chemotherapy. Am. J. Med., 63, 177-182.

19. Gehan, E.A. (1965). A generalized Wilcoxon test for comparing arbitrarily singly-censored samples. Biometrika, 52, 203-223.

20. Gérard-Marchant, R., I. Hamlin, K. Lennert, F. Rilke, A.G. Stansfeld, and J.A.M. van Unnik (1974). Classification of non-Hodgkin's lymphomas. Lancet, ii, 406-408.

21. Glatstein, E., Z. Fuks, D.R. Goffinet, and H.S. Kaplan (1976). Non-Hodgkin's lymphomas of stage III extent. Cancer, 37, 2806-2812.

22. Glatstein, E., S.S. Donaldson, S.A. Rosenberg, and H.S. Kaplan (1977). Combined modality therapy in malignant lymphomas. Cancer Treat. Rep., 61, 1199-1207.

23. Hellman, S., J.T. Chaffey, D.S. Rosenthal, W.C. Moloney, G.P. Canellos, and A.T. Skarin (1977). The place of radiation therapy in the treatment of non-Hodgkin's lymphomas. Cancer, 39, 843-851.

24. Jones, S.E., Z. Fuks, H.S. Kaplan, and S.A. Rosenberg (1973). Non-Hodgkin's lymphomas. V. Results of radiotherapy. Cancer, 32, 682-691.

25. Knospe, W.H., V. Loeb, and C.M. Huguley (1974). Bi-weekly chlorambucil treatment of chronic lymphocytic leukemia. Cancer, 33, 555-561.

26. Lauria, F., R. Frezza, M. Gobbi, P. Mazza, and S. Tura (1978). A five-years survey of MEV therapy for advanced non-Hodgkin's lymphomas. XVII Congress of the International Society of Hematology, Paris.

27. Lennert, K. in collaboration with N. Mohri, H. Stein, E. Kaiserling, and H.K. Müller-Hermelink (1978). Malignant lymphomas other than Hodgkin's disease. E. Uehlinger (Ed.), Handbuch der speziellen pathologischen Anatomie und Histologie, Vol. I/3B, Springer, Berlin-Heidelberg-New York, pp. 1-833.

28. McKelvey, E.M., J.A. Gottlieb, H.E. Wilson, A. Haut, R.W. Talley, R. Stephens, M. Lane, J.F. Gamble, S.E. Jones, P.N. Grozea, J. Gutterman, C. Coltman, and T.E. Moon (1976). Hydroxyldaunomycin (adriamycin) combination chemotherapy in malignant lymphoma. Cancer, 38, 1484-1493.

29. McKelvey, E.M., and T.E. Moon (1977). Curability of non-Hodgkin's lymphomas. Cancer Treat. Rep., 61, 1185- 1190.

30. Musshoff, K., and H. Schmidt-Vollmer (1975). Prognosis of non-Hodgkin's lymphomas with special emphasis on the staging classification. Z. Krebsforsch., 83, 323-341.

31. Pangalis, G.A., B.N. Nathwani, and H. Rappaport (1977). Malignant lymphoma, well differentiated lymphocytic. Cancer, 39, 999-1010.

32. Portlock, C.S., and S.A. Rosenberg (1977). Chemotherapy of the non-Hodgkin's
    lymphomas: The Stanford experience. Cancer Treat. Rep., 61, 1049-1055.

33. Rappaport, H. (1966). Tumors of the hematopoietic system. In Atlas of Tumor Pa-
    thology, Sect. III, Fasc. 8., Armed Forces Institute of Pathology,
    Washington, D.C., pp. 91-156.

34. Rappaport, H. (1977). In Roundtable discussion of histopathologic classifica-
    tion. Cancer Treat. Rep., 61, 1037-1048.

35. Rodriguez, V., F. Cabanillas, M.A. Burgess, E.M. McKelvey, M. Valdivieso, G.P.
    Bodey, and E.J. Freireich (1977). Combination chemotherapy ("CHOP-Bleo") in
    advanced (non-Hodgkin) malignant lymphoma. Blood, 49, 325-333.

36. Rosenberg, S.A. (1977). Validity of the Ann Arbor staging classification for the
    non-Hodgkin's lymphomas. Cancer Treat. Rep., 61, 1023-1027.

37. Schein, P.S., V.T. DeVita, S. Hubbard, B.A. Chabner, G.P. Canellos, C. Berard,
    and R.C. Young (1976). Bleomycin, adriamycin, cyclophosphamide, vincristine,
    and prednisone (BACOP) combination chemotherapy in the treatment of advanced
    diffuse histiocytic lymphoma. Ann. Intern. Med., 85, 417-422.

38. Silvestrini, R., A. Costa, M.G. Daidone, and F. Rilke (1978). Prognostic signi-
    ficance of the labeling index in non-Hodgkin   human malignant lymphomas.
    Antibiotics Chemother., 24, 105-111.

39. Skarin, A.T., D.S. Rosenthal, W.C. Moloney, and E. Frei (1977). Combination che-
    motherapy of advanced non-Hodgkin lymphoma with bleomycin, adriamycin, cyc-
    lophosphamide, vincristine, and prednisone (BACOP). Blood, 49, 759-770.

40. Stacher, A., R. Waldner, and H. Theml (Kieler Lymphomgruppe) (1976). Klinik der
    malignen Non-Hodgkin-Lymphome entsprechend der Kieler Klassifikation:Lympho-
    plasmozytoides Lymphom (LPL) und chronisch lymphatische Leukämie (CLL). In
    H. Löffler (Ed.), Maligne Lymphome und monoklonale Gammopathien. Häma-
    tologie und Bluttransfusion, Vol. 18, Lehmann, München, pp. 199-209.

41. Tubiana, M., P. Pouillart, M. Hayat, M. Schlienger, R. Gérard-Marchant, J.
    Schlumberger, J. Brugère, J.L. Amiel, and G. Mathé (1975). Results of ra-
    diotherapy in stages I and II of non-Hodgkin's lymphoma. Br. J. Cancer, 31,
    Supp. II, 402-412.

Non-Hodgkin's Lymphomas: Summary of Session 2

H. Kasdorf

Dep. Oncología, Fac. de Medicina, C. Correo 930, Montevideo, Uruguay

Exactly 5 years have elapsed since the First International Symposium on Non-Hodgkin Lymphomata was held in London (24), a meeting where a comprehensive view of the modern basic knowledge about this protean - disease was analized and discussed. Since then, many other meetings - have taken place, particularly the San Francisco Conference in 1976 (6). As a result of these and several other meetings we have now a clearer understanding of the many aspects of these diseases and, especially, - of the difficulties and obstacles which have to be overcome before a therapeutic breakthrough on a wide scale, as stated by Dr. Musshoff, can be claimed.

I) The observation of the natural history of the non-Hodgkin's lympho- mas (NHL) clearly recognizes two patterns of diseases, characterized - by a different biological behaviour and hence clinical evolution:a)slow onset, indolent course and a long median survival of six years or more b) rapid beginning, an often fulminating evolution with a median sur- vival of about one year or less. The response to present day treatments is equally dissimilar. Easy obtained remissions with moderate chemothe- rapy or even long survivals with no treatment at all in asymptomatic - patients in the first group against the need of an aggressive combina- tion of several drugs in the latter. Furthermore, the survival in non or partial responders is also significantly better in patients belon- ging to the more benign pattern. In accordance with the criteria used, this different biological behaviour has been expressed in various ways: favourable and unfavourable histology, nodular and diffuse pattern,low and high grade malignancy, good and poor risk, good and poor prognosis. There is however, an evident lack of correlation between the different concepts used. Besides, each biological entity is quite heterogeneous in itself and its subentities are not yet clearly defined. Though much has been learned in these years, it is the task of the coming years to identify, as precisely as possible, the various entities and subenti- ties, to group them in an easy, understandable and reproducible clas- sification and to define the type of treatments which offer the best possibilities.

What follows is an attempt to discuss the most important therapeutic - aspects presented at this panel in the context of tumours having a dif-

ferent biological behaviour. Equally important is to give to the general physician, in this still very complex and confusing chapter of oncology, a guideline which may be of use to him in his daily practice.

- NHL of favourable biology (corresponds preferentially to the lymphocytic lymphoma as defined by Rappaport (23); includes the majority
  of the lymphomas with a nodular pattern (23) and with a low grade -
  malignancy (14)).

There is no obvious evidence yet that with present day intensive -
treatments, one can really alter the natural history of these lymphomas. That is, if by improving the rate of overall response one -
can reach cure or prolong survival. In localized stages, as shown
by Dr. Bush and colleagues, the survival curve is not completely parallel to the survival curve of a matched normal population. The constant fall of the curve is more evident in advanced stages. But survival curves show that it is almost stage independent and that prog
nosis for advanced stages is not very different from that of locali
zed stages. If this is the current situation, one has to consider -
seriously which is the best treatment and select the one which offers
to the patient the best quality of survival with a minimum of complications. However, results from recent trials seem to indicate that
certain varieties tend to remain relapse-free for prolonged periods
of time and are therefore potentially curable (DLWD (16); NM (1,20);
NLPD (1,11)). If confirmed, they have to be treated aggressively.

a) Stages I and II localized[1]- Radiotherapy is the treatment of choice since it sterilizes the tumour in the irradiated field. Over 50%
of the patients so treated survive five years. The tendency to early
dissemination reduces the efficiency of a loco-regional treatment.
As present day systemic treatment modalities (chemotherapy, TBI) have noy proven to be able to erradicate the disease, it is doubtful
wether a systemic treatment as an adjuvant to radiotherapy is justified. Previous localized radical radiotherapy does not preclude other
treatments, therefore it makes the policy suggested by the Toronto
Group, to withhold systemic treatments until there is evidence of -
disseminated disease, very recommendable.

b) Stages II extensive,[1] III and IV - Above 50% of the patients in disseminated stages have an overall survival of five years; about 14%
of them are relapse-free at eight years (Chaffey). Patients with a
nodular pattern have more favourable prognosis than those with diffuse pattern (Bᵒrgsagel; Chaffey). The survival curves for all low
grade malignant types are about the same. However, minor differences
have been observed: in all series, centrocytic lymphomas are sligh-
tly less favourable; a significant better prognosis has been reported in the nodular variety of centroblastic-centrocytic as opposed
to the diffuse (21) but this difference has not been noticed by the
german investigators.

Usually there is no urgency to start a treatment, unless there is a
clinical situation which calls to it. This brings up the question of
the treatment philosophy for asymptomatic patients. As shown by Dr.

---

[1]Localized stage II is defined by the involvement of the primary site
(nodal and extranodal) and the contiguous regional nodes. Non-contiguous involvement is classified as extensive stage II and these patients have a high risk of disseminated disease.

Schwade, there are several trials going on to define if "watch and wait" policy with minimal palliative radiation therapy as needed, is more prudent than aggressive chemotherapy or long term single agent treatment. For patients with symptoms, it has been suggested that, when with an efficent treatment a CR can be obtained, the patient - will then have the benefit of a longer disease-free interval and e- ventually, a longer survival. This is still an unanswered problem - and needs further investigations. As mentioned, there are now some indications that the survival of several lymphomas with a favourable biology may be response related (1, 16, 20, 26). The multiple drug chemotherapy induces a higher rate of CR than does single agent che- motherapy but it has to be determined in which situations combined chemotherapy is superior. All combinations are equally effective and at the present time no one is better than the others (C-MOPP, BACOP, HOP, CHOP, MEV, COMA, etc.)

Several trials are testing the utility of sequential non-crossresis- tant drug combinations (Schwade) and the preliminary results repor- ted by Bonadonna (3) alternating CVP with ABP seem to be encouraging. The lack of cross resistance allows the use of another combination to induce a remission after relapse, partial remission or refracta- riness. The combinations under trial are CVP and ABP; B-COP and CHOP; COPA and CAP-Bleo.

Maintenance therapy seems to be limited to patients who have respon- ded only partially. However, as pointed out by Bender and De Vita(2), there is no evidence that maintenance therapy is superior to reinduc- tion at the time of progression of the disease.

TBI appears to be a most effective single agent modality, achieving the same cure rate than chemotherapy over an extended period of time with far less toxicity (4, 5, 15, 17), being therefore a useful al- ternative to combination chemotherapy (Chaffey). Its precise role re- mains to be established.

- NHL of unfavourable biology (corresponds to the histiocytic, mixed and undifferentiated lymphomas as defined by Rappaport (23) and to the high grade malignant lymphomas (14)).

These lymphomas can be cured by treatment, even in advanced stages in spite of their unfavourable natural history (8).

a) Stages I and II localized[1] - With involved field radiotherapy, a disease free survival of five or more years is commonly obtained in 40-60% of the cases (Bush, 15, 22, 25) and Fuller reports a projec- ted 69% at five years. Though the overall survival is about the same as with lymphomas of favourable biology, the relapse free rate is distintcly higher and remains stabilized the first two to three years after treatment, thus indicating cure.

It has not yet been firmly established if the addition of multidrug chemotherapy improves the overall result. Dr. Fuller, in laparotomy staged I and II peripheral presentations (axillar, neck, inguinal)

---

[1]Localized stage II is defined by the involvement of the primary site (nodal and extranodal) and the contiguous regional nodes. Non-conti- guous involvement is classified as extensive stage II and these pa- tients have a high risk of disseminated disease.

H. Kasdorf

of DH lymphomas, could not, in a small series of 24 patients, detect any difference in patients receiving IF radiotherapy only against IF radiotherapy plus CHOP-Bleo chemotherapy. Stanford's experience (13) until now shows that the employed adjuvant chemotherapy (CVP, CAT) has not improved the results when comparing against TLI. The Milan trial (19) is so far the first one to demonstrate a significant reduction of failure rate at three years from 56% to 27%,in a population consisting of 70% DH lymphomas, giving CVP four weeks after IF radiotherapy versus IF radiotherapy only. If confirmed, the adjuvant chemotherapy will permit to increase the percentage of cure in these lymphomas in apparently localized stages.

b) <u>Stages II extensive[1], III and IV</u> - For patients with an extensive stage II, the just mentioned preliminary results reported by Lattuada and coworkers (19) seem to be of particular importance since it has repeatedly been proved that the disease in this stage is much - more widespread than one can infer, even from laparotomy staged patients (9, 10).

For stages III and IV, aggressive high dose intermittent combination chemotherapy has improved five year survival rates from 20 to 40% - with a 20% relapse rate. A plateau has apparently been reached with present day chemotherapy and there are many trials under way to see if added radiotherapy proves to be of value to reach better results. Dr. Fuller reports in stage III DH lymphomas an estimated five year survival of 74% with initial and alternating CHOP-Bleo and IF radiotherapy, a result which promises more than the 65% survival obtained using combination chemotherapy only (12). For the abdominal presentation, a clear superiority over previous experience has been observed with a projected five year and disease free survival of 64% and 63% respectively. The Stanford trials (13) indicate that the addition of radiotherapy to CVP or CAT seems to be beneficial by increasing the survival figures from 24% (four years) to 47% (five years) and the relapse free period from 9% (at four years) to 24% (at five years).

Another way to possibly improve results is immunotherapy. A recently reported SWOG trial (18) tends to show the benefit of a significant better overall survival and overall response. The rate of complete and partial remissions is greater with chemotherapy plus BCG than with chemotherapy alone (CHOP-Bleo, COP-Bleo) but with no increase of the CR rate. This has to be confirmed by further studies before one can ascertain that added BCG to chemotherapy increases the survival or the duration of remission and therefore no recommendation can be made.

II) In their study of 981 cases seen between 1967 and 1975 at the Princess Margaret Hospital in Toronto, Dr. Bergsagel and coworkers analyzed, besides pathology, some clinical and biological parameters in relation to its prognostic value. Age appears to be an important factor, particularly for lymphocytic lymphomas where survival decreases progressively with increasing age. Old age may also be significant in histiocytic lymphomas where survival curves for patients over 60 years

---

[1]Localized stage II is defined by the involvement of the primary site (nodal and extranodal) and the contiguous regional nodes. Non-contiguous involvement is classified as extensive stage II and these patients have a high risk of disseminated disease.

show, with a follow-up of more than seven years, a definite lesser possibility of cure. The classical B symptoms and some biological parameters like the erithrocite sedimentation rate (above 40 mm/1st hour) -
and initial hemoglobin level (below 12 gm/100 ml) were found to clearly worsen the prognosis. In stage IV, the involvement of the liver significantly diminishes survival whereas the prognosis not distinctly -
changed with the involvement of other extranodal sites such as bone,
lung, spleen or skin. Other poor prognostic factors, not analyzed in
the Toronto material, have been recently observed in DH lymphomas and
reported by Fisher and colleagues (12). Great tumour masses (more than
10 cms.) and gastrointestinal or bone marrow involvement influence ne-
gatively the rate and durability of response. On the other hand, these
investigations did not find any statistical correlation between age -
and constitutional symptoms and response to chemotherapy. It is obvious that for the correct interpretation of future trials all these -
factors have to be considered.

In children, as shown by Dr. Murphy, obvious clinical and biological
factors of prognostic significance and therapeutic implications are:
the primary site of involvement, where head and neck and peripheral -
node presentations are more favourable than those in mediastinum and
abdomen; stage and the unfavourable characteristic of the presence of
B-cell surface markers.

III) The clinical usefulness of surface markers is still uncertain but
its investigation will improve the understanding of lymphoproliferative diseases. B- and T-cell markers have been found in lymphomas of
low and high degree malignancy and therefore did not allow a distinction to be made on that basis (Diehl). In adults, B-cells have been -
seen to be associated with a longer survival; however, as just mentioned
this is not the case in children (Murphy).

IV) Nobody doubts or questions the importance of staging to determine
the extent of the disease and the involvement of different sites. These requirements are needed for an adequate treatment and for a correct
evaluation of the treatment results. The more precise and accurate the
staging is, the greater the selection of the patients to be treated.
The results obtained for each stage with a given treatment will also
be better. Therefore, if the procedures used for staging two series of
patients are not equal, the results can and should not be compared. -
This most important fact has been brought forward by Dr. Bush and his
associates, reminding us that stage survival should not be confused -
with overall survival, which is really the only valid criteria to assess correctly the treatment results. This warning usually does not
apply to children where staging procedures are much less elaborate -
than in adults. Staging of prognostic and therapeutic value is obtained
by evaluating mainly clinical procedures (Murphy).

To conclude: the better survivals obtained in advanced stages of tu -
mours of unfavourable natural history and in childhood lymphomas distinctly show that a steady and promising progress is made in the difficult field of NHL. The correct identification of entities and sub -
entities of tumours with different biological behaviours and of tumours
which do not respond adequately to present day therapy is the challen-
ging problem which hopefully will be solved in the near future. It will
demand many carefully and thoughtfully designed prospective clinical
trials, as well as an agreement on the classification to be used.

REFERENCES

1 - Anderson, T., R.A. Bender, R.I. Fisher and others (1977). Combina
    tion chemotherapy in non-Hodgkin's lymphoma; the results of long
    term follow-up. Cancer Treat. Rep., 61, 1057-1066.
2 - Bender, R.A. and V.T. De Vita (1978). Non-Hodgkin's lymphoma. In
    M.J. Stagnet (Ed) Randomized Trials in Cancer, Raven Press, New
    York, pp. 77-102.
3 - Bonadonna, G., E. Villa, R. Canetta and others (1978). CTX, VCR,
    Pred. (CVP) alternated with ADM, BLM, Pred.(ABP) in advanced non-
    Hodgkin's lymphomas (NHL). Proc. Amer. Assoc. Ca. Res. 19, 216.
4 - Chaffey, J.T., D.S. Rosenthal, W.S. Moloney and others (1976). To-
    tal body irradiation as treatment for lymphosarcoma. Int. J. Radia
    tion Oncology Biol. Phys, 1, 399-405.
5 - Chaffey, J.T., S. Hellman, D.S. Rosenthal and others (1977). Total
    body irradiation in the treatment of lymphocitic lymphoma. Cancer
    Treat. Rep., 61, 1149-1152.
6 - Conference on non-Hodgkin's lymphomas, 30 september - 2 october -
    1976. Proceedings published in Cancer Treat. Rep., 61, S.E. Jones
    and J. Godden (Eds).
7 - Cox, J.D. (1978). Central lymphatic irradiation to low dose for ad-
    vanced nodular lymphoreticular tumors (non-Hodgkin's lymphoma). Ra
    diology, 126, 767-772.
8 - De Vita, V.T., G.P. Canellos, B.A. Chabner and others (1975). Ad-
    vanced diffuse histiocytic lymphoma, a potentially curable disea-
    se. Lancet, 1, 248-257.
9 - De Vita, V.T. (1977). Discussion and summary of symposium. In S.E.
    Jones and J. Godden (Eds) Proceedings of the Conference on non-Hodg
    kin's lymphomas. Cancer Treat. Rep., 61, 1032 and 1224.
10- De Vita, V.T., R.I. Fisher and R.C. Young (1977). Treatment of dif-
    fuse histiocytic lymphomas: new opportunities for the future. In H.
    J. Tagnon and M.J. Stagnet (Eds) Recent Advances in Cancer Treat-
    ment, Raven Press, pp. 39-54
11- Edzinli, E., W. Costello, R. Lenhard and others (1978). Survival
    of nodular versus diffuse pattern lymphocytic poorly differentia-
    ted lymphoma. Cancer, 41, 1990-1996.
12- Fisher, R.I., V.T. De Vita, B.L. Johnson and others (1977). Prog-
    nostic factors for advanced diffuse histiocytic lymphoma follow-
    ing treatment with combination chemotherapy. Ann. J. Med., 63, 177-
    182.
13- Glatstein, E., S.S. Donaldson, S.A. Rosenberg and others (1977).
    Combined modality therapy in malignant lymphomas. Cancer Treat.Rep.
    61, 1199-1207.
14- Gerard-Marchant, R., I. Hamlin, K. Lennert and others (1974). Clas-
    sification of non-Hodgkin's lymphomas. Lancet, 2, 406-408.
15- Hellman, S., J.T. Chaffey, D.S. Rosenthal and others (1977). The
    place of radiation therapy in the treatment of non-Hodgkin's lym-
    phomas. Cancer, 39, 843-851.
16- Icli, F., E.Z. Edzinli, W. Costello and others (1978). Diffuse -
    well-differentiated lymphocytic lymphoma (DLWD). Cancer, 42, 1936-
    1942.
17- Johnson, R.E., G.P. Canellos, R.C. Young and others (1978). Chemo-
    therapy (cyclophosphamide, vincristine, prednisone) versus radio-
    therapy (total body irradiation) for stages III and IV poorly dif-
    ferentiated lymphocytic lymphoma. Cancer Treat. Rep., 62, 321-325.
18- Jones, S.E. and S.E. Salmon (1977). Adjuvant chemotherapy with BCG
    in lymphomas. In S.E. Salmon and S.E. Jones (Eds) Adjuvant Thera-
    py of Cancer Elsenier/North Holland Biomedical Press, Amsterdam,

pp. 549-556
19- Lattuada, A., G. Bonadonna and others (1977). Adjuvant chemothera-
    py with CVP after radiotherapy in stage I-II non-Hodgkin's lympho-
    ma. In S.E. Salmon and S.E. Jones (Eds) Adjuvant Therapy of Cancer,
    Elsenier/North Holland Biomedical Press, Amsterdam, pp. 537-544.
20- Mc Kelvey, E.M., J.A. Gottlieb, H.E. Wilson and others (1976). Hy-
    droxildaunomycin (adriamycin) combination chemotherapy in malig-
    nant lymphoma. Cancer, 38, 1484-1493.
21- Meugé, C., B. Hoerni, A. De Mascarel and others (1978). Non-Hodg-
    kin malignant lymphomas. Clinico-pathologic correlations with the
    Kiel classification. Europ. J. Cancer, 14, 587-592.
22- Musshoff, K. and J. Slanina (1976). Maligne Systemerkrankungen.In
    E. Scherer (Ed) Strahlentherapie, Springer Verlag, Berlin, pp.705-
    788.
23- Rappaport, H. (1966). Tumors of the hematopoietic system. In Atlas
    of Tumor Pathology, section 3, fascicle 8, US Armed Forces Insti-
    tute of Pathology, Washington D.C.
24- Symposium on non-Hodgkin's lymphomata, 8-12 october 1973. Procee-
    dings published in Br. J. Cancer (1975), 31, Supp. II, M.J. Peck-
    ham (Ed).
25- Tubiana, M., P. Pouillart, M. Hoyat and others (1975). Results of
    radiotherapy in stages I and II of non-Hodgkin's lymphoma. Br. J.
    Cancer, 31, Supp. II, 402-412.
26- Young, R.C., R.E. Johnson, G.P. Canellos and others (1977). Advan-
    ced lymphocytic lymphoma: Randomized comparisons of chemotherapy
    and radiotherapy, alone or in combination. Cancer Treat. Rep., 61,
    1153-1159.

LIST OF ABBREVIATIONS USED

Institutions

SWOG - Southwestern Oncology Group

Remission

CR - Complete remission
PR - Partial remission

Radiation

IF - Involved field radiation therapy
TBI - Total body irradiation
TLI - Total lymphoid irradiation

Histological Types

DH - Diffuse histiocytic
DLWD - Diffuse lymphocytic well differentiated
NH - Nodular histiocytic
NLPD - Nodular lymphocytic poorly differentiated
NM - Nodular mixed

Drugs and Combinations

C-MOPP - Cyclophosphamide, Nit.Mustard, Vincristine, Procarbazine and
         Prednisone
BACOP - bis-chloroethyl nitrosourea (BCNU), Adriamycin, Cyclophospha

mide, Vincristine and Prednisone

HOP - Adriamycin, Vincristine and Prednisone

CHOP - Cyclophosphamide, Adriamycin, Vincristine and Prednisone

CHOP-Bleo- Cyclophosphamide, Adriamycin, Vincristine, Prednisone and Bleomycin

MEV - Methotrexate, Cyclophosphamide and Vincristine

COMA - Cyclophosphamide, Vincristine, Methotrexate and Cytosine-a-rabinoside

ABP - Adriamycin, Bleomycin and Prednisone

B-COP - bis-chloroethyl nitrosourea (BCNU), cyclophosphamide, Vincristine and Prednisone

COPA - Cyclophosphamide, Vincristine, Prednisone and Adriamycin

COP - Cyclophosphamide, Vincristine and Prednisone

CVP - Cyclophosphamide, Vincristine and Prednisone

COP-Bleo- Cyclophosphamide, Vincristine, Prednisone and Bleomycin

CAP-Bleo- Cyclophosphamide, Adriamycin, Procarbazine and Bleomycin

CAT - Cytosin arabinoside, Adriamycin and 6 thioguanine

Index

The page numbers refer to the first page of the article in which the index term appears.